T0362064

Imaging of Rheumatology

Editor

GIUSEPPE GUGLIELMI

RADIOLOGIC CLINICS OF NORTH AMERICA

www.radiologic.theclinics.com

Consulting Editor
FRANK H. MILLER

September 2017 • Volume 55 • Number 5

ELSEVIER

1600 John F. Kennedy Boulevard • Suite 1800 • Philadelphia, Pennsylvania, 19103-2899

http://www.theclinics.com

RADIOLOGIC CLINICS OF NORTH AMERICA Volume 55, Number 5
September 2017 ISSN 0033-8389, ISBN 13: 978-0-323-54570-9

Editor: John Vassallo (j.vassallo@elsevier.com)
Developmental Editor: Donald Mumford

Radiologic Clinics of North America (ISSN 0033-8389) is published bimonthly by Elsevier Inc., 360 Park Avenue South, New York, NY 10010-1710. Months of issue are January, March, May, July, September, and November. Periodicals postage paid at New York, NY and additional mailing offices. Subscription prices are USD 474 per year for US individuals, USD 831 per year for US institutions, USD 100 per year for US students and residents, USD 551 per year for Canadian individuals, USD 1062 per year for Canadian institutions, USD 680 per year for international individuals, USD 1062 per year for international institutions, and USD 315 per year for Canadian and international students/residents. To receive student and resident rate, orders must be accompanied by name of affiliated institution, date of term and the signature of program/residency coordinator on institution letterhead. Orders will be billed at individual rate until proof of status is received. Foreign air speed delivery is included in all *Clinics* subscription prices. All prices are subject to change without notice. **POSTMASTER:** Send address changes to *Radiologic Clinics of North America*, Elsevier Health Sciences Division, Subscription Customer Service, 3251 Riverport Lane, Maryland Heights, MO63043. **Customer Service: Telephone: 1-800-654-2452** (U.S. and Canada); **1-314-447-8871** (outside U.S. and Canada). **Fax: 1-314-447-8029. E-mail: journalscustomerservice-usa@ elsevier.com (for print support); journalsonlinesupport-usa@elsevier.com (for online support)**.

Reprints. For copies of 100 or more of articles in this publication, please contact the Commercial Reprints Department, Elsevier Inc., 360 Park Avenue South, New York, New York 10010-1710. Tel.: +1-212-633-3874; Fax: +1-212-633-3820; E-mail: reprints@elsevier.com.

Radiologic Clinics of North America also published in Greek Paschalidis Medical Publications, Athens, Greece.

Radiologic Clinics of North America is covered in *MEDLINE/PubMed (Index Medicus), EMBASE/Excerpta Medica, Current Contents/Life Sciences, Current Contents/Clinical Medicine, RSNA Index to Imaging Literature, BIOSIS, Science Citation Index,* and *ISI/BIOMED.*

Contributors

CONSULTING EDITOR

FRANK H. MILLER, MD
Chief, Body Imaging Section and Fellowship
Program, Medical Director of MRI, Professor,
Department of Radiology, Northwestern
University Feinberg School of Medicine,
Chicago, Illinois, USA

EDITOR

GIUSEPPE GUGLIELMI, MD
Professor, Department of Radiology, University
of Foggia, Department of Radiology, Casa
Sollievo della Sofferenza, Scientific Institute
Hospital, San Giovanni Rotondo, Foggia, Italy

AUTHORS

JOSE ACOSTA, MD
Department of Radiology, Hospital
Universitario Ramón y Cajal, Madrid, Spain

SONIA AIRALDI, MD
Radiologia III, IRCCS San Martino-IST,
DISSAL, Università degli studi di Genova,
Genova, Italy

GUSTAV ANDREISEK, MD, MBA
Department of Radiology, Kantonsspital
Münsterlingen, Münsterlingen, Switzerland;
University of Zurich, Zurich, Switzerland

**MARIA PILAR APARISI GÓMEZ, MBChB,
FRANZCR**
Department of Radiology, Auckland City
Hospital, Grafton, Auckland, New Zealand;
Department of Radiology, Hospital Nueve de
Octubre, Valencia, Spain

FRANCESCO ARRIGONI, MD
Diagnostic and Interventional Radiology,
Department of Biotechnological and Applied
Clinical Sciences, University of L'Aquila,
L'Aquila, Coppito, Italy

SAMMY BADR, MD, MSc
Division of Radiology and Musculoskeletal
Imaging, University Hospital of Lille, University
of Lille, Lille, France

ANTONIO BARILE, MD
Diagnostic and Interventional Radiology,
Department of Biotechnological and Applied
Clinical Sciences, University of L'Aquila,
L'Aquila, Coppito, Italy

ALBERTO BAZZOCCHI, MD, PhD
Diagnostic and Interventional Radiology,
Rizzoli Orthopaedic Institute, Bologna, Italy

JOHAN G. BLICKMAN, MD, PhD
Professor and Vice Chairman, Imaging
Sciences, University of Rochester Medical
Center, Rochester, New York, USA

JOHAN L. BLOEM, MD, PhD
Department of Radiology, Leiden University
Medical Center, Leiden, The Netherlands

LUCA BRUNESE, MD
Department of Medicine and Health Science
"V. Tiberio", University of Molise,
Campobasso, Italy

FEDERICO BRUNO, MD
Diagnostic and Interventional Radiology,
Department of Biotechnological and Applied
Clinical Sciences, University of L'Aquila,
L'Aquila, Coppito, Italy

CONSTANTINUS FRANCISCUS BUCKENS, MD, PhD
Department of Radiology, Academic Medical
Center, Universitair Medisch Centrum Utrecht,
Utrecht, The Netherlands

USA CAIN, MD
Resident Physician, Imaging Sciences,
University of Rochester Medical Center,
Rochester, New York, USA

VICTOR N. CASSAR-PULLICINO, MD, FRCR
Consultant Radiologist and Clinical Director,
Department of Diagnostic Imaging, The Robert
Jones and Agnes Hunt Orthopaedic and
District Hospital, NHS Foundation Trust,
Gobowen, Oswestry, United Kingdom

DIMITRIOU CHRISTOS, MD
Radiology Department, Hôpital Universitaire
des Enfants Reine Fabilola, Brussels, Belgium

PAOLA CIPRIANI, MD
Rheumatology Clinic, Department of
Biotechnological and Applied Clinical
Sciences, University of L'Aquila, L'Aquila,
Coppito, Italy

GIOVANNA STEFANIA COLAFATI, MD
Radiologia, IRCCS Ospedale Pediatrico
Bambino Gesù, Roma, Italy

ANNE COTTEN, MD, PhD
Division of Radiology and Musculoskeletal
Imaging, University Hospital of Lille, University
of Lille, Lille, France

PAOLA D'APRILE, MD
Department of Radiology, Ospedale San
Paolo, Bari, Italy

MARIA BEATRICE DAMASIO, MD
Radiologia, IRCCS Gaslini Children's Hospital,
Genova, Italy

FILIPPO DEL GRANDE, MD, MBA, MHEM
University of Zurich, Zurich, Switzerland;
Department of Radiology, Ospedale Regionale
di Lugano, Lugano, Switzerland

LUKAS FILLI, MD
Institute of Diagnostic and Interventional
Radiology, University Hospital Zurich,
University of Zurich, Zurich, Switzerland

GIULIA FRAUENFELDER, MD
Radiology Department, Università Campus
Bio-Medico, Rome, Italy

ROBERTO GIACOMELLI, MD
Rheumatology Clinic, Department of
Biotechnological and Applied Clinical
Sciences, University of L'Aquila, L'Aquila,
Coppito, Italy

FRANCESCO GIURAZZA, MD, PhD
Radiology Department, Università Campus
Bio-Medico, Rome, Italy

LAURENCE GOFFIN, MD
Pediatric Rheumatology Department, Hôpital
Universitaire des Enfants Reine Fabilola,
Brussels, Belgium

BOITSIOS GRAMMATINA, MD
Radiology Department, Hôpital Universitaire
des Enfants Reine Fabilola, Brussels, Belgium

CLAUDIO GRANATA, MD
Radiologia, IRCCS Gaslini Children's Hospital,
Genova, Italy

SIMON GREENWOOD, MBChB, MSc, MRCP, FRCR
Department of Diagnostic Imaging, The
Robert Jones and Agnes Hunt Orthopaedic
and District Hospital, NHS Foundation Trust,
Gobowen, Oswestry, United Kingdom

GIANLUIGI GUARNIERI, MD
Neuroradiology Department, Ospedale
Cardarelli, Naples, Italy

ALI GUERMAZI, MD, PhD
Professor, Department of Radiology,
Quantitative Imaging Center, Boston
University School of Medicine, Boston,
Massachusetts, USA

GIUSEPPE GUGLIELMI, MD
Professor, Department of Radiology, University of Foggia, Department of Radiology, Casa Sollievo della Sofferenza, Scientific Institute Hospital, San Giovanni Rotondo, Foggia, Italy

DAICHI HAYASHI, MD, PhD
Adjunct Research Assistant Professor, Department of Radiology, Quantitative Imaging Center, Boston University School of Medicine, Boston, Massachusetts, USA; Department of Radiology, Yale New Haven Health at Bridgeport Hospital, Bridgeport, Connecticut, USA

THIBAUT JACQUES, MD, MSc
Division of Radiology and Musculoskeletal Imaging, University Hospital of Lille, University of Lille, Lille, France

MOHAMED JARRAYA, MD
Adjunct Research Instructor, Department of Radiology, Quantitative Imaging Center, Boston University School of Medicine, Boston, Massachusetts, USA; Department of Radiology, Mercy Catholic Medical Center, Darby, Pennsylvania, USA

HERMAN M. KROON, MD, PhD
Department of Radiology, Leiden University Medical Center, Leiden, The Netherlands

NEAL LARKMAN, MD, MPH
Department of Radiology, Leeds Teaching Hospital Trust, Leeds, West Yorkshire, United Kingdom

PHU-QUOC LÊ, MD
Pediatric Rheumatology Department, Hôpital Universitaire des Enfants Reine Fabilola, Brussels, Belgium

GUILLAUME LEFEBVRE, MD
Division of Radiology and Musculoskeletal Imaging, University Hospital of Lille, University of Lille, Lille, France

ANTONIO LEONE, MD
Associate Professor, Institute of Radiology, Fondazione Policlinico Universitario A. Gemelli, Catholic University, School of Medicine, Rome, Italy

EVA LLOPIS, MD
Department of Radiology, Hospital de la Ribera, Alzira, Valencia, Spain

MARIO MAAS, MD, PhD
Professor, Division of Musculoskeletal Radiology, Department of Radiology, Academic Medical Center, Amsterdam, The Netherlands

GIANMICHELE MAGNANO, MD
Radiologia, IRCCS Gaslini Children's Hospital, Genova, Italy

CLARA MALATTIA, MD
Pediatria II, Reumatologia, IRCCS Gaslini Children's Hospital, Genova, Italy

STEFANO MARCIA, MD
Radiology Department, Ospedale Santissima Trinità, Cagliari, Italy

CARLO MARTINOLI, MD
Radiologia III, IRCCS San Martino-IST, DISSAL, Università degli studi di Genova, Genova, Italy

SALVATORE MASALA, MD
Musculoskeletal Interventional Radiology Department, Università Tor Vergata, Rome, Italy

CARLO MASCIOCCHI, MD
Diagnostic and Interventional Radiology, Department of Biotechnological and Applied Clinical Sciences, University of L'Aquila, L'Aquila, Coppito, Italy

PAUL MICHELIN, MD
Department of Radiology, CHRU de Rouen, Rouen, France

SIMONE MONTOYA, MD
Resident Physician, Imaging Sciences, University of Rochester Medical Center, Rochester, New York, USA

MARIO MUTO, MD
Neuroradiology Department, Ospedale Cardarelli, Naples, Italy

MICHELANGELO NASUTO, MD
Department of Radiology, University of Foggia, Foggia, Italy

MIKKEL ØSTERGAARD, MD, PhD, DMSc
Professor, Department of Rheumatology,
Copenhagen University Hospital at Hvidovre,
Hvidovre, Denmark

ATHENA PLAGOU, MD, PhD
Consultant Radiologist, Ultrasound Private
Institution, Athens, Greece

ALFONSO REGINELLI, MD
Department of Internal and Experimental
Medicine, Magrassi-Lanzara, Institute of
Radiology, Second University of Naples,
Naples, Italy

FRANK W. ROEMER, MD
Associate Professor, Department of
Radiology, Quantitative Imaging Center,
Boston University School of Medicine, Boston,
Massachusetts, USA; Department of
Radiology, University of Erlangen-Nuremburg,
Erlangen, Germany

ANDREY RUPASOV, DO
Resident Physician, Imaging Sciences,
University of Rochester Medical Center,
Rochester, New York, USA

PIERO RUSCITTI, MD
Rheumatology Clinic, Department of
Biotechnological and Applied Clinical
Sciences, University of L'Aquila, L'Aquila,
Coppito, Italy

**CLAUDIA SCHUELLER-WEIDEKAMM, MD,
MBA**
Associate Professor, Division of
Neuroradiology and Musculoskeletal
Radiology, Department of Biomedical Imaging
and Image-Guided Therapy, Vienna General
Hospital, Medical University of Vienna, Vienna,
Austria

PAOLO SIMONI, MD, PhD, MBA
Radiology Department, Hôpital Universitaire
des Enfants Reine Fabilola, Brussels, Belgium

IWONA SUDOŁ-SZOPIŃSKA, MD, PhD
Professor, Department of Radiology, National
Institute of Geriatrics, Rheumatology and
Rehabilitation, Department of Diagnostic
Imaging, Warsaw Medical University, Warsaw,
Poland

JAMES TEH, MD, MBBS, MRCP, FRCR
Consultant Radiologist, Department of
Radiology, Nuffield Orthopaedic Centre,
Oxford University Hospitals NHS Trust, Oxford,
United Kingdom

MAAIKE P. TERRA, MD, PhD
Division of Musculoskeletal Radiology,
Department of Radiology, Academic Medical
Center, Amsterdam, The Netherlands

PAOLO TOMÀ, MD
Radiologia, IRCCS Ospedale Pediatrico
Bambino Gesù, Roma, Italy

BADOT VALÉRIE, MD, PhD
Service de Rhumatologie et Médecine
Physique Rhumatologie Adulte et Pédiatrique,
Hôpital Erasme, Brussels, Belgium

SEBASTIAN WINKLHOFER, MD
Department of Neuroradiology, University
Hospital Zurich, University of Zurich, Zurich,
Switzerland

FEDERICO ZAOTTINI, MD
Radiologia III, IRCCS San Martino-IST,
DISSAL, Università degli studi di Genova,
Genova, Italy

MARCELLO ZAPPIA, MD
Department of Medicine and Health Science
"V. Tiberio", University of Molise,
Campobasso, Italy

Contents

asymptomatic. When resorbing, they become cloudy and less dense with an ill-defined shape and can migrate into adjacent structures.

Iwona Sudoł-Szopińska, Claudia Schueller-Weidekamm, Athena Plagou, and James Teh

Ultrasound imaging is currently performed in everyday rheumatologic practice. It is used for early diagnosis, to monitor treatment results, and to diagnose remission. The spectrum of pathologies seen in arthritis with ultrasound imaging includes early inflammatory features and associated complications. This article discusses the spectrum of ultrasound features of arthritides seen in rheumatoid arthritis and other connective tissue diseases in adults, such as Sjögren syndrome, lupus erythematosus, dermatomyositis, polymyositis, and juvenile idiopathic arthritis. Ultrasonographic findings in spondyloarthritis, osteoarthritis, and crystal-induced diseases are presented. Ultrasound-guided interventions in patients with arthritis are listed, and the advantages and disadvantages of ultrasound imaging are discussed.

Antonio Barile, Francesco Arrigoni, Federico Bruno, Giuseppe Guglielmi, Marcello Zappia, Alfonso Reginelli, Piero Ruscitti, Paola Cipriani, Roberto Giacomelli, Luca Brunese, and Carlo Masciocchi

The clinical diagnosis of rheumatoid arthritis is supported by imaging findings. MR imaging, in particular, can allow an early diagnosis to determine a target therapy that can stop or at least slow the disease progression.

Antonio Leone, Victor N. Cassar-Pullicino, Paola D'Aprile, Michelangelo Nasuto, and Giuseppe Guglielmi

This article provides an overview of the computed tomography (CT) and MR imaging appearances suggestive of spondyloarthritis, with a specific emphasis on the MR imaging findings of vertebral and sacroiliac involvement, and presents relevant clinical features that assist early diagnosis. CT is a sensitive imaging modality for the assessment of structural bone changes, but its clinical utility is limited. MR imaging is the modality of choice for early diagnosis, because of its ability to depict inflammation long before structural bone damage occurs, for monitoring of disease activity, and for evaluating therapeutic response.

Constantinus Franciscus Buckens, Maaike P. Terra, and Mario Maas

Crystalline-induced arthropathies impose substantial morbidity but can be challenging to diagnose, especially in early phases. The most common crystalline arthropathies are gout (monosodium urate deposition), calcium pyrophosphate dihydrate deposition, and hydroxyapatite deposition disease. Computed tomography (CT) and MR imaging provide 3-dimensional information on osseous structures, periarticular soft tissue, and tophi with superior spatial resolution. Dual-source CT (dual-energy CT [DECT]) offers the further advantage of selectively identifying crystalline deposits. CT, MR imaging, and DECT can be of value in problematic cases and can potentially be used for disease monitoring. Further research is necessary to elucidate their added value.

SAPHO and recurrent multifocal osteomyelitis are complex inflammatory conditions that clinical radiologists play an essential part in diagnosing. They present with a wide range of musculoskeletal and skin manifestations and exhibit several key diagnostic features that, when present, make the diagnoses unequivocal. The overall population group is young. Diagnostic delay is common with a relapsing and remitting clinical course and often subtle early radiologic findings. This article provides an up-to-date insight into both conditions, including their multifaceted pathogenesis, effective therapeutic options, and advanced imaging features, to arm radiologists with the knowledge required to make the diagnoses confidently in a timely manner.

This article clarifies the current role of MR imaging in the assessment of myopathies. Typical MR imaging findings are discussed for different forms of myopathies, including idiopathic inflammatory myopathies, muscular dystrophies, and congenital myopathies. The last section deals with advanced MR imaging techniques and their potential role in further characterization of muscular disease.

Juvenile idiopathic arthritis is an umbrella term covering several distinct categories that share common features. The European League Against Rheumatism and the Pediatric Rheumatology European Society have published a consensus article with recommendations to guide radiologists and clinicians in choosing the best imaging technique for each particular clinical setting. A reproducible, accurate, validated, and long-established scoring system to use in everyday practice for monitoring and predicting long-term response to therapy is still to be developed on MR imaging for each joint.

With technologic advances and the availability of sophisticated computer software and analytical strategies, imaging plays an increasingly important role in understanding the disease process of osteoarthritis (OA). Radiography has limitations in that it can visualize only limited features of OA, such as osteophytes and joint space narrowing, but remains the most commonly used modality for establishing an imaging-based diagnosis of OA. This article describes the roles and limitations of different imaging modalities and discusses the optimum imaging protocol, imaging diagnostic criteria of OA, differential diagnoses, and what the referring physician needs to know.

Patients affected by rheumatic conditions frequently present with spine degeneration and vertebral compression fractures, mainly related to the long-term therapies with glucocorticosteroids. A mini-invasive approach provided by interventional radiology techniques, especially vertebroplasty, plays a relevant role in the pain management of these patients; vertebroplasty represents the symptomatic treatment of fracture pain, so patients must always be included in a specific therapeutic workup of the rheumatic condition. This article describes patient selection criteria, technique, and outcomes of vertebroplasty in patients affected by rheumatic disease and secondary osteoporosis caused by glucocorticosteroids.

This article focuses on the imaging of 5 discrete entities with a common end result of disability: posttraumatic arthritis, a common form of secondary osteoarthritis that results from a prior insult to the joint; avascular necrosis, a disease of impaired osseous blood flow, leading to cellular death and subsequent osseous collapse; septic arthritis, an infectious process leading to destructive changes within the joint; complex regional pain syndrome, a chronic limb-confined painful condition arising after injury; and cases of cancer mimicking arthritis, in which the initial findings seem to represent arthritis, despite a more insidious cause.

Pediatric vasculitides are rare conditions that can represent a diagnostic challenge because symptoms are usually aspecific and variable. Symptoms are related to the size of the involved vessel, extension of disease, and organs affected. The outcome is closely linked to an early diagnosis and proper treatment. Diagnostic imaging allows visualization of the involvement of large-size and medium-size vessels and assesses end-organ changes and response to therapy, thus playing a pivotal role in the diagnosis and treatment. This article explores the general features of pediatric vasculitis and discusses the imaging approach and the most common diagnostic findings.

PROGRAM OBJECTIVE
The objective of the *Radiologic Clinics of North America* is to keep practicing radiologists and radiology residents up to date with current clinical practice in radiology by providing timely articles reviewing the state of the art in patient care.

TARGET AUDIENCE
Practicing radiologists, radiology residents, and other health care professionals who provide patient care utilizing radiologic findings.

LEARNING OBJECTIVES
Upon completion of this activity, participants will be able to:
1. Review topics in conventional radiology for various forms of arthritis.
2. Discuss the use of CT and MRI imaging in arthritis.
3. Recognize concepts in imaging oseteoarthritis, juvenile idiopathic arthritis, and childhood vasculitis, among other types.

ACCREDITATION
The Elsevier Office of Continuing Medical Education (EOCME) is accredited by the Accreditation Council for Continuing Medical Education (ACCME) to provide continuing medical education for physicians.

The EOCME designates this enduring material for a maximum of 15 *AMA PRA Category 1 Credit*(s)™. Physicians should claim only the credit commensurate with the extent of their participation in the activity.

All other health care professionals requesting continuing education credit for this enduring material will be issued a certificate of participation.

DISCLOSURE OF CONFLICTS OF INTEREST
The EOCME assesses conflict of interest with its instructors, faculty, planners, and other individuals who are in a position to control the content of CME activities. All relevant conflicts of interest that are identified are thoroughly vetted by EOCME for fair balance, scientific objectivity, and patient care recommendations. EOCME is committed to providing its learners with CME activities that promote improvements or quality in healthcare and not a specific proprietary business or a commercial interest.

The planning committee, staff, authors and editors listed below have identified no financial relationships or relationships to products or devices they or their spouse/life partner have with commercial interest related to the content of this CME activity:

Jose Acosta, MD; Sonia Airaldi, MD; Gustav Andreisek, MD, MBA; Maria Pilar Aparisi Gómez, MBChB, FRANZCR; Francesco Arrigoni, MD; Sammy Badr, MD, MSc; Antonio Barile, MD; Alberto Bazzocchi, MD, PhD; Maria Beatrice Damasio, MD; Johan G. Blickman, MD, PhD; Johan L. Bloem, MD, PhD; Luca Brunese, MD; Federico Bruno, MD; Usa Cain, MD; Victor N. Cassar-Pullicino, MD, FRCR; Dimitriou Christos, MD; Paola Cipriani, MD; Anne Cotten, MD, PhD; Paola D'Aprile, MD; Filippo Del Grande, MD, MBA, MHEM; Lukas Filli, MD; Anjali Fortna; Constantinus Franciscus Buckens, MD, PhD; Giulia Frauenfelder, MD; Roberto Giacomelli, MD; Francesco Giurazza, MD, PhD; Laurence Goffin, MD; Boitsios Grammatina, MD; Claudio Granata, MD; Simon Greenwood, MBChB, MSc, MRCP, FRCR; Gianluigi Guarnieri, MD; Giuseppe Guglielmi, MD; Daichi Hayashi, MD, PhD; Thibaut Jacques, MD, MSc; Mohamed Jarraya, MD; Herman M. Kroon, MD, PhD; Neal Larkman, MD, MPH; Phu-Quoc Lê, MD; Guillaume Lefebvre, MD; Antonio Leone, MD; Eva Llopis, MD; Mario Maas, MD, PhD; Gianmichele Magnano, MD; Clara Malattia, MD; Stefano Marcia, MD; Carlo Martinoli, MD; Salvatore Masala, MD; Carlo Masciocchi, MD; Paul Michelin, MD; Simone Montoya, MD; Mario Muto, MD; Michelangelo Nasuto, MD; Athena Plagou, MD, PhD; Alfonso Raginelli, MD; Andrey Rupasov, DO; Piero Ruscitti, MD; Claudia Schueller-Weidekamm, MD, MBA; Paolo Simoni, MD, PhD, MBA; Giovanna Stefania Colfati, MD; Mikkel Østergaard, MD, PhD, DMSc; Karthik Subramaniam; Iwona Sudoł-Szopińska, MD, PhD; James Teh, MD, MBBS, MRCP, FRCR; Maaike P. Terra, MD, PhD; Paolo Tomà, MD; Badot Valérie, MD, PhD; John Vassallo; Katie Widmeier; Sebastian Winklhofer, MD; Frederico Zattoni, MD; Marcello Zappia, MD.

The planning committee, staff, authors and editors listed below have identified financial relationships or relationships to products or devices they or their spouse/life partner have with commercial interest related to the content of this CME activity:

Ali Guermazi, MD, PhD has an employment affiliation with Boston Imaging Core Lab, LLC, and is a consultant/advisor for Pfizer Inc; TissueGene, Inc; OrthoTrophix, Inc; General Electric Company; Sanofi; EMD Serono, Inc; and AstraZeneca.
Frank W. Roemer, MD has stock ownership in Boston Imaging Core Lab, LLC.

UNAPPROVED/OFF-LABEL USE DISCLOSURE
The EOCME requires CME faculty to disclose to the participants:
1. When products or procedures being discussed are off-label, unlabelled, experimental, and/or investigational (not US Food and Drug Administration [FDA] approved); and
2. Any limitations on the information presented, such as data that are preliminary or that represent ongoing research, interim analyses, and/or unsupported opinions. Faculty may discuss information about pharmaceutical agents that is outside of FDA-approved labelling. This information is intended solely for CME and is not intended to promote off-label use of these

medications. If you have any questions, contact the medical affairs department of the manufacturer for the most recent pre-scribing information.

TO ENROLL
To enroll in the PET Clinics Continuing Medical Education program, call customer service at 1-800-654-2452 or sign up online at http://www.theclinics.com/home/cme. The CME program is available to subscribers for an additional annual fee of USD $315.

METHOD OF PARTICIPATION
In order to claim credit, participants must complete the following:
1. Complete enrolment as indicated above.
2. Read the activity.
3. Complete the CME Test and Evaluation. Participants must achieve a score of 70% on the test. All CME Tests and Evaluations must be completed online.

CME INQUIRIES/SPECIAL NEEDS
For all CME inquiries or special needs, please contact elsevierCME@elsevier.com.

RADIOLOGIC CLINICS OF NORTH AMERICA

THE CLINICS ARE AVAILABLE ONLINE!
Access your subscription at:
www.theclinics.com

Preface
Imaging in Rheumatology: An Update

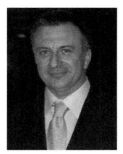

Giuseppe Guglielmi, MD
Editor

The role of imaging in rheumatology spans from the detection and characterization of macroanatomic and microanatomic changes in the joint and soft tissues in the pathophysiologic process to the use of the more advanced biomarkers of disease, targeting signs of early onset and disease activity.

The science of rheumatology is challenging and attractive for imaging professionals for three main reasons: First, the importance and "the beauty" of basic knowledge still central in daily practice, and the incentive for research and innovation; second, the current and future role of the different imaging techniques, as the whole range of imaging tools is involved in research and clinical practice; finally, the two-way interaction between the role of imaging in the definition and management of diseases and the evolution of the comprehension of pathophysiologic mechanisms. Imaging of rheumatologic diseases still relies on plain radiography, but has also evolved to the early detection of changes induced by diseases and to activity monitoring by ultrasound and MR imaging. The recognition of patterns and distribution of findings and the detection of either gross or tiny anatomic changes on radiography are still central. Furthermore, the availability of the use of new biomarkers at imaging methods in association with clinical data, and the perspective of the development of molecular diagnosis pathways, is being embraced in clinical practice; this is inspiring research and is aiding in the comprehension of rheumatologic diseases.

Imaging is essential in the diagnosis and staging of diseases as well as in assessing their activity and response to treatment, and this is crucial in driving treatment choices. Imaging positivity, what is radiologically visible and what is not, may represent the difference in the definition of the disease, or a cutoff between different entities, with significant clinical and prognostic implications.

This issue of the *Radiologic Clinics of North America* includes fifteen review articles covering different aspects of imaging in rheumatology, with the invaluable contribution of several internationally acclaimed and credited authors.

Radiologists should be confident with the clinical background and laboratory tests. The relationship between rheumatologist and radiologist should be close and open, and radiologists should be familiar with the clinical settings and how biohumoral markers of diseases are integrated into the diagnostic workup. One of the articles addresses what the rheumatologist is looking for and what the radiologist should know about diagnosis and treatment response, with the purpose of aiding at improving patient management and establishing a systematic approach to imaging analysis and reporting.

Classics like rheumatoid arthritis, spondyloarthritis, and crystals arthritis are revisited and updated, from the basic and still fundamental role of radiography to computed tomography and MR imaging and their new applications. The differential role of ultrasound in arthritis is presented and discussed. Special focus articles have been included: on SAPHO and recurrent

Radiol Clin N Am 55 (2017) xv–xvi
http://dx.doi.org/10.1016/j.rcl.2017.06.001
0033-8389/17/

multifocal osteomyelitis, on pediatric vasculitis, juvenile arthritis, and other pediatric rheumatologic disorders. Imaging of myopathies is the subject of a dedicated review article.

Other rheumatologic-related disease and misleading findings or pathologic entities are described to address specific questions and differential diagnosis concerns.

Current imaging techniques in osteoarthritis are also comprehensively reviewed in a specific article.

At the end of the issue, a review is given to summarize and provide a "take-home" message for interventions and therapy in rheumatology.

Finally, I would like to acknowledge Dr Alberto Bazzocchi, MD, PhD, from the Diagnostic and Interventional Radiology, the "Rizzoli" Orthopaedic Institute, Bologna, Italy, who significantly collaborated with me in the selection of authors and topics for this issue.

Giuseppe Guglielmi, MD
Department of Radiology
University of Foggia
Viale L. Pinto 1
71100 Foggia, Italy

Department of Radiology
Scientific Institute "Casa Sollievo della Sofferenza" Hospital
Viale Cappuccini 1
San Giovanni Rotondo
Foggia 71013, Italy

E-mail address:
giuseppe.guglielmi@unifg.it

What the Rheumatologist Is Looking for and What the Radiologist Should Know in Imaging for Rheumatoid Arthritis

James Teh, MD, MBBS, MRCP, FRCR[a],*,
Mikkel Østergaard, MD, PhD, DMSc[b]

KEYWORDS

- Rheumatoid • Arthritis • Inflammatory • Imaging • Ultrasound • MR Imaging • Rheumatologist
- Radiologist

KEY POINTS

- The early diagnosis and treatment of patients with rheumatoid arthritis is the key to preventing irreversible joint damage.
- Plain radiographs are insensitive to early detection of synovitis and joint damage; in recent years, there has been an increasing reliance on ultrasound and MR imaging.
- A clear understanding between the rheumatologist and radiologist is essential to ensure that the patient is investigated efficiently and effectively.
- This article outlines what the rheumatologists is looking for and what the radiologist should know when imaging patients with inflammatory arthritis in the clinical setting.

INTRODUCTION

In recent years, the development of biologic disease-modifying antirheumatic drugs has greatly improved the treatment and prognosis of patients with inflammatory arthritis. Novel treatment regimes aim to suppress joint inflammation, minimize structural damage, and thus prevent disability.[1] The early implementation of treatment, and its optimal adjustment, requires early diagnosis and accurate monitoring of disease activity. In addition, accurate prognostic markers are required to select the appropriate treatment regime.

A good understanding between rheumatologists and radiologists is required to ensure that investigations are carried out in an efficient,

cost-effective way, with careful attention to the patient's individual needs, using locally available equipment and expertise. This article outlines what the rheumatologist is looking for and what the radiologist should know in the clinical imaging of inflammatory arthritis.

DIAGNOSIS

Does the Patient Have Inflammatory Changes and/or Structural Changes?

In suspected inflammatory arthritis, the clinical question is usually whether or not there is synovitis, and if so is there structural change? In early rheumatoid arthritis, the spectrum of disease includes synovitis, tenosynovitis, bone marrow

Disclosure Statement: The authors have nothing to disclose.
[a] Department of Radiology, Nuffield Orthopaedic Centre, Oxford University Hospitals NHS Trust, Windmill Road, Oxford OX3 7LD, UK; [b] Department of Rheumatology, Copenhagen University Hospital at Hvidovre, Kettegaard alle 30, Hvidovre 2650, Denmark
* Corresponding author.
E-mail address: jamesteh1@gmail.com

Radiol Clin N Am 55 (2017) 905–916
http://dx.doi.org/10.1016/j.rcl.2017.04.001
0033-8389/17/© 2017 Elsevier Inc. All rights reserved.

edema, bone erosions, and bursitis. To answer this question effectively, several supplemental questions should be answered, including: Which imaging modality should be used? Is there synovitis? Is there tenosynovitis? Are the findings in this patient indicative of structural damage in the future or functional decline? Is there bone marrow edema? Are there bone erosions? and Which regions should be imaged?

Which imaging modality should be used?

Radiographs Radiographs are inexpensive and easily available, allowing wide coverage of affected regions with a reasonable level of reproducibility. In addition, there are validated assessment methods and scoring systems allowing longitudinal comparisons.[2] The disadvantages of radiographs are that it uses ionizing radiation, and is insensitive for soft tissue inflammation and early bony change. Radiographs, therefore, have a limited role in the early diagnosis of rheumatoid arthritis. The earliest radiographic findings of disease are of periarticular soft tissue swelling and juxtaarticular osteopenia. Early erosions typically occur at the junction between the cartilage and periosteal synovial membrane insertion and the bone (the so-called bare area). The joint space may initially be widened owing to the presence of a joint effusion or synovitis, but as cartilage destruction occurs, the joint space may narrow. Eventually, the joint is destroyed and there is joint subluxation and in some cases bony fusion.

Although radiographs have a low sensitivity, they have a high specificity for making a diagnosis of rheumatoid arthritis if erosions are present. In clinical practice, radiographs of the hands are typically obtained at presentation, because, if erosions are seen, they immediately classify the patient as having aggressive disease (**Fig. 1**). Radiographs also serve as a useful baseline, and may reveal a pattern of disease that suggests an alternative diagnosis such as psoriasis. Radiographs can also depict chondrocalcinosis, which may suggest gout or calcium pyrophosphate disease.

MR imaging MR imaging is more sensitive than clinical examination and radiographs for the detection of inflammatory and destructive joint changes in early rheumatoid arthritis.[3] MR imaging can assess all the structures involved in arthritic disease, that is, synovial membrane, fluid collections, cartilage, bone, ligaments, tendons, and tendon sheaths. Its multiplanar capability and excellent soft tissue contrast resolution makes MR imaging a very sensitive examination for joint inflammation, allowing for the assessment of

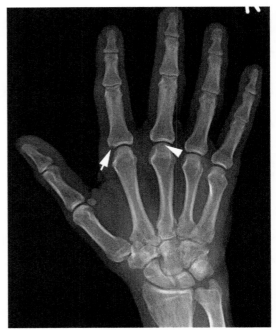

Fig. 1. Plain radiograph demonstrating early erosions (*arrows*) at the metacarpophalangeal joints.

structural changes and disease activity.[4] It is, however, a relatively expensive modality, which is time consuming and sometimes not well-tolerated by patients.

In clinical practice, the use of MR imaging for the detection of early inflammation depends on many factors, including local practice, cost, ease of access, and the degree of uncertainty of diagnosis. Its use will therefore vary between institutions, but radiologists should be aware that this modality offers the most comprehensive assessment of inflammatory arthritis in any particular joint.

Ultrasound imaging Ultrasound (US) imaging, with its multiplanar capability and excellent soft tissue resolution, allows for the delineation of inflammatory and structural changes in inflammatory arthritis. The use of Doppler allows a real-time assessment of neovascularity in joints, which correlates with histopathological findings.[5] US imaging can assess several regions relatively quickly, and with comparative ease and less expense when compared with MR imaging. However, because US imaging cannot penetrate bone, certain areas are not assessable. Furthermore, US imaging is highly operator dependent, and differing results may be obtained according to the training and ability of the sonographer. Finally, the findings, and changes therein may be difficult to quantify.

In clinical practice, US imaging plays a very important role in the early diagnosis of arthritis, because it is readily available and can be easily deployed in clinic to determine if there is active inflammation.

Is there synovitis?

Synovial inflammation is manifest by increased synovial vascularity, capillary leakage, and joint effusion. Joint swelling in rheumatoid arthritis reflects inflammation of the synovial membrane and is characterized by both innate (eg, monocytes, mast cells, and innate lymphoid cells) and adaptive immune cells (eg, T helper and B cells) infiltrating the synovial compartment. The inflammatory milieu ultimately triggers an osteoclastic response that results in bony erosions.[6] Synovitis occurs early in the natural history of rheumatoid arthritis and is considered to be a strong predictor of erosions. Disease activity in a joint also correlates well with synovial vascularity.

OMERACT (Outcome Measures in Rheumatoid Arthritis Clinical Trials) is an international, multidisciplinary group established with the aim of developing and validating outcome measures for rheumatology clinical trials. OMERACT has developed standardized techniques, joint pathology definitions, and scoring systems for the use of imaging MR imaging in rheumatoid arthritis. The OMERACT definition of synovitis on MR imaging is an area in the synovial compartment that shows above normal, postgadolinium enhancement of a thickness greater than the width of the normal synovium.[7] The width of normal synovium is not defined, however. A joint effusion may be seen in association with synovial thickening, but does not demonstrate the rapid enhancement after intravenous gadolinium. On delayed imaging, contrast may diffuse into the joint effusion, and therefore effusions and synovitis may be impossible to differentiate. The use of intravenous gadolinium increases the sensitivity for detection of synovitis and tenosynovitis[8] and bone marrow edema.[9] In clinical practice, the administration of gadolinium is often omitted, with a reliance on fat-suppressed T2-weighted sequences or short tau inversion recovery imaging for the assessment of synovitis. This means, however, that the radiologist is unable to accurately differentiate with certainty between effusion and synovial hypertrophy. It has been shown that not using intravenous contrast results in a decrease in sensitivity, specificity and intrareader and interreader reliability with regard to synovitis.[8,10] The radiologist needs to be aware that an effusion per se, although a good indicator of joint disease is nonspecific with regard to disease activity in rheumatoid arthritis.

OMERACT defines synovitis on US imaging as hypoechogenic, thickened intraarticular tissue that is nondisplaceable and poorly compressible and that may exhibit Doppler signals.[11] Increased Doppler signal is correlated with disease activity (**Fig. 2**). Joint effusions, in contrast, appear to be anechoic, with increased through transmission and compressibility, with no Doppler signal. There is a high concordance between Doppler US imaging and contrast-enhanced MR imaging for the detection of synovitis in rheumatoid arthritis wrist and finger joints, indicating that the imaging findings reflect a similar pathologic phenomenon.[12]

Both MR imaging and US imaging are more sensitive than clinical assessment for detecting synovitis, and both can demonstrate subclinical synovitis. When no synovitis is present in the peripheral joints, both modalities have a strong negative predictive value for rheumatoid arthritis, which is an important clinical consideration.

Is there tenosynovitis?

Tenosynovitis is commonly seen in patients with early rheumatoid arthritis, and is often bilateral. In the wrist, the flexor and extensor digitorum tendons are typically involved, and in the fingers the index and middle flexor tendons are involved most frequently. Tenosynovitis may occur in isolation, and may be the only feature in early rheumatoid arthritis.

On MR imaging, tenosynovitis is demonstrated as thickening of the synovial sheath or fluid within the sheath, with high signal on T2-weighted images[13] (**Fig. 3**). After intravenous gadolinium injection, there is rapid enhancement of synovial hypertrophy, but not of fluid within the sheath. Tendinosis may be evident on MR imaging because tendon thickening with heterogeneous increased intratendinous signal on T2-weighted images. There may be enhancement with intravenous gadolinium on T1-weighted MR imaging.

On US imaging, tenosynovitis is demonstrated as hypoechoic thickening of the synovial sheath

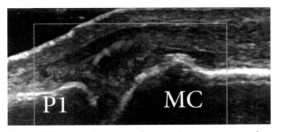

Fig. 2. Ultrasound image of the index metacarpophalangeal joint demonstrating moderate active synovitis with increased power Doppler signal. MC, metacarpal; P1, proximal phalanx.

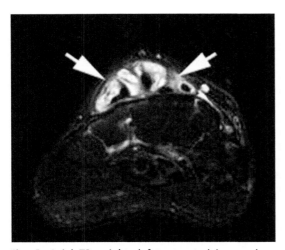

Fig. 3. Axial T2-weighted fat-saturated image demonstrating extensor digitorum tenosynovitis with synovial hypertrophy surrounding the tendons (arrows).

with increased vascularity on Doppler interrogation.[11] On US imaging, tendinosis is demonstrated as tendon thickening with hypoechoic change and loss of the normal fibrillar pattern. On Doppler, there is typically increased vascularity.

Are the findings in this patient indicative of structural damage in the future or functional decline? Is there bone marrow edema?

MR imaging signal alterations in the subchondral bone marrow of patients with rheumatoid arthritis have been shown histologically to represent the formation of inflammatory infiltrates, including lymphocytes and osteoclasts.[14,15] Therefore, bone marrow "edema" on MR imaging corresponds with inflammation rather than representing increased water content per se. This finding has primarily been thought to be secondary to external inflamed synovium, but there is evidence that the cellular infiltrate might also mediate the development of bone erosions from the subchondral bone toward the joint surface.[16] Bone marrow changes cannot be demonstrated on radiographs, computed tomography (CT) scans, or US imaging. On MR imaging, bone marrow edema is identified as a poorly defined area of low signal within bone on T1-weighted images, with high signal on T2-weighted fat-suppressed or short tau inversion recovery images (Fig. 4).[7]

The presence of bone marrow edema in rheumatoid arthritis is associated with a high risk of progression to bone erosions and thus irreversible joint damage over time. Bone edema scored on MR imaging scans of the dominant carpus at presentation has been shown to predict radiographic joint damage of the hands and feet 5 to 6 years later in patients with rheumatoid arthritis.[17,18] One study found that bone marrow edema was associated with a 6.5-fold risk of erosions at that site within 1 year.[19] Bone marrow edema can be used as a clinical tool to predict medium-term functional disability and can therefore help to determine which patients need early and aggressive therapeutic management to avoid subsequent joint damage and disability.[20,21] Bone marrow edema seems to be a stronger predictor of future erosions than synovial volumes. Nevertheless, irrespective of the modality of examination of joints, the presence of synovitis has also been shown to be predictive for subsequent structural and functional deterioration.[20–23]

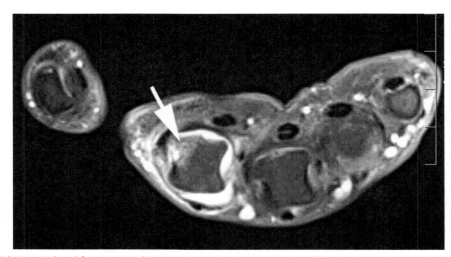

Fig. 4. Axial T2-weighted fat-saturated image demonstrating synovitis of the index metacarpophalangeal joint. There is bone marrow edema of the metacarpal head (arrow).

Are there bone erosions?

Bone erosion is an important pathologic feature of rheumatoid arthritis and is associated with disease severity and poor functional outcome.[24] Most erosions develop in the first 2 years of the disease, and frequently occur within 6 months in aggressive disease.[25] The carpal bones—particularly the capitate, ulnar styloid, the radial aspect of the index and middle finger metacarpal bones, and the lateral aspect of the little finger metacarpal bone—are most frequently involved with bone erosions. Once they are established, bone erosions rarely repair.[26]

OMERACT defines an erosion on MR imaging as a sharply marginated bone lesion, with a juxtaarticular location and typical signal characteristics, which is visible in at least 2 planes with a cortical break seen in at least 1 plane.[7] On T1-weighted images the low signal intensity of cortical bone is lost and the normal fatty marrow signal is replaced. Rapid gadolinium enhancement suggests the presence of active, hypervascularized pannus within the erosion. Active erosions enhance with gadolinium differentiating them from intraosseous fluid-filled cystic lesions. MR imaging has been shown in several studies to be superior to radiographs for the detection of erosions, and can visualize lesions 6 to 12 months before they show up on radiographs.[19,23,27]

US imaging is a reliable technique that detects more erosions than radiography, especially in early rheumatoid arthritis.[28] On US imaging, bone erosions are seen as intraarticular discontinuities of the bone surface that are visible in 2 perpendicular planes (**Fig. 5**). On Doppler imaging, the presence of high signal within the bone erosions is due to proliferative, hypervascularized pannus tissue.[29] US imaging has been shown to have a comparable sensitivity as MR imaging in detecting bone erosions in metacarpophalangeal joints, but is limited by the fact that ultrasound cannot penetrate bone, and therefore erosions at certain location are

not accessible by US imaging, particularly in the more complicated joints, for example, the wrist joint.[27,30]

Tomosynthesis has been developed from conventional tomography and involves collecting a number of projected images at different angles using a digital detector, allowing reconstruction at various depths.[31] The detection of erosions is improved because there is less projectional overlapping than on conventional radiographs. Using multidetector CT scanning as the gold standard, tomosynthesis has been shown to be far superior to conventional radiography for the depiction of bone erosions of the hands and wrists.[32] This technique, however, is not widely available, and involves ionizing radiation; however, it is a potential tool for the early detection of erosions.

CT scanning provides high-resolution multiplanar imaging allowing excellent definition of the bony anatomy. It is thus considered the reference standard for imaging of erosions.[27,30] It does, however, confer a significant radiation dose and is not recommended for routine clinical practice. Erosion scores derived from CT scans of the wrist have been shown to be significantly higher than erosion scores from MR imaging scans of the same region.[33] In this study, both modalities identified erosions in 87% of cases. In 9% of cases, CT imaging detected lesions not seen on MR imaging, and in 4% of cases MR imaging detected lesions not seen on CT imaging.

In clinical practice, if radiographs are negative but structural damage is suspected, either MR imaging or US imaging can be used to detect whether erosions are present.

Which regions should be imaged?

Choosing the regions to be imaged requires careful consideration. The target areas for early joint involvement in rheumatoid arthritis are the hands and feet, particularly the wrists and the metacarpophalangeal joints or metatarsophalangeal joints.

Typically, the most symptomatic extremity, the dominant extremity, or both are examined together, when using US imaging or MR imaging. US imaging allows several joints to be assessed relatively easily and quickly compared with MR imaging, and so may be preferable if numerous joints require analysis. With a large field, the small joints of the hand are not well-assessed, so generally whole-body MR imaging is not appropriate for the assessment of rheumatoid arthritis. Nevertheless, whole body MR imaging at 3 T has been shown to be able to identify inflammation and structural damage in the peripheral and axial skeleton in rheumatoid arthritis, providing an option for an MR imaging joint count.[34]

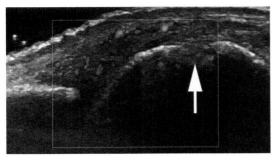

Fig. 5. Ultrasound image of the metacarpal head demonstrating an erosion (*arrow*).

DIFFERENTIAL DIAGNOSIS

What Is the Difference Between Classification and Diagnostic Criteria?

Both rheumatologists and radiologists should be aware of the difference in diagnostic and classification criteria. Diagnostic criteria are a set of signs, symptoms, and tests developed for use in clinical practice to guide the care of individual patients.[35] They must, therefore, reflect all the possible different features of the disease across a spectrum of severity and disease heterogeneity. Classification criteria in contrast are standardized definitions that are primarily intended to enable clinical studies to have uniform cohorts for research. They need to define (relatively) homogenous groups that can be compared across different studies and regions. Classification is, therefore, not synonymous with diagnosis. Whereas diagnosis has the ultimate aim of being correct for an individual patient, the goal of classification is to maximize homogeneous populations for study purposes. Clinicians can, therefore, diagnose conditions in patients who have not met classification criteria definitions. Classification criteria can and are often used to support the diagnosis.

What Is the Differential Diagnosis? What Features Help in Making a Diagnosis?

Rheumatoid arthritis is one of the most common chronic autoimmune inflammatory diseases affecting around 0.5% to 1.0% of the population.[36] Although it primarily involves the joints, it should be considered a multisystem disorder, with occasional extraarticular manifestations such as interstitial lung disease and vasculitis.[37] In rheumatoid arthritis, the typical patient presents with symmetrically tender and swollen peripheral joints, morning joint stiffness, and increased serum inflammatory markers. This presentation is, however, nonspecific. Other causes of arthritis need to be considered, such as reactive arthritis, osteoarthritis, psoriatic arthritis, infectious arthritis, and connective tissue diseases. Indeed, more than 150 forms of arthritis have been recognized.[38] Nevertheless, in clinical practice the majority of cases of hand arthritis can be covered by a handful of diagnoses, namely osteoarthritis, rheumatoid arthritis, calcium pyrophosphate deposition disease, psoriatic arthritis, and gout. In many patients, no specific diagnosis can be made at the initial presentation, and the diagnosis of exclusion is undifferentiated arthritis.

The most recent American College of Rheumatology classification criteria for rheumatoid arthritis were developed using cohorts and case scenarios of patients with early arthritis.[39] The new criteria, classifies "definite rheumatoid arthritis" based on the confirmed presence of synovitis in at least 1 joint, the absence of an alternative diagnosis better explaining the synovitis, and amassing a total score of 6 or greater (of a possible 10) from the individual scores in 4 domains: number and site of involved joints (range, 0–5), serologic abnormality (range, 0–3), elevated acute phase response (range, 0–1), and symptom duration (range, 0–1). The criteria allow for sensitive assessment of joint involvement (tender or swollen joints, or joints positive by ultrasound or MR imaging can be classified as involved joints).

Analyzing which anatomic structures are affected—the synovium, cartilage, or enthesis—can effectively narrow the differential diagnosis.[38] For example, in rheumatoid arthritis inflammation is more frequent in the synovial membrane than at the enthesis, whereas the opposite is true for seronegative spondyloarthritides, such as psoriatic arthritis. With the increasing use of MR imaging and US imaging in early inflammatory arthritis, there has been interest in whether or not these imaging modalities improve the specificity of diagnosis. In 1 study, the inclusion of the MR imaging criterion "bilateral joint enhancement" (ie, bilateral synovitis in hands/wrists) as an adjunct to the 1987 American College of Rheumatology criteria for establishing a diagnosis of rheumatoid arthritis increased the baseline sensitivity for rheumatoid arthritis from 77% to 96% and increased the diagnostic accuracy from 83% to 94%.[40] In a group of patients with rheumatoid arthritis, systemic lupus erythematosus and primary Sjögren syndrome with hand arthritis, metacarpophalangeal joint bone edema was found much more commonly in rheumatoid arthritis patients (71%) than non-rheumatoid arthritis patients (5%).[41] MR imaging evidence of bone edema in the metatarsophalangeal and wrist joints has also been found to be an independent predictor of future rheumatoid arthritis in patients with early undifferentiated arthritis.[42]

In psoriasis, there is a predilection for the distal interphalangeal joints and the disease is more often asymmetrical, as opposed to rheumatoid arthritis, where there is typically a symmetric distribution of disease involving the metacarpophalangeal joints.[43] In patients with psoriatic arthritis, there is often predominant tenosynovial involvement in the hands, particularly the flexor tendons. This is often associated subcutaneous soft tissue edema contributing to dactylitis. Periarticular bone marrow edema is often extracapsular related to enthesitis. Erosions may be morphologically similar to rheumatoid arthritis, but may be associated with distinctive bone proliferation and periostitis. This is often better appreciated on radiographs than MR imaging.

Gout is a form of inflammatory arthropathy characterized by acute attacks of synovitis associated with the deposition of monosodium urate crystals in the soft tissues or joints.[44] Chronic gout is manifest by the presence of gouty tophi, with punched out erosions in the peripheral and axial skeleton. There is a predilection for the first metatarsophalangeal joint, which may offer a clue as to the diagnosis. Radiographs have limited use in the early diagnosis of gout, because the erosions may only manifest after many years. On US imaging, the recognition of gouty aggregates may allow a specific diagnosis. Several patterns have been described, ranging from punctiform spots in the synovium through to large aggregates (**Fig. 6**). The double contour sign, indicating the presence of gout crystals on the articular cartilage, is highly specific.[45] The OMERACT US imaging study group has defined US imaging elementary lesions and validated an assessment system.[46] On MR imaging, gouty tophi are typically of medium to high signal on T2-weighted images and low signal on T1-weighted images.[47] Erosions and bone edema may be indistinguishable from other forms of inflammatory arthritis. Dual-energy CT is a valuable new tool for the diagnosis of gout. Images are acquired simultaneously at 2 different energy levels, providing 2 datasets, which can be analyzed using a 3-dimensional material decomposition algorithm that allows characterization of uric acid (**Fig. 7**).[48]

MONITORING
Is the Patient in Remission?

An important treatment goal in inflammatory arthritis is to suppress disease activity and achieve a state of remission to prevent joint damage, thus maintaining function and avoiding disability.[49] Remission refers to a state of disease inactivity, but there is no universally agreed definition. Remission implies absence of disease, with no

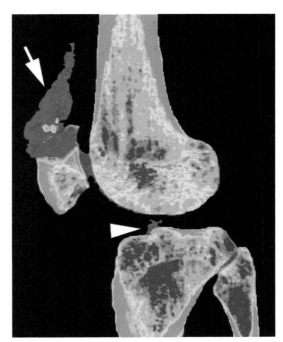

Fig. 7. Dual energy computed tomography color-coded image demonstrating brown gout deposits in the quadriceps tendon (*arrow*), and also within the knee joint (*arrowhead*). There is erosion of the superior pole of the patella.

signs or symptoms of active disease, but this is not synonymous with "cure," which implies that the disease process will not return.[50] It should be recognized that clinical remission does not equate to remission on imaging.[51,52] Imaging may show evidence of progression of joint damage despite apparent remission.[53,54] Subclinical synovitis with ongoing synovial inflammation or bone marrow edema on imaging may indicate that therapy needs to be continued or escalated. However, there is ongoing uncertainty as to whether or not imaging should be relied on to determine treatment.

There is good evidence that targeting low-disease activity or remission (ie, systematic monitoring of disease activity) in the management of rheumatoid arthritis conveys better outcomes than routine care.[1,55] The American College of Rheumatology has proposed 2 different definitions of remission for rheumatoid arthritis for use in clinical trials: either the compilation of 4 individual measures (tender joint count, swollen joint count, C-reactive protein and patient global assessment) or an index-based alternative (Simplified Disease Activity Index).[56] It is an important research question whether these composite measures of remission are equivalent to relying on imaging alone for

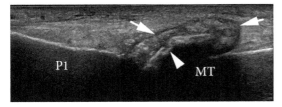

Fig. 6. Ultrasound image of the first metatarsophalangeal joint demonstrating synovitis (*long arrows*) with gout aggregates (small echogenic foci) and an erosion (*arrowhead*). MT, metatarsal; P1, proximal phalanx.

remission. Two recent studies have found that aiming for sonographic remission in early rheumatoid arthritis does not seem to provide any benefit over targeting clinical remission,[57,58] but this remains an area of controversy. Studies of patients in clinical remission and studies using MR imaging are still awaited[59] and will have important implications for the use of advanced imaging to assess clinical outcomes.

Has the Inflammatory Activity in This Patient Improved? Is There Any Structural Progression in This Patient?

The assessment of disease activity and therapeutic response predominantly relies on clinical assessment and serum markers of inflammation, although increasingly imaging has been used. For an imaging modality to be an effective technique for monitoring disease, it ideally needs to be reproducible, quantifiable, and sensitive to change. Serial examinations should ideally be performed on the same equipment using similar parameters and positioning. Essentially the rheumatologist wants to know if there is active inflammation and if there has been structural progression, that is, erosions.

Many of the detailed quantification methods described in papers on imaging for clinical trials are too time consuming, and unnecessary, for every day clinical practice. Imaging that is tailored toward an individual patient may also differ in frequency and modality from imaging geared toward study populations.

Using radiographs

Radiographs have no useful role in the assessment of synovial inflammation per se. In the routine clinical management of rheumatoid arthritis and clinical trials, radiographic evaluation focuses on joint space narrowing and bone erosions in hands, wrists, and forefeet as measures of structural joint damage. Validated scoring methods of radiological damage (including the Larsen method, the Sharp method and van der Heijde and Genant modifications) are available and are used extensively in clinical trials.[2,60] For clinical practice, the less time-consuming Simple Erosion Narrowing Score, based on counting joints with bone erosions and joints with joint space narrowing, is an option,[61] but is rarely used.

Using MR imaging

Early contrast enhancement of the synovium can be quantitatively assessed by dynamic-contrast enhanced MR imaging, by analyzing enhancement curves or using computer-aided detection.[62,63] Color maps allow for the assessment of enhancement patterns that can evaluate the degree of disease activity. These quantitative methods of synovitis quantification correlate closely to histopathologic synovitis. Automated volume quantification of various synovitis and other pathologies may also be a future option.[64] These techniques may be very useful in the context of clinical trials, where defined endpoints are critical; however, they are generally not used in routine clinical practice Fig. 8.

Semiquantitative scoring has been the most frequently used technique in clinical trials. The OMERACT Rheumatoid Arthritis MRI Scoring System (RAMRIS) involves semiquantitative assessment of synovitis, bone erosions, and bone edema in the hands and wrists.[7] The technique was developed and validated through iterative multicenter studies under OMERACT and European League against Rheumatism (EULAR) umbrella. The EULAR–OMERACT group has also produced an rheumatoid arthritis MR imaging reference image atlas, allowing comparison with standard reference images of activity and damage.[65] RAMRIS has been validated through controlled studies showing very good intrareader reliability, good interreader reliability, and a high level of sensitivity to change. When readers are trained and calibrated, the technique is suitable for monitoring inflammation and structural damage.

Synovitis is scored on a 0 to 3 semiquantitative scale, where 0 = normal, 1 = mild, 2 = moderate, and 3 = severe, with each point representing one-third of the maximum volume of the enhancing tissue in the synovial compartment.

Bone marrow edema is scored corresponding to the proportion of each bone that contains edema, using a 0 to 3 scale, where 0 = no edema, 1 = 1% to 33% of the bone is edematous, 2 = 34% to 66% of the bone is edematous, and 3 = 67% to 100% of the bone is edematous. Sum scores of synovitis, erosion, and edema can be calculated by summation of individual joint scores, as a total sum or separately in the wrist and second to fifth metacarpophalangeal joints, respectively.

A scoring system for tenosynovitis has also been developed.[13] Using a combined score of synovitis, tenosynovitis and bone edema has been shown to be more sensitive to change than conventional biomarkers and clinical measures, as well as the individual MR imaging parameters separately.[50]

Using ultrasound imaging

US imaging has great potential for use in clinical practice as an outcome measure in inflammatory arthritis[66]; however, compared with MR imaging there are fewer data regarding its validity,

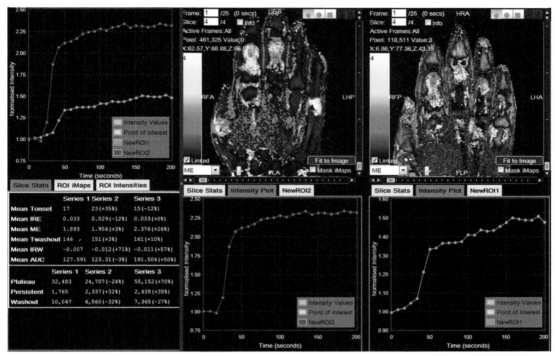

Fig. 8. Baseline and follow-up dynamic contrast-enhanced MR imaging scans. Inflammation in the joints is visible through the color-coded maps. The degree of inflammation is encoded in a heat map: yellow = high inflammation; red = lower inflammation. Curves show contrast enhancement for each region of interest (ROI). Numbers show volume of enhancing pixels. Reduction in follow-up examination (*right*) indicates reduced inflammation and, therefore, treatment response. (*Courtesy of* Dynamika, Image Analysis Group.)

reproducibility, and responsiveness to change, making follow-up studies difficult to interpret. Nevertheless, several studies have shown that US imaging is a reliable technique for following up patients with rheumatoid arthritis.[67–69] The semiquantitative scale most commonly used for synovitis is as follows: grade 0, no flow in the synovium; grade 1, single vessel signal; grade 2, confluent vessel signals in less than one-half the area of the synovium; grade 3, vessel signals in more than on-e-half the area of the synovium.[12] Several different techniques have been proposed for quantitatively assessing synovitis.[70–72] Quantifying power Doppler by measuring the fraction of color pixels in the region of interest and evaluating the changes over time has also been suggested.[73] It is apparent that differences between US imaging units, ultrasonographers, and scanning technique need to taken into account, and methodologies standardized. The follow-up assessment of structural damage in joints is difficult in US imaging mainly because of issues regarding exact probe repositioning.[74] In clinical practice, the question that is typically asked is simply whether or not there is active synovitis or progressive joint damage after treatment, and as such both MR imaging

and US imaging are useful tools. Most reports do not offer a quantitative evaluation in the routine clinical setting, but MR imaging readers and ultrasonographers should at least aim to give a semiquantitative report on whether or not there has been an improvement in the degree of inflammation, and whether or not there is structural damage.

REFERENCES

1. Smolen JS, Landewé R, Breedveld FC, et al. EULAR recommendations for the management of rheumatoid arthritis with synthetic and biological disease-modifying antirheumatic drugs: 2013 update. Ann Rheum Dis 2014;73:492–509.

2. van der Heijde DM. Plain X-rays in rheumatoid arthritis: overview of scoring methods, their reliability and applicability. Baillieres Clin Rheumatol 1996; 10(3):435–53.

3. McQueen FM. A vital clue to deciphering bone pathology: MRI bone oedema in rheumatoid arthritis and osteoarthritis. Ann Rheum Dis 2007;66(12): 1549–52.

4. Sudoł-Szopińska I, Jurik A, Eshed I, et al. Recommendations of the ESSR arthritis subcommittee for

the use of Magnetic Resonance Imaging in musculo-skeletal rheumatic diseases. Semin Musculoskelet Radiol 2015;19(04):396–411.

5. Walther M, Harms H, Krenn V, et al. Correlation of power Doppler sonography with vascularity of the synovial tissue of the knee joint in patients with oste-oarthritis and rheumatoid arthritis. Arthritis Rheum 2001;44(2):331–8.

6. Redlich K, Hayer S, Ricci R, et al. Osteoclasts are essential for TNF-alpha-mediated joint destruction. J Clin Invest 2002;110(10):1419–27.

7. Østergaard M, Peterfy C, Conaghan P, et al. OMER-ACT Rheumatoid Arthritis Magnetic Resonance Im-aging Studies. Core set of MRI acquisitions, joint pathology definitions, and the OMERACT RA-MRI scoring system. J Rheumatol 2003;30(6):1385–6.

8. Østergaard M, Conaghan PG, O'Connor P, et al. Reducing invasiveness, duration, and cost of mag-netic resonance imaging in rheumatoid arthritis by omitting intravenous contrast injection – Does it change the assessment of inflammatory and destruc-tive joint changes by the OMERACT RAMRIS? J Rheumatol 2009;36(8):1806–10.

9. Stomp W, Krabben A, van der Heijde D, et al. Aiming for a simpler early arthritis MRI protocol: can Gd contrast administration be eliminated? Eur Radiol 2015;25(5):1520–7.

10. Stomp W, Krabben A, van der Heijde D, et al. Aiming for a shorter rheumatoid arthritis MRI protocol: can contrast-enhanced MRI replace T2 for the detection of bone marrow oedema? Eur Radiol 2014;24(10):2614–22.

11. Wakefield RJ, Balint PV, Szkudlarek M, et al. Muscu-loskeletal ultrasound including definitions for ultraso-nographic pathology. J Rheumatol 2005;32(12):2485–7.

12. Szkudlarek M, Klarlund M, Narvestad E, et al. Ultra-sonography of the metacarpophalangeal and prox-imal interphalangeal joints in rheumatoid arthritis: a comparison with magnetic resonance imaging, con-ventional radiography and clinical examination. Arthritis Res Ther 2006;8(2):R52.

13. Haavardsholm EA, Østergaard M, Ejbjerg BJ, et al. Introduction of a novel magnetic resonance imaging tenosynovitis score for rheumatoid arthritis: reliability in a multireader longitudinal study. Ann Rheum Dis 2007;66(9):1216–20.

14. Jimenez Boj E, Nöbauer Huhmann I, Hanslik Schnabel B, et al. Bone erosions and bone marrow edema as defined by magnetic resonance imaging reflect true bone marrow inflammation in rheumatoid arthritis. Arthritis Rheum 2007;56(4):1118–24.

15. McQueen FM, Gao A, Ostergaard M, et al. High-grade MRI bone oedema is common within the surgical field in rheumatoid arthritis patients undergoing joint replacement and is associated with osteitis in sub-chondral bone. Ann Rheum Dis 2007;66(12):1581–7.

16. Schwarz EM, Looney RJ, Drissi MH, et al. Autoimmu-nity and bone. Ann N Y Acad Sci 2006;1068(1):275–83.

17. Hetland ML, Ejbjerg B, Hørslev-Petersen K, et al. MRI bone oedema is the strongest predictor of sub-sequent radiographic progression in early rheuma-toid arthritis. Results from a 2-year randomised controlled trial (CIMESTRA). Ann Rheum Dis 2009;68(3):384–90.

18. McQueen FM, Benton N, Perry D, et al. Bone edema scored on magnetic resonance imaging scans of the dominant carpus at presentation predicts radio-graphic joint damage of the hands and feet six years later in patients with rheumatoid arthritis. Arthritis Rheum 2003;48(7):1814–27.

19. McQueen FM, Stewart N, Crabbe J, et al. Magnetic resonance imaging of the wrist in early rheumatoid arthritis reveals a high prevalence of erosions at four months after symptom onset. Ann Rheum Dis 1998;57(6):350–6.

20. Baker JF, Conaghan PG, Emery P, et al. Relationship of patient-reported outcomes with MRI measures in rheumatoid arthritis. Ann Rheum Dis 2016;76:486–90.

21. Benton N, Stewart N, Crabbe J, et al. MRI of the wrist in early rheumatoid arthritis can be used to predict functional outcome at 6 years. Ann Rheum Dis 2004;63(5):555–61.

22. Dougados M, Devauchelle-Pensec V, Ferlet JF, et al. The ability of synovitis to predict structural damage in rheumatoid arthritis: a comparative study between clinical examination and ultrasound. Ann Rheum Dis 2012;72(5):665–71.

23. Boyesen P, Haavardsholm EA, Ostergaard M, et al. MRI in early rheumatoid arthritis: synovitis and bone marrow oedema are independent predictors of subsequent radiographic progression. Ann Rheum Dis 2011;70(3):428–33.

24. Bombardier C, Barbieri M, Parthan A, et al. The rela-tionship between joint damage and functional disability in rheumatoid arthritis: a systematic review. Ann Rheum Dis 2012;71(6):836–44.

25. Bird P, Kirkham B, Portek I, et al. Documenting dam-age progression in a two-year longitudinal study of rheumatoid arthritis patients with established dis-ease (the DAMAGE study cohort): is there an advan-tage in the use of magnetic resonance imaging as compared with plain radiography? Arthritis Rheum 2004;50(5):1383–9.

26. Møller Døhn U, Boonen A, Hetland ML, et al. Erosive progression is minimal, but erosion healing rare, in patients with rheumatoid arthritis treated with adali-mumab. A 1 year investigator-initiated follow-up study using high-resolution computed tomography as the primary outcome measure. Ann Rheum Dis 2009;68(10):1585–90.

27. Dohn UM, Ejbjerg BJ, Hasselquist M. Detection of bone erosions in rheumatoid arthritis wrist joints

with magnetic resonance imaging, computed tomography and radiography. Arthritis Res 2008;10:R25.

28. Wakefield RJ, Gibbon WW, Conaghan PG. The value of sonography in the detection of bone erosions in patients with rheumatoid arthritis. Arthritis Rheum 2000;43(12):2762–70.

29. Jahns R. Evaluation of pannus and vascularization of the metacarpophalangeal and proximal interphalangeal joints in rheumatoid arthritis by high-resolution ultrasound (multidimensional linear array). Arthritis Rheum 1999;42(11):2303–8.

30. Døhn UM, Ejbjerg BJ, Court Payen M, et al. Are bone erosions detected by magnetic resonance imaging and ultrasonography true erosions? A comparison with computed tomography in rheumatoid arthritis metacarpophalangeal joints. Arthritis Res Ther 2006;8(4):R110.

31. Duryea J, Dobbins JT, Lynch JA. Digital tomosynthesis of hand joints for arthritis assessment. Med Phys 2003;30(3):325–33.

32. Canella C, Philippe P, Pansini V, et al. Use of Tomosynthesis for Erosion Evaluation in Rheumatoid Arthritic Hands and Wrists. Radiology 2011;258(1):199–205.

33. Perry D, Stewart N, Benton N, et al. Detection of erosions in the rheumatoid hand; a comparative study of multidetector computerized tomography versus magnetic resonance scanning. J Rheumatol 2005; 32(2):256–67.

34. Axelsen MB, Eshed I, Duer-Jensen A, et al. Wholebody MRI assessment of disease activity and structural damage in rheumatoid arthritis: first step towards an MRI joint count. Rheumatology (Oxford) 2014;53(5):845–53.

35. Aggarwal R, Ringold S, Khanna D, et al. Distinctions between diagnostic and classification criteria? Arthritis Care Res 2015;67(7):891–7.

36. Silman AJ, Pearson JE. Epidemiology and genetics of rheumatoid arthritis. Arthritis Res 2002; 4(Suppl 3):S265–72.

37. Smolen JS, Aletaha D, McInnes IB. Rheumatoid arthritis. Lancet 2016;388(10055):2023–38.

38. Watt I. Basic differential diagnosis of arthritis. Eur Radiol 1997;7(3):344–51.

39. Aletaha D, Neogi T, Silman AJ, et al. 2010 rheumatoid arthritis classification criteria: an American College of Rheumatology/European League Against Rheumatism collaborative initiative. Ann Rheum Dis 2010;69(9):1580–8.

40. Sugimoto H, Takeda A, Hyodoh K. Early-stage rheumatoid arthritis: prospective study of the effectiveness of MR imaging for diagnosis. Radiology 2000; 216(2):569–75.

41. Boutry N, Hachulla E, Flipo R-M, et al. MR imaging findings in hands in early rheumatoid arthritis: comparison with those in systemic lupus erythematosus and primary Sjögren syndrome. Radiology 2005; 236(2):593–600.

42. Duer-Jensen A, Hørslev-Petersen K, Hetland ML, et al. Bone edema on magnetic resonance imaging is an independent predictor of rheumatoid arthritis development in patients with early undifferentiated arthritis. Arthritis Rheum 2011;63(8):2192–202.

43. Coates LC, Hodgson R, Conaghan PG, et al. MRI and ultrasonography for diagnosis and monitoring of psoriatic arthritis. Best Pract Res Clin Rheumatol 2012;26(6):805–22.

44. Neogi T, Jansen TLTA, Dalbeth N, et al. 2015 Gout Classification Criteria: an American College of Rheumatology/European League Against Rheumatism collaborative initiative. Ann Rheum Dis 2015;74: 2557–68.

45. Lai K-L, Chiu Y-M. Role of ultrasonography in diagnosing gouty arthritis. J Med Ultrasound 2011; 19(1):7–13.

46. Terslev L, Gutierrez M, Christensen R, et al. Assessing elementary lesions in gout by ultrasound: results of an OMERACT patient-based agreement and reliability exercise. J Rheumatol 2015;42(11):2149–54.

47. McQueen FM, Doyle A, Dalbeth N. Imaging in gout: what can we learn from MRI, CT, DECT and US. Arthritis Res Ther 2011;13(6):246.

48. Choi HK, Al-Arfaj AM, Eftekhari A, et al. Dual energy computed tomography in tophaceous gout. Ann Rheum Dis 2009;68(10):1609–12.

49. Ranganath VK, Motamedi K, Haavardsholm EA, et al. Comprehensive appraisal of magnetic resonance imaging findings in sustained rheumatoid arthritis remission: a substudy. Arthritis Care Res 2015;67(7):929–39.

50. Haavardsholm EA, Lie E, Lillegraven S. Should modern imaging be part of remission criteria in rheumatoid arthritis? Best Pract Res Clin Rheumatol 2012; 26(6):767–85.

51. Brown AK, Conaghan PG, Karim Z, et al. An explanation for the apparent dissociation between clinical remission and continued structural deterioration in rheumatoid arthritis. Arthritis Rheum 2008;58(10): 2958–67.

52. Gandjbakhch F, Conaghan PG, Ejbjerg B, et al. Synovitis and osteitis are very frequent in rheumatoid arthritis clinical remission: results from an MRI study of 294 patients in clinical remission or low disease activity state. J Rheumatol 2011;38(9):2039–44.

53. Mulherin D, Fitzgerald O, Bresnihan B. Clinical improvement and radiological deterioration in rheumatoid arthritis: evidence that the pathogenesis of synovial inflammation and articular erosion may differ. Br J Rheumatol 1996;35(12):1263–8.

54. Molenaar ETH, Voskuyl AE, Dinant HJ, et al. Progression of radiologic damage in patients with rheumatoid arthritis in clinical remission. Arthritis Rheum 2004;50(1):36–42.

55. Goekoop-Ruiterman YPM, de Vries-Bouwstra JK, Kerstens PJSM, et al. DAS-driven therapy versus

routine care in patients with recent-onset active rheumatoid arthritis. Ann Rheum Dis 2010;69(01):65–9.

56. Felson DT, Smolen JS, Wells G, et al. American College of Rheumatology/European League Against Rheumatism provisional definition of remission in rheumatoid arthritis for clinical trials. Arthritis Rheum 2011;63(3):573–86.

57. Haavardsholm EA, Aga A-B, Olsen IC, et al. Ultrasound in management of rheumatoid arthritis: ARCTIC randomised controlled strategy trial. BMJ 2016;354:i4205.

58. Dale J, Stirling A, Zhang R, et al. Targeting ultrasound remission in early rheumatoid arthritis: the results of the TaSER study, a randomised clinical trial. Ann Rheum Dis 2016;75(6):1043–50.

59. Østergaard M, Møller-Bisgaard S. Rheumatoid arthritis: is imaging needed to define remission in rheumatoid arthritis? Nat Rev Rheumatol 2014;10(6):326–8.

60. Boini S, Guillemin F. Radiographic scoring methods as outcome measures in rheumatoid arthritis: properties and advantages. Ann Rheum Dis 2001;60(9):817–27.

61. Oude Voshaar MAH, Schenk O, Klooster Ten PM, et al. Further simplification of the simple erosion narrowing score with item response theory methodology. Arthritis Care Res 2016;68(8):1206–10.

62. Kubassova O, Boesen M, Cimmino MA, et al. A computer-aided detection system for rheumatoid arthritis MRI data interpretation and quantification of synovial activity. Eur J Radiol 2010;74(3):e67–72.

63. Hodgson RJ, O'connor P, Moots R. MRI of rheumatoid arthritis image quantitation for the assessment of disease activity, progression and response to therapy. Rheumatology 2008;47(1):13–21.

64. Conaghan PG, Østergaard M, Bowes MA, et al. Comparing the effects of tofacitinib, methotrexate and the combination, on bone marrow oedema, synovitis and bone erosion in methotrexate-naive, early active rheumatoid arthritis: results of an exploratory randomised MRI study incorporating semiquantitative and quantitative techniques. Ann Rheum Dis 2016;75(6):1024–33.

65. Ostergaard M. An introduction to the EULAR-OMERACT rheumatoid arthritis MRI reference image atlas. Ann Rheum Dis 2005;64(Suppl 1):i3–7.

66. Wakefield RJ, D'Agostino MA, Naredo E, et al. After treat-to-target: can a targeted ultrasound initiative improve RA outcomes? Postgrad Med J 2012;88(1042):482–6.

67. D'Agostino MA, Wakefield RJ, Berner-Hammer H, et al. Value of ultrasonography as a marker of early response to abatacept in patients with rheumatoid arthritis and an inadequate response to methotrexate: results from the APPRAISE study. Ann Rheum Dis 2015;75(10):1763–9.

68. Scheel AK, Hermann KGA, Ohrndorf S, et al. Prospective 7 year follow up imaging study comparing radiography, ultrasonography, and magnetic resonance imaging in rheumatoid arthritis finger joints. Ann Rheum Dis 2006;65(5):595–600.

69. Naredo E, Collado P, Cruz A, et al. Longitudinal power Doppler ultrasonographic assessment of joint inflammatory activity in early rheumatoid arthritis: predictive value in disease activity and radiologic progression. Arthritis Rheum 2007;57(1):116–24.

70. Teh J, Stevens K, Williamson L, et al. Power Doppler ultrasound of rheumatoid synovitis: quantification of therapeutic response. Br J Radiol 2003;76(912):875–9.

71. Fukae J, Kon Y, Henmi M, et al. Change of synovial vascularity in a single finger joint assessed by power doppler sonography correlated with radiographic change in rheumatoid arthritis: comparative study of a novel quantitative score with a semiquantitative score. Arthritis Care Res 2010;62(5):657–63.

72. Kamishima T, Tanimura K, Henmi M, et al. Power Doppler ultrasound of rheumatoid synovitis: quantification of vascular signal and analysis of interobserver variability. Skeletal Radiol 2009;38(5):467–72.

73. Terslev L, Ellegaard K, Christensen R, et al. Head-to-head comparison of quantitative and semi-quantitative ultrasound scoring systems for rheumatoid arthritis: reliability, agreement and construct validity. Rheumatology (Oxford) 2012;51(11):2034–8.

74. Teh J. Applications of Doppler Imaging in the musculoskeletal system. Curr Probl Diagn Radiol 2006;35(1):22–34.

Conventional Radiology in Rheumatoid Arthritis

Eva Llopis, MD[a],*, Herman M. Kroon, MD, PhD[b],
Jose Acosta, MD[c], Johan L. Bloem, MD, PhD[b]

KEYWORDS

- Rheumatoid arthritis • Peripheral arthropathies • Conventional radiology • Inflammation

KEY POINTS

- Rheumatoid arthritis (RA) is a polyarticular disease with bilateral and symmetric distribution.
- Small joints of the feet, wrists, and hands are frequently involved, especially metacarpal phalangeal joint (MCP), metatarsal phalangeal joint (MTP), and proximal interphalangeal joint.
- Periarticular osteoporosis and soft tissue swelling are the earliest radiographic signs. Erosions in specific sites are key for the radiologic diagnostis of RA.
- In the clinical practice, conventional radiography is still the method of choice for the evaluation of progression RA disease.
- Advanced RA disease causes subluxation, deformities, ulnar deviation of the MCP, lateral deviation of the MTP, and carpal collapse.

INTRODUCTION

With the change of treatment paradigm and the introduction of early aggressive therapies including biologicals and chemotherapy, the face of rheumatoid arthritis (RA) has changed fundamentally within the last decade. The focus of imaging has shifted from visualizing joint and bone destruction to early diagnosis before joints and bones are severely affected. Imaging of soft tissue features and bone marrow changes using ultrasound (US) and magnetic resonance (MR) has result in a new field of clinical research, aimed at determining the not yet defined place of imaging techniques in early diagnosis. Therefore, has also change the place of conventional radiographs. In addition to the conventional role of radiography in visualizing late sequelae that can be used in (surgical) treatment planning, radiographs have remained important in differential diagnosis in patients presenting with possible RA, visualizing complications of RA, and also, albeit less so, in monitoring (absence) of progressive disease during treatment. The reasons are that radiographs are very useful in differentiating RA from other clinical entities, and that radiographs have high specificity, provide a quick overview of all symptomatic joints, and are low-cost procedures. Unfortunately, the interpretation of conventional radiology can be considered a vanishing art. This article mainly focuses on conventional radiology of the wrist and hand in RA, but briefly reviews other joints, such as the feet, hip, knees, or cervical spine.[1–3]

PATHOLOPHYSIOLOGY

Imaging reflects pathophysiology of RA. The advantage of MR over conventional radiography is that it allows detection of the entire spectrum

Disclosure Statement: The authors have nothing to disclose.
[a] Department of Radiology, Hospital de la Ribera, Carretera Corbera km1, Alzira, Valencia 46600, Spain;
[b] Department of Radiology, Leiden University Medical Center, Albinusdreef 2, Leiden 233 ZA, The Netherlands;
[c] Department of Radiology, Hospital Universitario Ramon y Cajal, Carretera de Colmenar Viejo KM 9, 100, Madrid 28034, Spain
* Corresponding author.
E-mail address: Evallopis@gmail.com

of changes in all tissues that occur in RA. Synovium and probably bone marrow are the target tissues of RA. Therefore, synovial joints, synovial tendon sheaths, and bone marrow are the primary structures involved. Secondary cartilage, cortical bone, and ligaments can be involved. Cartilage covers bone surface except in a bare area at the insertion of the capsule. The contact between the synovium and the bone not protected by cartilage or cortex makes this area the more susceptible area for developing small bone erosions.

The synovium has 2 layers separated by fat: the outer layer is fibrous and is continued with the periosteum; the inner layer has A cells from bone marrow and B cells from mesenchymal origin that have capacity for phagocytosis. There is no cell layer between the synoviocytes and the joint cavity, making the interchange of synovial fluid easier. Synovial hyperplasia and hyperemia lead to production of various cytokines, such as tumor necrosis factors and interleukin. Together with infiltration of the synovial tissue by macrophages, fibroblasts, and lymphocytes, this starts the process of destruction of tissue, including bone, by increasing the production of enzymes, mainly metalloproteinases, that increase inflammation and bone destruction, thus starting and maintaining a vicious circle.[4]

DIAGNOSIS OF RHEUMATOID ARTHRITIS

RA is a chronic systemic inflammatory disease characterized by synovial hyperplasia, autoantibody production (rheumatoid factor [RF] and anticitrullinated protein antibody [ACCP]), secondary cartilage and bone destruction, and systemic disease. There are no accurate criteria to diagnosis early RA. Early diagnosis is based on a combination of clinical, serologic, and imaging tests (Table 1). Unfortunately, the diagnosis cannot be based only on serologic tests. RF is only positive in 50% of the patients during the first 6 months; when the disease is more advanced, it becomes positive in 85% of the patients. RF is unspecific and can be positive in other diseases, such as reactive arthritis, other autoimmune diseases, infections, or malignancies, as well as in healthy subjects. Newer antibodies, especially ACCP, have higher specificity for RA and also are related to a poorer prognosis. However, 20% of the patients remain seronegative, and early diagnosis is also based on clinical examination and imaging techniques. Moreover, RF and ACCP are not used to monitor the disease because once positive they remain so. Erythrocyte sedimentation rate (ESR) and C-reactive protein (CRP) measure

Table 1 2010 the American College of Rheumatology/ European League Against Rheumatism classification criteria for rheumatoid arthritis	
Joint distribution	
1 large joint	0
2–10 large joints	1
1–3 small joints (with or without involvement of large joints)	2
4–10 small joints (with or without involvement of large joints)	3
>10 joints (at least 1 small joint)	5
Serology	
Negative RF and negative ACPA	0
Low-positive RF or low-positive ACPA	2
High-positive RF or high-positive ACPA	3
Symptom duration	
<6 wk	0
>6 wk	1
Acute phase reactants	
Normal CRP and normal ESR	0
Abnormal CPR or abnormal ESR	1

ACR/EULAR classification criteria are valid for a patients having at least 1 joint with definitive clinical synovitis not explained by another disease. Score of 6 or more is needed for a classification of definite diagnosis of RA.

Joint distribution refers to any swollen or tender joint excluding DIP of hand and feet, first MTP, and first CMC.
Small joints are MCP, PIP, MTP 2 to 5, thumb IP, and wrist.
Large joints are shoulder, elbow, hip, knees, and ankles.
Abbreviations: ACPA, anticitrullinated protein antibodies; CMC, carpometacarpal joint.

inflammation activity and are used to monitor the patient's disease.[2,3,5]

In 2010, the American College of Rheumatology (ACR) and the European League Against Rheumatism (EULAR) published updated criteria to classify the RA. However, classification is not the same as diagnosis. Classification serves to define more homogeneous populations especially for research purposes, whereas diagnosis aims at being correct at the level of the individual patient. Because of the difficulty in making an early diagnosis, this classification system is used also in the diagnostic process. Before this system can be used, the patient has to fulfill one entry criterion, that is, the presence of at least one small joint with clinical synovitis, with the exception of the first metacarpalphalangeal joint, the first carpo-metacarpal, and all distal interphalangeal joints (DIPs). Thereafter, the 2010 ACR/EULAR criteria can be used. All types of imaging studies can be used to confirm the clinical diagnosis of synovitis as defined in the ACR/EULAR 2010 criteria. For the late diagnosis of RA, or advanced disease, the presence of erosions visualized with radiographs can be used to make a specific diagnosis of RA according to the 2010 ACR/EULAR criteria.[2,3]

RADIOLOGIC DIAGNOSIS

In clinical practice, RA diagnosis and follow-up are based on conventional radiographs, although its limitation compared with US or MR is well known. The role of MR and US in clinical practice still needs to be determined. In a research setting, US and MR have many advantages, especially higher sensitivity. However, the cost-effectiveness together with lower specificity because of overlap in early diagnosis with other inflammatory disease, but also with an asymptomatic population, provides that conventional radiographs are still considered in clinical practice the main radiologic method for the diagnosis and follow-up of RA.[6–8]

Radiologic evaluation should be based on a general and regional analysis and will allow a diagnostic approach (see Table 1; Fig. 1). Analysis should start with the location and distribution of radiologic findings. RA is a polyarticular disease with typically bilateral and symmetric involvement of the peripheral joints and less frequently the cervical spine. On radiographs, the authors evaluate the distribution of the disease, soft tissue, bone density, joint space, erosions, bone proliferation, and deformities. The analysis of these parameters will narrow down the differential diagnosis.[1,4,9–11]

For the diagnosis of RA, the involvement of small and large joints should, clinically or radiographically, be defined or ruled out.[2,4,9–11]

Distribution

RA is a polyarticular disease, involving more than 3 joints, with a bilateral and symmetrical distribution. Small joints, hand, wrist, foot, or cervical spine, are commonly involved in RA, especially proximal ones, such as metacarpal phalangeal joint

A

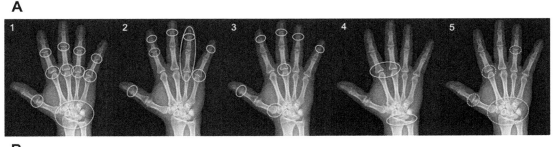

B

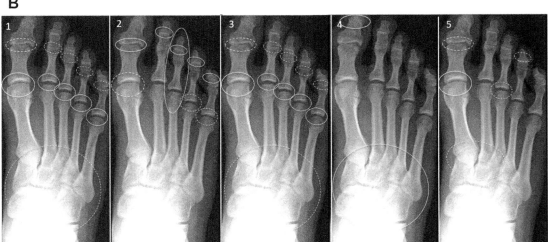

Fig. 1. (A) Different distribution of hand and wrist involvement, being ___ frequently involvement joints and _ _ _ less frequently involved. (1) RA; (2) psoriasis; (3) osteoarthrosis; (4) CPPD deposit; (5) gout. (B). Different distribution of the feet being ___ frequently involvement joints and _ _ _ less frequently involved. (1) RA; (2) psoriasis; (3) reactive arthritis; (4) diabetes; (5) gout.

(MCP), metatarsal phalangeal joint (MTP), and proximal interphalangeal joint (PIP); but larger joints, like shoulder, elbow, hip, knee, and ankle, can be involved (see **Fig. 1**). The first carpometacarpal joint, first MTP, and DIPs are excluded from the classification system because of their frequent involvement in osteoarthritis. For equivalent joints in the feet, the same criteria apply. Although DIPs can be involved in RA, they are more frequently and specifically involved in osteoarthritis or psoriasis.[2,9–11]

Soft Tissue Swelling

One of the earliest radiographic signs of RA is the presence of symmetric or fusiform periarticular soft tissue swelling, which is secondary to joint effusion and synovitis. Discrete swelling of the joints especially in the small joints is difficult to assess on conventional radiographs (**Fig. 2**). However, conventional radiographs are sensitive for effusions and bursitis in large joints that can be easily depicted by separation of fat pats, which surround the joints, and displacement of soft tissue structures (**Figs. 3** and **4**). The absence of calcification will help to differentiate RA from crystal deposit arthropathies.

Soft tissue swelling in the later stages of the disease should be differentiated from rheumatoid nodules. A rheumatoid nodule consists of fibroid necrosis in the center with histiocytes in the periphery. Rheumatoid nodules are frequently seen in the subcutaneous soft tissues close to pressure points and prominent bones, such as the extensor surfaces of the forearm or the hands and feet. These soft tissue lesions can be easily diagnosed as rheumatoid nodules when there is radiographic evidence of arthritis in the adjacent joint (**Fig. 5**). Similar to RA, tophaceous gout may result in the formation of nodular asymmetrical soft tissue masses that may contain densities caused by urate crystal depositions; the high density allows differential diagnosis with RA[2,4,9–12] (**Fig. 6**).

Calcific deposits within rheumatoid nodules and within periarticular subcutaneous tissue have occasionally been described. In all such cases, the possibility of mixed connective tissue disease or collagen vascular overlap syndromes must be considered.[10]

Osteoporosis

Osteopenia caused by osteoporosis is an early sign of RA with 2 different forms, periarticular close to the affected joints and generalized.[13,14]

Generalized osteoporosis affects both the axial and the appendicular skeleton. The pathophysiology is still not completely understood, but it has been associated with longstanding disease, immobilization, production of proinflammatory cytokines, and also the intake of steroids by patients suffering from RA.[15] Especially at risk are older patients, and/or postmenopausal patients, patients with long disease duration, patients with elevated RF, and those who have been treated with corticosteroids. Osteoporosis has an overall prevalence of 26.5% in patients with RA. Osteoporosis in these patients increases their risk of hip and vertebral fractures. The recent more aggressive treatment of RA has not been accompanied by a reduction of osteoporosis; therefore, in patients with increased risk, dual-energy x-ray absorptiometry should be performed to diagnose generalized osteoporosis.[14–22]

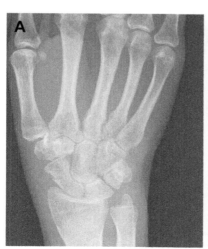
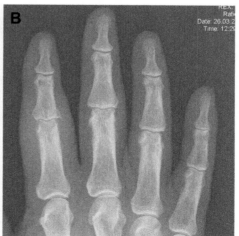

Fig. 2. (*A*) Wrist radiograph showing soft tissue swelling and periarticular osteoporosis. (*B*) Hand radiograph soft tissue swelling in the second and third fingers with early cartilage loss in the PIP.

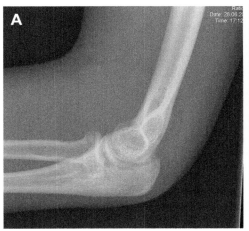
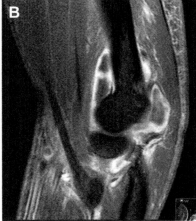

Fig. 3. (A) Lateral elbow plain film showing joint effusion in the posterior and anterior recesses with displacement of the fat pats. (B) Correponding sagittal spin echo (FSE) T1-weighted image with fat saturation after Gadolinium injection confirming the joint effusion and synovial enhancement.

Periarticular osteoporosis is the first osseous morphologic sign that occurs before development of erosions and joint space narrowing[14–22] (Fig. 7). Periarticular osteoporosis in RA is different from that in osteoarthritis and is characterized by hyperemia around the joint, synovial inflammation, and recruitment of various signaling pathways, which also result in an increase of osteoclast activity in the periarticular trabecular bone. Periarticular osteoporosis appears before corticosteroid treatment.[14,19] It has been demonstrated that a decrease of hand bone mineral density in 1 year follow-up was a marker of worse prognosis and greater joint damage. It can thus be used as a biological marker. Immobilization can cause osteoporosis, but the location is different, as this is especially located more distally.[20–22]

Erosions

Erosions are small cortical interruptions with exposure of cancellous bone, and they are key in diagnosing RA. They develop early, start in the bare area zone as mentioned earlier, and extend

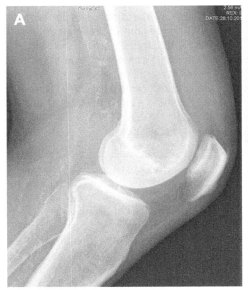
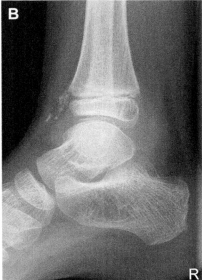

Fig. 4. (A) Lateral knee plain film with joint effusion on the suprapatellar recess. (B) Lateral ankle plain film showing tibiotalar effusion displacing the anterior and posterior recesses.

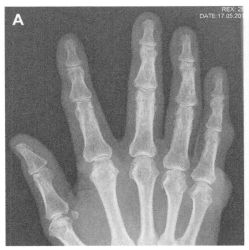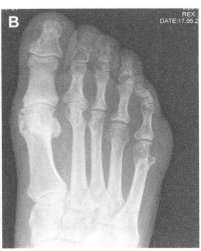

Fig. 5. (A) Hand radiograph film rheumatoid nodules in the lateral radial side of the PIP and MCP joints of the second finger, and ulnar lateral side of the PIP and MCP joints of the fifth finger. (B) Foot radiograph demonstrates rheumatoid nodule in the lateral side of the MTP joint of the fifth toe adjacent to a lateral side erosion on the MT head. Other erosions are nicely seen in the first, second and third metatarsal heads.

toward the center. Erosions also occur in the attachment of the tendons and ligaments on bone, the enthesis, but also can be seen in specific sites, such as the ulnar styloid, MCP, MTF, or PIP (**Figs. 8** and **9**) When present in joints, the proximal side is usually more affected. Bone erosions are only detected on conventional radiographs when a substantial amount of bone is destroyed and are therefore detected relatively late on

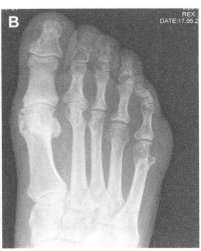

Fig. 6. Magnified hand radiograph of a gout arthropathy. Notice periarticular calcified nodules in the MCF and PIP of the fingers; in the second finger MCP joint, the nodule is close to an overhanging erosion.

conventional radiographs, especially compared with computed tomography (CT) or MR.[2,4,9–11]

However, true erosions have to be distinguished from pseudoerosions. Pseudoerosions can be secondary to ligament insertions, vascular foramen, mucoid cysts, or secondary to overlap in complex anatomic areas that create radiologic pitfalls. The knowledge of the normal location of pseudoerosions will help to make appropriate diagnosis. Wawer and colleagues[23,24] studied pseudoerosions of the wrist and hand, demonstrating that they are more frequent on the distal ulnar portion of the capitate, hamate, the bases of the third, fourth, and fifth metacarpals, and in the MCP joints. US, CT, and MR can detect true erosions in patients with normal radiographs.

In chronic patients, progressive erosions may fuse, resulting in pencil-in-cup deformity of the MCPs and MTPs (**Fig. 10**).[2]

Subchondral Cyst

Subchondral cysts are pseudocysts that probably develop secondary to extension of pannus either through defects in cartilage or by penetration of the chondroosseous junction, thus creating a pathway for fluid to pass, creating a cystic cavity. They are really pseudocysts because they do not have an epithelial lining. The term of geode is usually used when they are large. The term comes from the geological term for hollow rock lined with crystals. Subchondral cysts are usually open to the

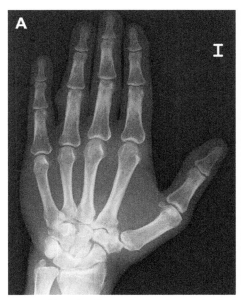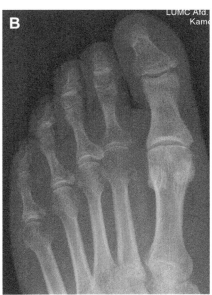

Fig. 7. (A) Wrist and hand radiograph showing periarticular osteoporosis in the MCP and PIP. (B) Foot radiograph demonstrating periarticular osteoporosis of the MTP joint of the second toe.

joint; however, often fibrous tissue or debris can close its communication. They have been related to physical activity, secondary to intraarticular hyperpression. In large joints, these pseudocysts are usually larger. They represent a risk factor to develop subchondral fractures especially in load sites such as in the hip or the knee[25,26] (Fig. 11).

Cysts can be incidental or associated with repetitive osseous microtrauma, usually without secondary findings such as bone marrow edema on MR. The cysts can be found in the metacarpal heads, more frequent in the attachment of the radial collateral ligament in the second, third, and fourth fingers. They are related to compressive forces in areas with higher pressure during grasping. In the wrist, they can also be found in

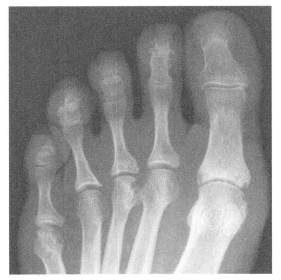

Fig. 8. Foot radiograph of an early phase of RA showing marginal erosions of the MTP joints of the first, third, fifth MTP joints with soft tissue swelling adjacent to the MTP joint of the 5th toe.

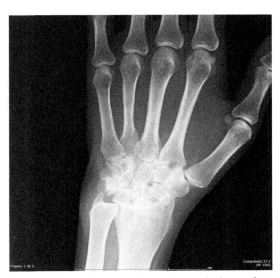

Fig. 9. Wrist radiograph of an advanced phase of RA with pancarpal involvement. Note the erosions in the ulnar styloid, scaphoid, and triquetrum.

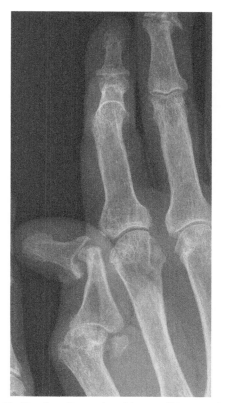

Fig. 10. Hand radiograph with pencil-in-cup deformity in the IP of the first finger and Boutonniere deformity of the PIP of the second finger.

the midcapitate at the attachment site of the extrinsic radioscaphocapitate ligament. Other cysts can be secondary to impaction syndromes or related to ligaments or tendons attachments. The characteristic location permits the differentiation of cysts and pseudocysts related to RA (**Fig. 12**).[27–31]

Loss of Joint Space

Progressive loss of joint space is secondary to the destruction of cartilage by the inflammatory exudates of the hypertrophic synovitis and is usually concentric and bilateral. Because evaluation of this feature is time consuming and subjective, new methods have been developed for automatic quantification. These new methods are especially useful for follow-up. Computed-based semiquantitative automatic or completely automatic measurements of the joint space of fingers, wrist, and toes, reducing operator dependence, have been used for osteoarthrosis and RA[31–34] (**Fig. 13**).

Osteitis

Osteitis can be identified only with MR imaging. Marrow edema and enhancement of subcortical bone are frequent collateral findings with joint involvement. It may precede subcortical cysts and erosions but may also regress without any subsequent damage to the bone. There is no

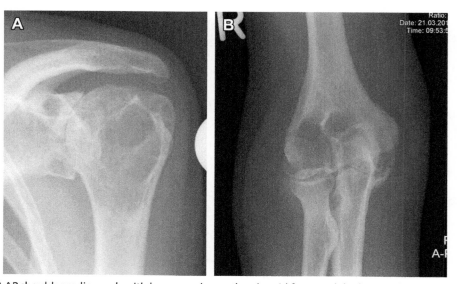

Fig. 11. (A) AP shoulder radiograph with large geodes on the glenoid fossa and the lesser tuberosity with marked uniform decrease of the joint space. (B) AP elbow radiograph demonstrating large geodes in the epicondyle, capitellum, radial side of the ulnar tuberosity together with marginal erosions on the ulnar side.

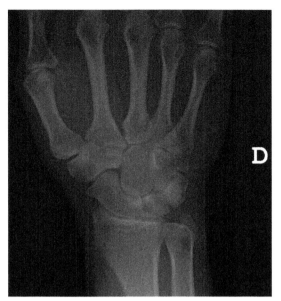

Fig. 12. AP wrist radiograph of a patient with lunate intraosseous ganglion cyst.

necessary relation to osteoporosis on conventional film radiographs.[4]

Osteolysis

In advanced stages, the inflammatory process may lead to massive erosions and bone mutilation as well as destruction of the soft tissue structures of and around the joint (**Fig. 14**).[4,9–11]

IMAGING FOLLOW-UP

RA may show different patterns of progression: linear progression, rapid onset with a later plateau, slow onset with acceleration, and nonprogressive.[35] It has been also demonstrated that there is strong relation between joint damage and later disability, and when the maximum damage scores exceed 33%, the relation becomes lineal[36–38] (see **Fig. 13**).

The methods that have been used to measure the progression of RA are considerable. Radiographs are still the preferred method for the evaluation of RA progression in clinical practice. Of course, radiographs also have several limitations, such as technical and positioning issues, the floor effect (erosions and joint space narrowing may occur late in the course of the disease), and the ceiling effect (radiographic progression continues even after the highest damage score has been assigned). Radiographs are readily available, can be interpreted without significant variability, and can compare at the same time in different joints.

Single-reading, paired-reading blinded to treatment and timing, and paired reading with chronologic ordered have been used. Single-reading methods are less reliable than paired readings. Paired reading blinded to sequence may have greater power to test treatment, but chronologically paired reading provides more sensitive assessment of damage especially in long-term studies.[36–38]

The 2 major scoring systems for RA are the Larsen and the Sharp systems and its modified scoring systems. The advantage of the modified Sharp system is that it allows scoring of hands and feet, grading the progression of erosions and joint space narrowing.[39,40]

However, use of any of the different scoring systems is subjective, tedious, and time consuming. Moreover, the problem of demonstration of a reduction in joint structural damage is challenging because of the low progression rate also in the placebo groups. The inability to detect synovial hypertrophy on radiographs should be kept in mind in order to avoid wrong conclusions.[40–42] Other methods such as US or MR have been used to assess progression, but the cost-effectiveness and the predictive value have yet to be determined.[36–38]

WRIST AND HAND
Technique

Radiographs of the wrist and hand are used for diagnosis, staging, and follow-up. First, the important step is to have good-quality high-resolution radiographs. Standard wrist radiographs include posteroanterior (PA) and lateral projection. However, in RA, an oblique semisupinated view is also recommended (see **Fig. 17**). Additional projections such as oblique view, radial, and ulnar deviation are usually not required for RA. The PA view is obtained with the arm abducted 90° from the truck and the forearm flexed at 90° to the arm and with the wrist in neutral position to avoid overlap of the ulnar styloid.[1,4,11]

The semisupinated anteroposterior (AP) oblique view, also called the Norgaard view or ball catchers view (**Fig. 15**), is optimal for the evaluation of early erosive changes and shows the pisiform, palmar aspect of the triquetrum, palmar ulnar surface of the hamate, and the profiles of the pisiform-triquetral joint to best advantage.

The lateral view should be obtained also in neutral position. It is, however, less useful for RA, unless ligament destruction has occurred and dislocation of the wrist has to be ruled out. On the lateral projection, the long axis of the third

926

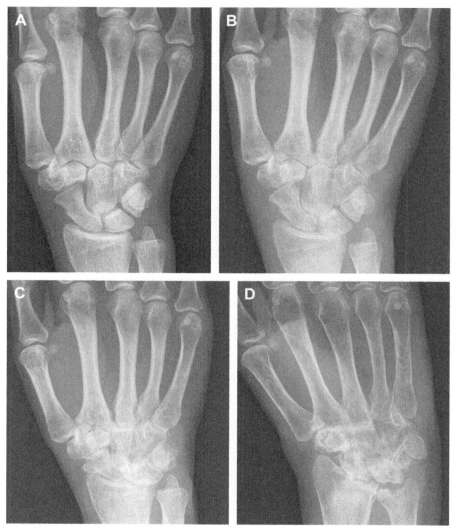

Fig. 13. Development of cartilage loss and progressive destruction of the wrist within time. (A) Early stage normal plain film. (B) Osteoporosis periarticular and minimal loss of the joint space. (C) Joint space is markedly decrease and carpal collapse is starting. (D) Carpal collapse with loss of the normal alignment, lunate hamate ankylosis, and ulnar displacement of the carpus.

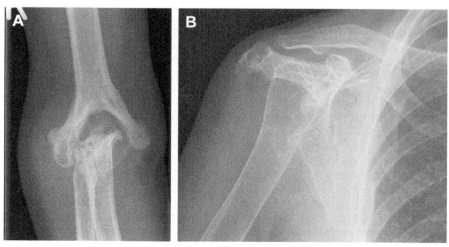

Fig. 14. (A) AP radiograph shows severe osteolysis of the elbow. (B) AP radiograph of the shoulder with lysis of the humeral head and distal clavicular osteolysis and generalized osteoporosis.

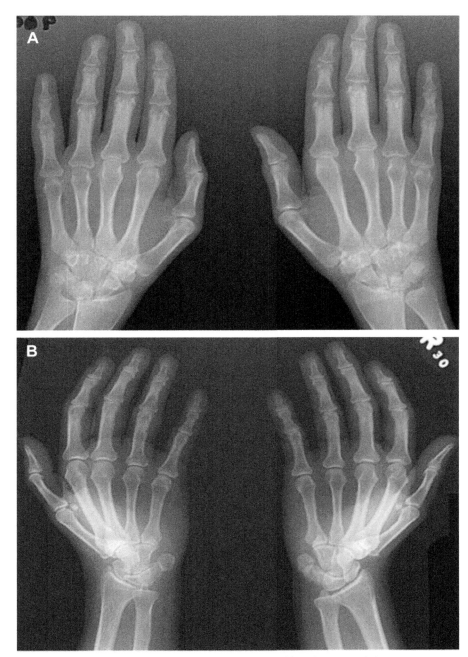

Fig. 15. (A) PA bilateral wrist and hand radiograph. (B) Wrist and hand Norgaard view.

metacarpal should be parallel with the long axis of the radius, while the pisiform projects over the dorsal pole of the scaphoid.[1,4,11]

Early Radiographic Findings

Early radiologic findings include bilateral and symmetric periarticular osteoporosis, early erosions, and soft tissue swelling. On the PA view, early erosions have predilection for some specific locations; the MCP and PIP joints especially of the second and third finger, the waist of the scaphoid, the waist of the capitate, the articulation of the hamate with the base of the 3 metacarpal base, the trapezoid with the trapezium, the radial styloid, and the ulnar styloid.

The DIP joints are typically spared. If the disease progresses, the changes affect all the joints and bones; pancarpal involvement results, with loss of cartilage and joint space[2,4,10,11] (see **Figs. 2, 7, 8,** and **12**).

Periarticular osteoporosis is predominant in the distal articular surface of the MCP joints.[4] It has been described as a predictive factor for the development of joint space loss and erosions (see **Fig. 7**). However, because of the lack of sensitivity and the difficulties in assessing this during follow-up, some investigators have advocated the use of other techniques such as digital x-ray radiogrammetry, dual x-ray absorptiometry, or quantitative ultrasonography for monitoring periarticular osteoporosis.[12–20]

Radiographic Progression and Late Sequelae

Longstanding RA with progressive disease causes bone destruction, ligament deficiency, and rupture as well as deficiency of tendons causing subluxation, deformities, and carpal instability. Late onset RA shows no radiographic differences with early onset RA.[43]

Radioscaphoid and radiolunate have the most severe progression of all joints. The progression of the MCP joints follows a predictable pattern from the radial to the ulnar site, starting in each joint in the dominant hand (**Fig. 16**).[43,44]

Chronic synovitis of the MCP and MTP capsule and periarticular connective tissues will lead to instability of the joints. The common presentations are palmar subluxation and ulnar drift or deviation. Weakness of the connective tissue inhibits resistance to the palmar force exerted by the flexor muscle. There is an increased pressure on the collateral ligament, and therefore, the proximal phalanx moves to the palmar side, creating a subluxed MCP joint and secondary to that a reduction of the normal palmar concavity.[45]

RA patients with progressive disease have a gradual shifting of the fingers (or toes) toward the ulnar side, called ulnar deviation or ulnar drift (**Fig. 17**). Ulnar deviation occurs because of 3 different mechanisms: asymmetry in the slope of the metacarpal heads, a prevailing ulnar force of the digital and interosseous muscles, and ulnar traction on the palmar plate by the connections of the deep transverse ligament and the hypothenar muscles. The resulting increased torque forces together with the chronic synovitis, leading to joint dislocation, increased by the extensor tendon rupture.[45]

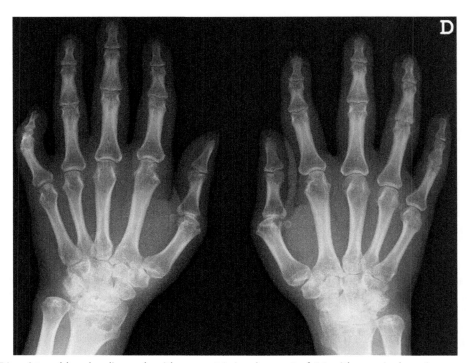

Fig. 16. PA wrist and hand radiograph with symmetric involvement of RA with marginal erosions especially on the MCP and radiocarpal joints.

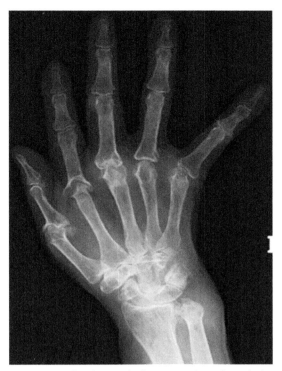

Fig. 17. Hand radiograph demonstrating ulnar deviation of the third, fourth, and fifth fingers MCP joints and pencil-and-cup deformity in the MCP joint of the first and second finger.

Characteristic deformities of the fingers are boutonniere and swan neck deformities. Boutonniere deformity is a flexion contracture of the PIP secondary to progressive synovitis of the joint followed by elongation and interruption of the central slip of the extensor tendon, subluxation of the lateral bands, and contracture of the retinacular ligaments. The flexion deformity of the PIP joint is compensated by the hyperextension in the DIP (see Fig. 10).[46,47]

Swan neck deformity consists of hyperextension in the PIP with secondary flexion in the DIP. Disruption or weakening of any of the stabilizing collateral ligaments, palmar plate, superficial flexor tendon, or retinacular ligaments secondary to progressive synovitis causes extension in the PIP joint.[48]

Instability of the wrist is related to weakening of the interosseous ligaments, especially the scapholunate ligament with secondary dorsal deviation, dorsal intercalated segment instability (DISI), deformity (Fig. 18).

RA in the wrist may start a cascade of events, more specifically wrist deformity, caput ulnae syndrome, and ultimately collapse. Wrist deformity is secondary to progressive synovitis in

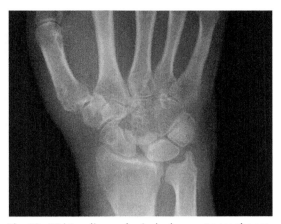

Fig. 18. Wrist radiograph nicely demonstrates the scapholunate increase of space secondary to tear of the ligament.

the radiocarpal and distal radioulnar joint (with erosions in ulnar styloid, ulnar head, and the scaphoid), and synovitis involving the carpal ligament complex. Caput ulnae syndrome is secondary to destruction of the distal radioulnar joint that causes abnormal dorsal location of the ulnar styloid and the ulnar head, supination of the carpus of the radius that impinges on the extensor tendons causing tenosynovitis, synovitis, and progressive degeneration of the tendon with subsequently rupture of the ulnar-sided extensor tendons. Wrist collapse is end-stage RA with destruction of the carpal bones, dissociation of the radioulnar joint, radial deviation of the metacarpals, and ulnar deviation of the fingers (see Figs. 13B and 16).[4,10,11]

ANKLE AND FOOT

Approximately 90% of the patients with RA will have involvement of the foot and ankle at some point of their disease. The forefoot is the most frequently involved of these. It has been published that erosions might occur first in the feet.[41] All the joints and the surrounding soft tissues may be affected.[49]

As in other joints, periarticular soft tissue swelling is an early sign. Periarticular osteoporosis is more difficult to detect. As the disease advances, erosions and joint space narrowing will appear (see Fig. 7B; Fig. 19).

Biomechanics can be altered secondary to degeneration of ligaments and tendons, but also secondary to osteoporotic insufficiency fractures and coexisting mechanical abnormalities, such as flat foot (Fig. 20).

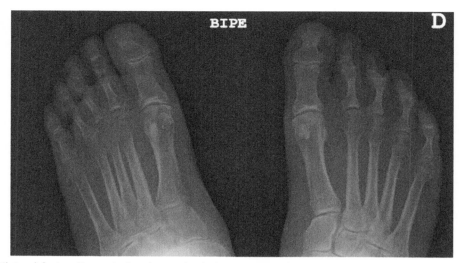

Fig. 19. Bilateral feet radiograph showing periarticular osteoporosis.

Indirect radiologic signs of involvement of surrounding soft tissue structures can be seen, such as lengthening of the Achilles tendon secondary to Achilles tendinopathy or retrocalcaneal bursitis.

Forefoot

The first locations where RA affects the forefoot are the lateral metatarsophalangeal joints, starting in the proximal metatarsal head. Erosions of the fifth MTP joint usually start on the lateral side and in the other MTP joints on the medial side. The plantar plate of the second and third MTP joints can be destroyed by synovial pannus. Then, the MT head might become medially and inferior dislocated, whereas the proximal phalange (PP) laterally and dorsally are dislocated[11,49] (Fig. 21).

In the plantar structures, degeneration of the transverse ligament will cause a decrease of the plantar arch and widening of the forefoot.

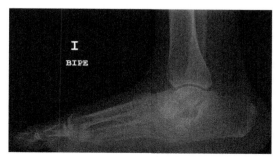

Fig. 20. Lateral standing foot radiograph of patient with RA and flat foot showing midfoot collapse.

In the first MTP, the sesamoid can be eroded or displaced by the synovial mass.[50] Hallux valgus is frequent and usually progresses with time. PIPs can be affected, especially the first PIP (see Figs. 23–25).

Midfoot

Midfoot involvement is common; the talocalcaneonavicular joint especially is frequently affected. Radiographic joint space narrowing and secondary osteophytes are the main features and occur more frequently than swelling and erosions. Tibialis posterior tendon is commonly affected, resulting in secondary flat foot and hindfoot valgus (see Fig. 20).[49]

Hindfoot

In the hindfoot, synovial proliferation is frequently present in the subtalar joints, displaying a soft tissue mass in the posterior recess. Posteriorly located erosions and progressive deformity can occur. Tibiotalar swelling is less frequent, but when present is seen, on lateral projection, as a teardrop-shaped soft tissue density displacing the anterior fat pad, superior to the talar neck. Lateral foot radiographs may demonstrate a retrocalcaneal bursitis, which may obliterate the normal pre-Achilles fat triangle of Kager. This may occasionally be associated with erosive change at the posterior calcaneus[49,51] (Fig. 22). Identical findings may be present in ankylosing spondylitis and reactive arthritis. Plantar calcaneal erosions mimic those seen in psoriatic arthritis (Fig. 23).[52]

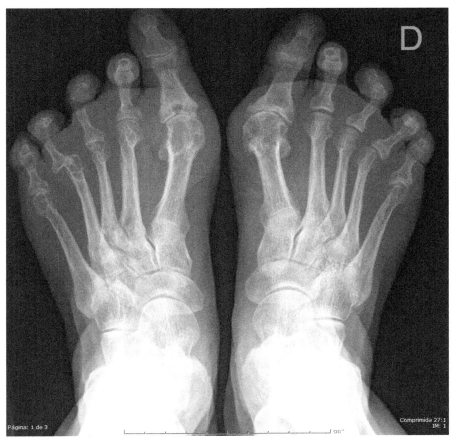

Fig. 21. AP feet radiograph of advance RA of the forefoot, erosions, and loss of the joint spaces are seen on the MTP joints with lateral deviation on the right foot and dislocation of the MTP joint of the fourth toe.

ELBOW

The elbow is frequently involved in RA. Erosions normally start in the humeral radial joint and extend toward the humeral ulnar joint. Decrease of the joint space in the elbow occurs late after the erosions probably because of the absence of weight-bearing that protects articular cartilage (see **Figs. 3, 11,** and **14**). The radiologic sign of the sail, because of its triangular shape simulating a boat sail, is the key to recognizing elbow effusion. On a lateral radiograph, an effusion causes displacement of the anterior and posterior fat pads surrounding the distal humerus. Olecranon bursitis may be seen as a "mass" at the olecranon bursa (**Fig. 24**).[4,10,11,51,53]

KNEE

The knee is the most frequent large joint involved by RA. Joint effusion and popliteal synovial cyst are seen early in the disease (see **Fig. 4**A). The effusion is easy to detect on lateral knee radiographs as a well-defined increased soft tissue density in the suprapatellar recess, with obliteration and anterior displacement of the posterior margin of the quadriceps tendon.

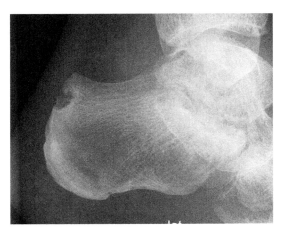

Fig. 22. Lateral calcaneus view showing nice erosion on the posterior tuberosity in a patient with RA.

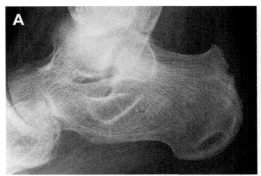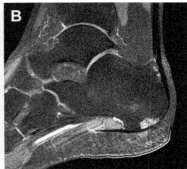

Fig. 23. (A) Lateral calcaneous view of a patient with psoriasis showing erosion on the posterior tuberosity, with the corresponding (B) MR on sagittal T1 fat saturation after gadolinium injection that demonstrates enthesitis of the Achilles and plantar fascia insertion.

Once erosive change begins, all 3 compartments of the knee demonstrate uniform cartilage loss, erosions, and subchondral cyst formation (**Figs. 25** and **26**). Patellar tendon ruptures occasionally occur.[52]

HIP

RA of the hip causes bilateral and symmetric concentric decrease of the joint space with axial migration of the femoral head. This result combined with acetabular remodeling in protusio acetabuli deformity. These 2 features can help to distinguish RA from osteoarthritis. The latter is characterized by nonuniform joint space narrowing (preferential narrowing in the superior and lateral compartments), subchondral sclerosis, osteophytes. Fibrous ankyloses is the late state of RA of the hip (**Figs. 27** and **28**) Iliopsoas bursitis may cause an anteriorly located soft tissue mass.[51,52]

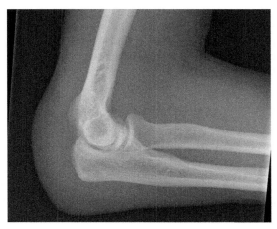

Fig. 24. Lateral elbow view demonstrates posterior soft tissue swelling, olecranon bursitis.

SHOULDER

The primary structures affected by RA around the shoulder are the glenohumeral joint, rotator cuff, and distal end of the clavicle (**Fig. 29**). The acromioclavicular joint can show early radiologic signs of RA involvement, such as lysis of the distal clavicula and erosion of the coracoclavicular ligament insertion (see **Fig. 14; Fig. 30**).[54]

Marginal erosions can be found at the humeral head adjacent to the greater tuberosity, at the capsular insertion, and on the anatomic neck of the humerus.

The rotator cuff is frequently torn. The chronicity of the rotator cuff tear is so prominent in patients with RA that they often develop the elevated humeral head and mechanical erosion at the undersurface of the acromion. A similar finding might be also associated with ankylosing spondylitis or hyperparathyroidism.[11,51]

TEMPOROMANDIBULAR JOINT

The temporomandibular joint is affected in more than 50% of patients with RA. Swelling, loss of joint pace, flattening of bone, and osseous erosions are the radiologic changes that lead to a decreased and abnormal range of motion and problems of occlusion. When occurring at an early age, even mandibular growth problems and facial deformity may ensue.[4,55]

CERVICAL SPINE

With the advent of aggressive, effective treatment in early stages of RA, extensive manifestations of RA in the cervical spine have decreased substantially.[56] Still, after the hands and feet, the cervical spine, with its many synovial joints, is the third most commonly affected region by RA.[57] The

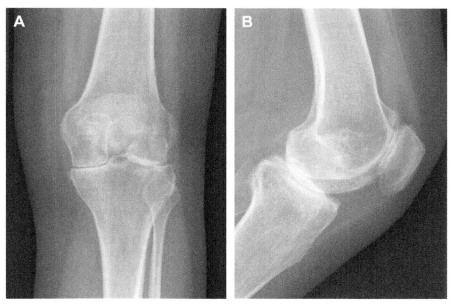

Fig. 25. (A) AP knee and (B) lateral view radiographs with RA involvement, osteoporosis, uniform decrease of the joint space and joint effusion.

pathophysiology with synovial inflammation, secondary ligamentous and osseous destruction is the same as in the small joints of the hands and feet. The ensuing (potential) instability secondary to this destruction and close relationship of these structures to the medulla oblongata, spinal cord, and vertebral vessels is a worrisome component of RA. Although severe neurologic and even fatal complications of subluxations have been described extensively, it is remarkable how poor the correlation is of marked destruction on imaging and clinical symptoms. Up to 50% of patients with marked RA manifestations in the cervical spine may be asymptomatic.[58] When symptoms are present, pain is the major symptom. This overall paucity of symptoms is thought to be secondary

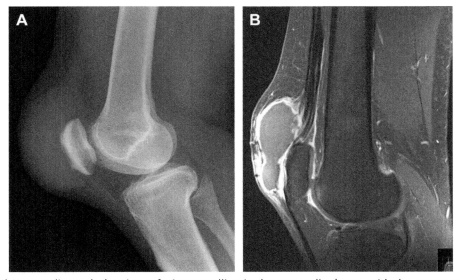

Fig. 26. (A) Knee radiograph showing soft tissue swelling in the prepatellar bursa, with the corresponding MR. (B) Sagittal view (FSE T1-weighted image with fat saturation after Gd). Notice the peripheral enhancement of the prepatellar bursa.

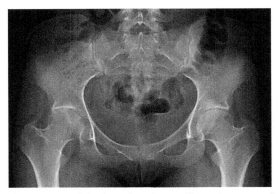

Fig. 27. AP pelvis view showing uniform decrease of the joint space, small erosions, and coxa profunda.

to compensating mechanisms, such as decrease (erosions) of bone mass, creating more space, and fixation of structures lacking ligamentous support by pannus. In addition to inflammation, the spine is also affected by the generalized osteoporosis that is associated with RA, secondary osteoarthritis, and an increased risk of infection. All 3 of these may cause radiographically detectable abnormalities. As in other parts of the body, radiographs are less sensitive than MR in depicting soft tissue manifestations of RA, and less sensitive to MR and CT in demonstrating osseous sequelae of RA. However, flexion and extension radiographs taken in the upright position are more informative

than MR or CT in displaying dynamic instability in the cervical spine.

More specifically, radiographs may show erosions at the C1-2 level with destruction of the transverse ligament resulting in atlantoaxial subluxation, and subaxial subluxation. Development of pannus is most frequent, but cannot be detected directly on conventional radiographs. The second most common findings are erosions that can be seen on conventional radiographs, although with lower sensitivity than CT or MR. Erosions can occur in all synovial joints in the spine and are even seen in advanced disease in spinous processes and in discs in combination with vertebral endplates (Figs. 31 and 32).

Although anterior subluxation of C2 relative to C1 is the most frequent subluxation detected on radiographs, subluxation may also be lateral, vertical, rotatory, and/or subaxial (see Fig. 32). Anterior atlantoaxial subluxation is diagnosed on the lateral radiograph. Measurements may be inaccurate because of many factors, including rotation and erosions of the dens, but a distance between atlas and dens of more than 3 mm is defined as abnormal. A distance of 9 mm or more has been associated with a higher prevalence of neurologic symptoms.[56] Flexion views showing an increase of this distance, even when the distance is 3 mm or less in the neutral position, are useful in showing

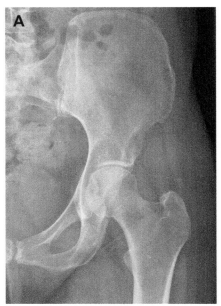
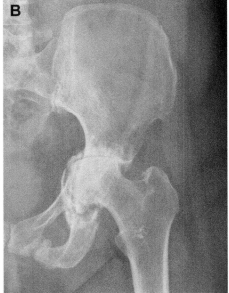

Fig. 28. Progression within time of hip involvement. (A) Normal radiograph (2010) and (B) (2016) with marked acetabular protrusion and fracture of the acetabular bone. Note the fracture of the pubic ischiopubic rami.

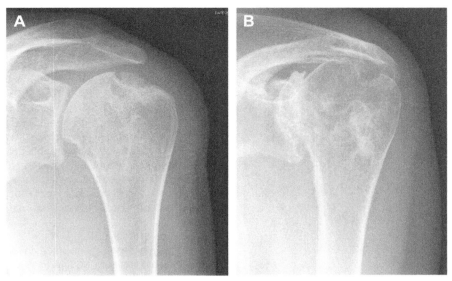

Fig. 29. (*A*) Shoulder AP radiograph showing early changes with erosion in the upper and lower part of the humeral head. (*B*) Shoulder AP radiograph advanced destruction of the humeral head and glenoid with a decrease of the joint space, large erosions, and superior migration of the humeral head as an indirect sign of rotator cuff tear.

mechanical instability. An increase of the atlantoaxial distance only during flexion has been described in approximately two-thirds of patients.[56] A posterior atlantodens interval of 14 mm is abnormal and indicates potential cord compromise. Posterior subluxation can occur when there are severe erosions of the dens allowing the atlas to move posterior over the destroyed dens. Posterior subluxation is diagnosed when the anterior margin of C2 is anterior to the posterior margin of the anterior arch of C1 on the lateral radiograph in neutral position and/or in extension.

Vertical subluxation is the second most common subluxation. It may cause neurologic symptoms in its severe form (cranial settling) and may even be fatal. There are several methods[59–61] to describe the relationship between the tip of the dens and the base of the skull. A commonly use criterion for basilar invagination is the tip of the dens being 5 mm above McGregor's line. When this distance reaches 8 to 10 mm, the prevalence of neurologic complications increases substantially. As mentioned before, these measurements become inaccurate when there are severe erosions present (Fig. 33).

Lateral atlantoaxial subluxation is considered to be present when the distance between C1-2 is 2 mm or more asymmetrical on the AP open mouth view. Rotatory subluxation can be diagnosed with there is asymmetry of the lateral mass relative to the dens.

Subaxial disease has received less attention than disease at the atlantoaxial level, but also is an important cause for neurologic complications.[62] The reasons for spinal stenosis are largely similar for RA and degenerative disease. Shared frequent causes are hypertrophy of flavum ligament and disc disease. There are, however, also differences. Features of RA are the presence of inflammatory tissue, the absence of osteophyte formation, erosions of the synovial joints, discs, and endplates (extending from the uncovertebral joints), and even spinous processus.[57,63] The last

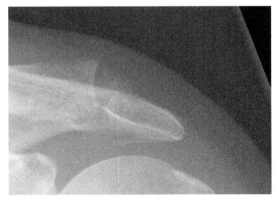

Fig. 30. Acromioclavicular radiograph demonstrates erosions and osteolysis of the distal clavicle.

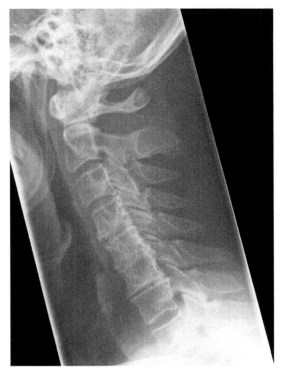

Fig. 31. Lateral cervical spine view. Small erosions on the endplates, with a decrease of the intervertebral space in C4-C5, C5-C6, and C6-C7.

4 of these 5 features can be detected on radiographs. Subaxial subluxation can also develop secondary to destruction of these structures and is diagnosed when there is a 3-mm or greater distance between the anterior margin of a vertebral body relative to the underlying vertebral body.

DIFFERENTIAL DIAGNOSIS

A large variety of conditions must be considered in the differential diagnosis of RA. Systemic rheumatic diseases such as systemic lupus erythematosus, Sjogren syndrome, dermatomyositis, or overlap syndromes have associated systemic features not seen in RA. In these entities, deformities and dislocations are usually related to loosening and degeneration of the periarticular structures and tendons, and therefore, they do not show periarticular osteoporosis, erosions, or loss of the joint space.[2,9–11]

Reactive arthritis of the hands or feet is commonly asymmetric, and the involvement of the fingers or toes surrounding tissues (tenosynovium, enthesis, and soft tissues) gives the appearance of sausage fingers or toes. Oligoarthritis of large joints, especially the knee or ankle, cause diagnostic problems, because this may also be a presentation of RA. Reactive arthritis normally is HLA B27 positive and frequently displays sacroilitis.[2,9–11]

Lyme arthritis should be in the differential diagnosis in patients that have traveled to endemic areas. They usually involve larger joints and are preceded by history of erythema migrans.

Psoriatic arthritis has some features that set it apart from RA. Psoriasis is characterized by an asymmetrical distribution, erosions located in DIP and PIP joints, bone proliferation, enthesis involvement, and normal mineralization. The lack of bone

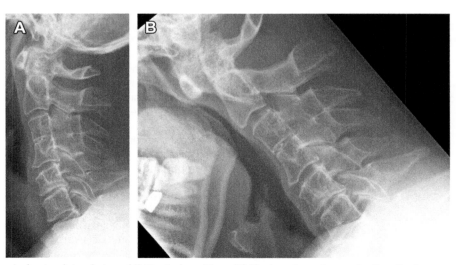

Fig. 32. Cervical spine lateral view. (*A*) Neutral position. (*B*) Flexion view, demonstrating the increase of the atlantoodontoid space with flexion of the cervical space. Patient has fusion in C3-C4 and lower cervical spine degenerative changes associated.

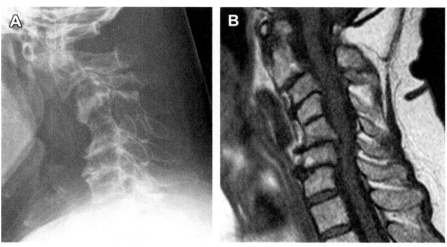

Fig. 33. (A) Cervical spine lateral view, with vertical subluxation and subaxial subluxations. (B) Corresponding sagittal FSE T1-weighted image. Note that on MR, the subluxations are not visible.

proliferation in RA will help to differentiate it from psoriasis. Especially when RF or ACCP is positive in a patient without skin lesions, and with bilateral symmetric involvement, an erroneous diagnosis of RA can be made. Psoriatic arthritis can precede cutaneous symptoms, sometimes making the specific diagnosis difficult; time is needed to allow an accurate diagnosis to be made[2,9–11,64] (see Fig. 23; Figs. 34–36).

Detection of synovial fluid urate crystals or calcium pyrophosphate dehydrate deposition (CPPD) crystals will allow the diagnosis of crystal deposition arthritis. One of the advantages of radiographs over MR is the ability to detect subtle calcifications. Detection of calcifications together with the characteristic radiographic appearance of gout (pararticular erosions with sclerotic rim, dense nodules, normal osseous mineralization, and normal joint space), the classic locations (first MTF joint, Lisfranc) allows a correct diagnosis of gout to be made. The key for the diagnosis of CPPD arthropathy is the presence of chondrocalcinosis[2,9–12] (Fig. 37).

The pattern of hand osteoarthritis is different from the RA pattern, especially because of the preferential involvement of DIP joints in osteoarthritis, the Heberden nodules around the DIP

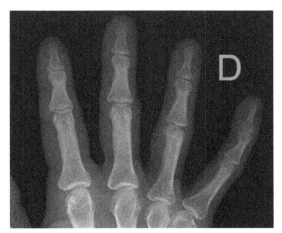

Fig. 34. Psoriatic arthritis nicely showing second finger diffuse soft tissue swelling, sausage finger.

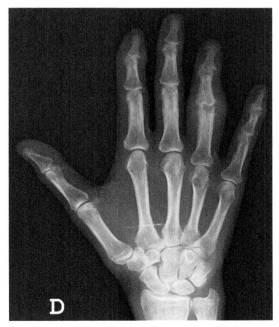

Fig. 35. Psoriatic arthritis with asymmetrical involvement of the DIP of the second, fourth, and fifth fingers.

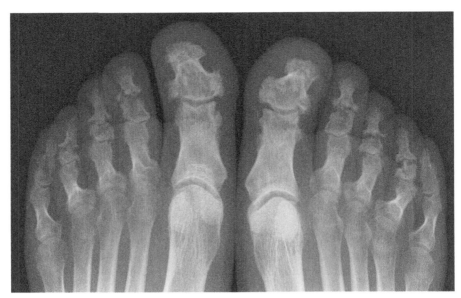

Fig. 36. Forefeet radiograph AP view demonstrating involvement of the PIP with marginal erosions, periostitis.

joints, narrowing of the joint spaces, and presence of osteophytes and absence of erosions in the proximal joints of the second to fifth rays. Erosions and cysts do occur in osteoarthritis, but they are located in the DIP joints and in the first carpometa-carpal joint[2,9–11] (**Fig. 38**).

Hemochromatosis is a disorder that causes increased intestinal iron absorption and secondary iron deposits in liver, pancreas, heart, and carti-lage. Approximately 50% of the patients will develop arthritis secondary to iron deposits in the joints. Radiologic manifestations are similar to those of RA or CPPD arthropathy. Findings are bone enlargement, joint space narrowing,

subchondral cysts with sclerotic borders, osteo-porosis, and osteophytes, with typically a hook or beak shape. They can also have CPPD deposits and chondrocalcinosis. The distribution of hemo-chromatosis is polyarticular, usually symmetric

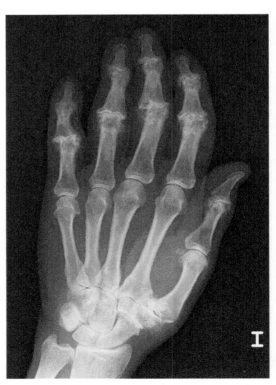

Fig. 37. Wrist radiograph of chondrocalcinosis with calcifications of the soft tissues, triangular fibrocarti-lage, scapholunate and lunotriquetal ligaments.

Fig. 38. Wrist and hand view of erosive osteoarthritis with severe involvement of the PIP and DIP joints.

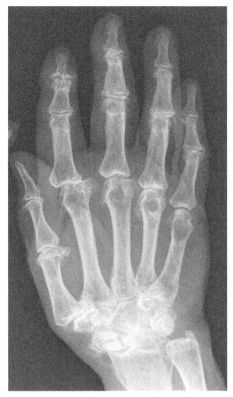

Fig. 39. Wrist and hand radiograph of hemochromatosis with characteristic hooklike osteophytes along the second, third, and fourth radial aspect of the metacarpal heads.

involvement, especially in the MCP, PIP of the second and third finger. The absence of soft tissue effusion, ulnar deviation and the location of the erosions helps to differentiate hemochromatosis arthropathy from RA[65] (**Fig. 39**).

REFERENCES

1. Loredo RA, Sorge DG, Garcia G. Radiographic evaluation of the wrist: a vanishing art. Semin Roentgenol 2005;40(3):248–89.
2. Aletaha D, Neogi T, Silman AJ, et al. 2010 Rheumatoid arthritis classification criteria: an American College of Rheumatology/European League Against Rheumatism collaborative initiative. Arthritis Rheum 2010;62(9):2569–81.
3. Smolen JS, Aletaha D, McInnes IB. Rheumatoid arthritis. Lancet 2016;388(10055):2023–38.
4. Sommer OJ, Kladosek A, Weiler V, et al. Rheumatoid arthritis: a practical guide to state-of-the-art imaging, image interpretation, and clinical implications. Radiographics 2005;25(2):381–98.
5. De Rycke L, Peene I, Hoffman IE, et al. Rheumatoid factor and anticitrullinated protein antibodies in

rheumatoid arthritis: diagnostic value, associations with radiological progression rate, and extra-articular manifestations. Ann Rheum Dis 2004; 63(12):1587–93.
6. Mangnus L, van Steenbergen HW, Reijnierse M, et al. Magnetic resonance imaging-detected features of inflammation and erosions in symptom-free persons from the general population. Arthritis Rheumatol 2016;68(11):2593–602.
7. Stomp W, Krabben A, van der Heijde D, et al. Are rheumatoid arthritis patients discernible from other early arthritis patients using 1.5T extremity magnetic resonance imaging? a large cross-sectional study. J Rheumatol 2014;41(8):1630–7.
8. Østergaard M, Haavardsholm EA. Imaging: MRI in healthy volunteers - important to do, and do correctly. Nat Rev Rheumatol 2016;12(10):563–4.
9. Jacobson JA, Girish G, Jiang Y, et al. Radiographic evaluation of arthritis: inflammatory conditions. Radiology 2008;248(2):378–89.
10. Resnick D, Kransdorf M. Bone and joint imaging. Rheumatoid arthritis and the seronegative spondyloarthropathies: radiographic and pathologic concepts. Chapter 15. 3rd edition. Philadelphia: Elsevier. p. 220–1.
11. Brower A, Fleming DJ. Arthritis in black and white. Philadelphia: W.B. Saunders; 1997.
12. Neogi T, Jansen TL, Dalbeth N, et al. 2015 Gout Classification Criteria: an American College of Rheumatology/European League Against Rheumatism collaborative initiative. Arthritis Rheumatol 2015; 67(10):2557–68.
13. Meirer R, Müller-Gerbl M, Huemer GM, et al. Quantitative assessment of periarticular osteopenia in patients with early rheumatoid arthritis: a preliminary report. Scand J Rheumatol 2004;33(5):307–11.
14. Böttcher J, Pfeil A. Diagnosis of periarticular osteoporosis in rheumatoid arthritis using digital X-ray radiogrammetry. Arthritis Res Ther 2008;10(1):103.
15. Gough AK, Lilley J, Eyre S, et al. Generalised bone loss in patients with early rheumatoid arthritis. Lancet 1994;344(8914):23–7.
16. Fouque-Aubert A, Chapurlat R, Miossec P, et al. A comparative review of the different techniques to assess hand bone damage in rheumatoid arthritis. Joint Bone Spine 2010;77(3):212–7.
17. Haugeberg G, Uhlig T, Falch JA, et al. Bone mineral density and frequency of osteoporosis in female patients with rheumatoid arthritis: results from 394 patients in the Oslo County rheumatoid arthritis register. Arthritis Rheum 2000;43(3):522–30.
18. Hauser B, Riches PL, Wilson JF, et al. Prevalence and clinical prediction of osteoporosis in a contemporary cohort of patients with rheumatoid arthritis. Rheumatology (Oxford) 2014;53(10):1759–66.
19. Shimizu S, Shiozawa S, Shiozawa K, et al. Quantitative histologic studies on the pathogenesis of

periarticular osteoporosis in rheumatoid arthritis. Arthritis Rheum 1985;28(1):25–31.

20. Hoff M, Haugeberg G, Odegård S, et al. Cortical hand bone loss after 1 year in early rheumatoid arthritis predicts radiographic hand joint damage at 5-year and 10-year follow-up. Ann Rheum Dis 2009;68(3):324–9.

21. Harrison BJ, Hutchinson CE, Adams J, et al. Assessing periarticular bone mineral density in patients with early psoriatic arthritis or rheumatoid arthritis. Ann Rheum Dis 2002;61(11):1007–11.

22. Haugeberg G, Green MJ, Quinn MA, et al. Hand bone loss in early undifferentiated arthritis: evaluating bone mineral density loss before the development of rheumatoid arthritis. Ann Rheum Dis 2006; 65(6):736–40.

23. Døhn UM, Ejbjerg BJ, Court-Payen M, et al. Are bone erosions detected by magnetic resonance imaging and ultrasonography true erosions? A comparison with computed tomography in rheumatoid arthritis metacarpophalangeal joints. Arthritis Res Ther 2006;8(4):R110.

24. Wawer R, Budzik JF, Demondion X, et al. Carpal pseudoerosions: a plain X-ray interpretation pitfall. Skeletal Radiol 2014;43(10):1377–85.

25. Lowthian PJ, Calin A. Geode development and multiple fractures in rheumatoid arthritis. Ann Rheum Dis 1985;44(2):130–3.

26. Bancroft LW, Peterson JJ, Kransdorf MJ. Cysts, geodes, and erosions. Radiol Clin North Am 2004; 42(1):73–87.

27. Schrank C, Meirer R, Stabler A, et al. Morphology and topography of intraosseous ganglion cysts in the carpus: an anatomic, histopathologic, and magnetic resonance imaging correlation study. J Hand Surg 2003;28A:52–61.

28. Resnick D, Niwayama G, Coutts RD. Subchondral cysts (geodes) in arthritic disorders. Pathologic and radiographic appearance of the hip joint. AJR Am J Roentgenol 1977;128:799–806.

29. Williams HJ, Davies AM, Allen G, et al. Imaging features of intraosseous ganglia: a report of 45 cases. Eur Radiol 2004;14(10):1761–9.

30. Williams M, Lambert RG, Jhangri GS, et al. Humeral head cysts and rotator cuff tears: an MR arthrographic study. Skeletal Radiol 2006;35:909–14.

31. Huo Y, Vincken KL, van der Heijde D, et al. Automatic quantification of radiographic finger joint space width of patients with early rheumatoid arthritis. IEEE Trans Biomed Eng 2016;63(10): 2177–86.

32. Sharp JT, Angwin J, Boers M, et al. Computer based methods for measurement of joint space width: update of an ongoing OMERACT project. J Rheumatol 2007;34(4):874–83.

33. Sharp JT, Angwin J, Boers M, et al. Multiple computer-based methods of measuring joint space

width can discriminate between treatment arms in the COBRA trial – update of an ongoing OMERACT project. J Rheumatol 2009;36(8):1825–8.

34. van 't Klooster R, Hendriks EA, Watt I, et al. Automatic quantification of osteoarthritis in hand radiographs: validation of a new method to measure joint space width. Osteoarthritis Cartilage 2008; 16(1):18–25.

35. Scott DL. Radiological progression in established rheumatoid arthritis. J Rheumatol Suppl 2004;69: 55–65.

36. Ory PA. Interpreting radiographic data in rheumatoid arthritis. Ann Rheum Dis 2003;62(7):597–604.

37. Scott DL, Pugner K, Kaarela K, et al. The links between joint damage and disability in rheumatoid arthritis. Rheumatology (Oxford) 2000;39:122–32.

38. van der Heijde D. Radiographic progression in rheumatoid arthritis: does it reflect outcome? Does it reflect treatment? Ann Rheum Dis 2001;60(Suppl III):iii47–50.

39. Boonen A, van der Heijde D. Conventional x-ray in early arthritis. Rheum Dis Clin North Am 2005; 31(4):681–98.

40. Landewé R, van der Heijde D. Radiographic progression in rheumatoid arthritis. Clin Exp Rheumatol 2005;23(5 Suppl 39):S63–8.

41. Brower A. Use of the radiograph to measure the course of rheumatoid arthritis. Arthritis Rheum 1990;33(3):316–24.

42. Landewé RB, Connell CA, Bradley JD, et al. Is radiographic progression in modern rheumatoid arthritis trials still a robust outcome? Experience from tofacitinib clinical trials. Arthritis Res Ther 2016;18(1):212.

43. Mueller RB, Kaegi T, Finckh A, et al. Is radiographic progression of late-onset rheumatoid arthritis different from young-onset rheumatoid arthritis? Results from the Swiss prospective observational cohort. Rheumatology (Oxford) 2014;53(4):671–7.

44. Leak RS, Rayan GM, Arthur RE. Longitudinal radiographic analysis of rheumatoid arthritis in the hand and wrist. J Hand Surg Am 2003;28(3):427–34.

45. Bielefeld T, Neumann DA. The unstable metacarpophalangeal joint in rheumatoid arthritis: anatomy, pathomechanics, and physical rehabilitation considerations. J Orthop Sports Phys Ther 2005;35(8): 502–20.

46. Rizio L, Belsky MR. Finger deformities in rheumatoid arthritis. Hand Clin 1996;12(3):531–40.

47. Ferlic DC. Boutonniere deformities in rheumatoid arthritis. Hand Clin 1989;5(2):215–22.

48. Dreyfus JN, Schnitzer TJ. Pathogenesis and differential diagnosis of the swan-neck deformity. Semin Arthritis Rheum 1983;13(2):200–11.

49. McKie SJ, O'Connor PJ, McKie SJ, O'Connor PJ. Imaging of the foot and ankle in rheumatoid arthritis. In: Helliwell P, Woodburn J, Redmond A, et al, editors. The foot and ankle in rheumatoid arthritis.

Philadelphia: Churchill Livingstone Elsevier; 2007. p. 99–112.

50. Resnick D, Niwayama G, Feingold ML. The sesamoid bones of the hands and feet: participators in arthritis. Radiology 1977;123(1):57–62.

51. Manaster BJ, May DA, Disler DG. Chapter 17 - Musculoskeletal imaging: The requisites in radiology. Rheumatoid arthritis and juveline rheumatoid arthritis. Third edition. Philadelphia: Mosby Elsevier; 2007. p. 292.

52. Weissman B. Imaging of arthritis and metabolic bone disease, imaging of rheumatoid arthritis. 1st edition. Philadelphia: Elsevier; 2009. Chapter 20.

53. Lehtinen JT, Kaarela K, Belt EA, et al. Radiographic joint space in rheumatoid elbow joints. A 15-year prospective follow-up study in 74 patients. Rheumatology (Oxford) 2001;40(10):1141–5.

54. Kieft GJ, Dijkmans BAC, Bloem JL, et al. Magnetic resonance imaging of the shoulder in patients with rheumatoid arthritis. Ann Rheum Dis 1990;49:7–11.

55. Voog U, Alstergren P, Eliasson S, et al. Inflammatory mediators and radiographic changes in temporomandibular joints of patients with rheumatoid arthritis. Acta Odontol Scand 2003;61(1):57–64.

56. Younes M, Belghali S, Kriaa S, et al. Compared imaging of the rheumatoid cervical spine: prevalence study and associated factors. Joint Bone Spine 2009;76(4):361–8.

57. Zikou AK, Alamanos Y, Argyropoulou MI, et al. Radiological cervical spine involvement in patients with rheumatoid arthritis: a cross sectional study. J Rheumatol 2005;32:801–6.

58. Bouchaud-Chabot A, Liote F. Cervical spine involvement in rheumatoid arthritis. Joint Bone Spine 2002; 69:141–54.

59. McGregor M. The significance of certain measurements of the skull in the diagnosis of basilar impression. Br J Radiol 1948;21:171–8.

60. Ranawat CS, O'Leary P, Pellici P, et al. Cervical spine fusion in rheumatoid arthritis. J Bone Joint Surg Am 1979;61:1003–10.

61. Kauppi M, Sakaguchi M, Konttinen YT, et al. A new method of screening for vertical atlantoaxial dislocation. J Rheumatol 1990;17:167–72.

62. Reijnierse M, Dijkmans BA, Hansen B, et al. Neurologic dysfunction in patients with rheumatoid arthritis of the cervical spine: predictive value of clinical, radiographic and MR imaging parameters. Eur Radiol 2001;11:467–73.

63. Kroft LJM, Reijnierse M, Kloppenburg M, et al. Rheumatoid arthritis: epidural enhancement as an underestimated cause of subaxial cervical spinal stenosis. Radiology 2004;231:57–63.

64. Ory PA, Gladman D, Mease PJ. Psoriatic arthritis and imaging. Ann Rheum Dis 2005;64:ii55–7.

65. Lonardo A, Neri P, Mascia MT, et al. Hereditary hemochromatosis masquerading as rheumatoid arthritis. Ann Ital Med Int 2001;16:46–9.

Conventional Radiology in Spondyloarthritis

Alberto Bazzocchi, MD, PhD[a],*, Maria Pilar Aparisi Gómez, MBChB, FRANZCR[b,c], Giuseppe Guglielmi, MD[d,e]

KEYWORDS

- Radiography • Spondylarthritis • Spondylitis • Ankylosing • Arthritis • Psoriatic
- Reactive • Diagnostic imaging

KEY POINTS

- Spondyloarthritides represent a group of inflammatory rheumatic diseases with negative rheumatoid factor. Clinically, 2 large subgroups are defined, axial spondyloarthritis (axSpA) and peripheral spondyloarthritis (pSpA), with some overlap.
- The presence of sacroiliitis represents the most characteristic feature of these disorders.
- Radiography is the recommended first method for diagnosis of sacroiliitis and to monitor structural axial and peripheral changes that predict severity of outcome.
- Nonradiographic xSpA (nr-axSpA) is a new classification concept that includes patients without radiographic signs of sacroiliitis who satisfy clinical criteria for diagnosis of axial SpA (axSp).

INTRODUCTION

The term, *spondyloarthritis (SpA)*, refers to a group of closely related inflammatory rheumatic diseases, comprising ankylosing SpA (AS), psoriatic arthritis (PsA), reactive arthritis (ReA), enteropathic-related SpA, and undifferentiated SpA.[1,2]

By definition, SpA patients have a negative rheumatoid factor, hence the term seronegative SpA; all SpA subgroups typically show a familiar clustering and are strongly associated with the HLA-B27 gene.[2,3]

Based on their clinical presentation, 2 large SpA subtypes can be identified, axSpA and pSpA, with some overlap between these 2 subtypes: patients with axSpA demonstrate a predominant involvement of the axial skeleton, reflecting inflammation of the sacroiliac joints (SIJs) and/or the spine; patients with pSpA show a predominant involvement of the peripheral joints, consisting of peripheral arthritis, enthesitis, and dactylitis.[2,3] This approach, which allows a better description of the presenting disease, has important clinical implications, because therapeutic strategies differ for axSpA versus pSpA.[2] Because specific therapy is available, early diagnosis and therapeutic intervention are crucial to modify disease progression.[2,4,5] The diagnosis of an early SpA can be challenging, however, because clinical presentation is frequently heterogeneous and no specific distinguishing feature is available; in daily

The authors have no commercial or financial conflict of interest or funding sources related to the present work.

[a] Diagnostic and Interventional Radiology, Rizzoli Orthopaedic Institute, Via G. C. Pupilli 1, Bologna 40136, Italy; [b] Department of Radiology, Auckland City Hospital, 2 Park Road, Grafton, Auckland 1023, New Zealand; [c] Department of Radiology, Hospital Nueve de Octubre, Calle Valle de la Ballestera, 59, Valencia 46015, Spain; [d] Department of Radiology, University of Foggia, Viale Luigi Pinto 1, Foggia 71100, Italy; [e] Department of Radiology, Scientific Institute, Casa Sollievo della Sofferenza Hospital, Viale Cappuccini 1, San Giovanni Rotondo, Foggia 71013, Italy
* Corresponding author.
E-mail address: abazzo@inwind.it

radiologic.theclinics.com

practice, the diagnosis of SpA is usually made based on a combination of positive family history, clinical symptoms, physical examination, laboratory parameters, and suggestive findings at imaging investigations.[2,6]

CLASSICAL TYPES: PREVALENCE AND EPIDEMIOLOGY
Ankylosing Spondylitis

Overall, the prevalence of AS ranges from 0.1 to 1.4, with the highest prevalence in northern Europe; the disease generally presents in late adolescence or in early adulthood, whereas the presentation after the age of 40 is unusual.[7] Men are more often affected than women with a male-to-female ratio of 3:1.[8] Morning stiffness and low

back pain are the most common presenting symptoms; younger patients may experience also peripheral symptoms, such as heel pain (Table 1).[7,9]

The prevalence of HLA-B27 in a population has a significant impact on the occurrence of AS. HLA-B27–negative individuals, however, may develop typical AS. For whites, 90% to 95% of AS patients are HLA-B27 positive. HLA-B27 positivity can be considered a risk factor for development of sacroiliitis and progression to AS.[10,11]

Psoriatic Arthritis

It has been estimated that between 1% and 6% of the population in the Western countries have some degree of psoriasis vulgaris. There is no known gender predilection. Peak incidence is between

Table 1
Characteristics of the most common spondyloarthritides

Features	Ankylosing Spondylitis	Psoriatic Arthritis	Reactive Arthritis	Enteropathic Arthritis
Prevalence	0.1%–0.2%	0.2%–0.4%	0.1%	Rare
Age of apparition	20–30	35–45	20–30	Any
Male:female	3:1	1:1	5:1	1:1
Spine involvement	Symmetric sacroiliitis (100%) Delicate marginal syndesmophytes Lumbar spine and lower thoracic spine involved initially	Asymmetric sacroiliitis Bulky marginal syndesmophytes Cervical spine involvement most commonly	Asymmetric sacroiliitis Bulky marginal syndesmophytes	Symmetric sacroiliitis Delicate marginal syndesmophytes
Peripheral arthritis	Asymmetric lower extremities	Any joint	Asymmetric lower extremities	Asymmetric lower extremities
Enthesitis	Common	Very common	Very common	Less common
Dactylitis	Uncommon	Common	Common	Uncommon
Dermatologic manifestations	Nonspecific	Psoriasis	Keratoderma Blennorrhagica Circinate balanitis	Erythema nodosum Pyoderma gangrenosum
Uveitis	Occasional	Occasional	Common	Occasional
Other manifestations	Aortic regurgitation Conduction defects Upper lobe pulmonary fibrosis IgA nephropathy Amyloidosis Prostatitis Oral ulcers	Aortic regurgitation Conduction defects Pitting onicholisis Amyloidosis Oral ulcers	Aortic regurgitation Conduction defects Onycholisis Diarrhea Amyloidosis Urethritis, cervicitis Oral ulcers	Aortic regurgitation Conduction defects Clubbing nails Crohn disease Ulcerative colitis Nephrolithiasis Oral ulcers
Familial aggregation	Common	Common	Common	Common
HLA-B27	90%	40%	80%	30%

Data from Kataria RK, Brent LH. Spondyloarthropathies. Am Fam Physician 2004;69(12):2853–60.

35 years and 45 years of age. Up to 15% of these patients develop clinically and radiologically variable degrees of PsA (in some series up to 20% of the patients) (see **Table 1**).[12]

According to the literature, in 20% to 30% of cases, there are no psoriatic skin changes on onset of arthritic symptoms.[13] This rate is likely to be overestimated, however, given many patients are not investigated by experienced dermatologists.[14]

Besides skin and bones, other typical sites of involvement are the tendons at the entheses.

Patients often present with diffuse swelling of 1 of more digits (dactylitis). After the sudden apparition of symptoms, the course of the disease is variable.

Psoriatic SpA accounts for almost 20% of the seronegative spondyloarthritides. Genetic association with HLA-B27 antigen has been identified.

In HIV-infected patients, PsA is 40 times more common than in general population.[12]

The severity of the arthritis usually does not correlate with the severity of the skin involvement.

Reactive Arthritis

ReA is an aseptic arthritis that is triggered by an infectious agent located outside the joint. It usually develops 1 week to 4 weeks after a genitourinary or gastrointestinal tract infection. Typical agents involved are *Chlamydia, Ureaplasma, Shigella, Salmonella, Yersinia,* and *Campylobacter* species.[15] The symptom triad of arthritis, conjunctivitis, and urethritis after a triggering infection is classically known as Reiter syndrome.

Incidence and prevalence are difficult to determine, given the variability in the use of criteria to make the diagnosis in different series and that there could be substantial underestimation because mild, self-limited cases may never be recognized.

The predominant feature of ReA is an asymmetric lower limb predominant oligoarthritis (4 or fewer affected joints). Extra-articular symptoms, including urethritis and conjunctivitis, represent more severe disease. This is only observed in approximately 30% of cases.[15]

As an approximation, the incidence follows the prevalence of HLA-B27 in the population. In individuals with ReA, the prevalence of HLA-B27 is approximately 50%,[16] reported to be as much as 80% in other sources (see **Table 1**).[17]

The disease is more common in those between 20 years and 40 years old. There is a slight male predominance, attributed specifically to *Chlamydia*-associated ReA. Enteric infection–associated ReA affects man and woman with equal

frequency. Among HIV-positive individuals, the incidence of ReA is at least 10 times greater than in normal population.

Enteropathic Arthritis

SpA is seen in up to 20% of patients with inflammatory bowel disease, such as Crohn disease and ulcerative colitis.[18]

There is no significant difference in incidence by genders.

Association with HLA-B27 is reported to up to 30% of cases.

Typically, the arthritis affects the lower limbs in an asymmetric pattern. Onset is sudden, and the pattern is migratory. The initial symptoms subside in 6 weeks to 8 weeks, but recurrence is common; 10% of patients are estimated to develop chronic arthritis.

In up to 20% of affected patients, the associated SpA shows as SpA that is indistinguishable from idiopathic AS.

The exacerbations of peripheral arthritis and inflammatory bowel disease tend to coincide, whereas axial disease is independent of activity of bowel disease.[17]

Undifferentiated Spondyloarthritis

The term, *undifferentiated SpA*, describes manifestations of the disease that do not meet criteria to be classified into any of the spondyloarthritides, discussed previously.

Most patients have nonspecific symptoms, such as inflammatory back pain, buttock pain, enthesitis, dactylitis, and even extra-articular manifestations. In general, they respond well to nonsteroidal anti-inflammatory drugs (NSAIDs) and have good prognosis. If severe forms develop, approach to treatment is similar to that of AS.[17]

DIAGNOSIS
The Concept of Radiographic and Nonradiographic Spondyloarthritis

To cover the entire spectrum of the disease, in 2009 the classification criteria recently developed by the Assessment of SpondyloArthritis International Society (ASAS) highlighted a specific new entity, nr-axSpA.[19–22] This group includes patients without signs of sacroiliitis on conventional radiographs but who satisfy clinical criteria for diagnosis for axSpA (ie, HLA-B27 positive and 2 other SpA features) (**Box 1**) as well as patients with active inflammation in the SIJ detected by MR imaging.[20,23] Nr-axSpA can be considered an early stage of axSpA: progression is reported in approximately 10% of cases over 2 years, although the characteristics of the subgroup of patients who develop radiographic signs of sacroiliitis have not yet been determined.[23,24]

Few data are available on the incidence, prevalence, and proportion of patients classified or diagnosed as nr-axSpA[17]; moreover, these data derive mainly from noninterventional cohorts and anti–tumor necrosis factor (TNF) treatment trials; thus, they are not generalizable to axSpA patients in general.[23] Even if most clinical features show no significant differences in patients with radiographic axSpA (r-axSpA) and nr-axSpA, 3 main differentiating features have been observed among the 2 subgroups: the opposite male-to-female ratio, the presence of objective evidences of inflammation (ie, C-reactive protein [CRP] levels and/or positive MR imaging findings), and the degree of limitation in spinal mobility.[23,24] Both 2:1 and 1:2 male-to-female ratios have been observed, respectively, among patients with

r-axSpA and nr-axSpA.[23–27] Recently, a positive association was found between male gender and the evidence of SIJ abnormalities on radiograph or MR imaging in axSpA patients, suggesting that men may develop radiographic structural changes sooner and more frequently.[23,28,29] Other important differences have been reported in the proportion of patients with objective signs of inflammation: the level of CRP (biochemical parameter) and the amount and the extension of inflammatory spinal lesions on MR imaging are significantly lower in patients with nr-axSpA compared with patients with r-axSpA.[23,25,30] Moreover a radiographic progression of the disease occurs more frequently if objective evidence of inflammation (ie, CRP levels and/or positive MR imaging findings) is present.[23,29] Lastly, data from treatment trials also indicate that patients with nr-axSpA have fewer limitations in spinal mobility in comparison with patients with radiographic disease and that the impairment of spinal mobility increases with the duration of the disease, likely the result of development of structural changes at the spine.[23,24,31,32] No significant difference was found in terms of level of disease activity, pain, and patient global assessment between the 2 subgroups.[23,24]

Despite the differences discussed previously, at diagnosis it is not necessary to make a distinction between r-axSpA and nr-axSpA; the 2 subgroups are similar in terms of clinical presentation and have an almost identical response rate to TNF.[24]

The Role of Conventional Radiology, from Past to Modern Times

Imaging of the SIJ is a unifying diagnostic tool for the seronegative SpA.[9] The different types differ greatly from one another, but all of them can affect the entire axial and appendicular skeleton. The presence of sacroiliitis represents the most characteristic feature of these disorders, and, in absence of sacroiliitis, the involvement of other sites of both axial and appendicular skeleton is rare.[9]

According to the new criteria for SpA classification of the ASAS, conventional radiography still plays a pivotal role in diagnosis of axSpA. Radiographic assessment of the SIJs is recommended as the first imaging method to diagnose sacroiliitis as part of axSpA, according to ASAS and European League Against Rheumatism (EULAR) recommendation.[33] (ASAS classification criteria for axSpA and pSpA are summarized in **Boxes 1** and **2**).

The SIJ is assessed on AP images of the pelvis.[34,35] The SIJ has a complex anatomy and

In most circumstances, the standard AP pelvis film alone yields the diagnosis of sacroiliitis, with no need of dedicated imaging for the SIJ. The ASAS recommends the whole pelvis with the hip joints be included as part of the initial evaluation of patients with suspected SpA.[20,34] Hip joints are affected in 25% of patients with SpA and, according to several studies, involvement of the hip is strongly associated with cervical disease and higher scores for spinal change at radiology.[34,35,42–44]

According to the modified New York criteria, 5 stages of radiographic changes in the SIJ can be identified (**Box 3, Table 2**).[45] These structural damage in the SIJ could be probably best recognized with CT; however, there is no established scoring system for sacroiliitis on CT and the high dose of ionizing radiation makes this technique unsuitable for evaluating progression of the disease over time.[46]

Early sacroiliitis is often difficult to identify and because the progression of radiographic damage is generally slow, the delay between the onset of the first symptoms and the diagnosis can be up to 10 years.[2,47] Moreover, pelvic radiographs are able to detect structural changes that are the consequences of the inflammation (erosions and sclerosis) rather than the inflammation itself.[2] The identification of early sacroiliitis is dramatically improved by the introduction of MR imaging, a technique that is able to detect inflammation of the SIJ in patients without evidence of abnormalities on conventional radiography.[48] Despite the

---

Box 2

Assessment of Spondyloarthritis International Society diagnostic criteria for peripheral spondyloarthritis

Peripheral arthritis and/or enthesitis and/or dactylitis PLUS

≥1 SpA feature OR	≥2 other SpA features
• Uveitis	• Arthritis
• Psoriasis	• Enthesitis (heel)
• Crohn disease/ ulcerative colitis	• Dactylitis
• Preceding infection	• Inflammatory back pain
• HLA-B27 positive	• Family history of SpA
• Sacroiliitis on imaging	

Data from Rudwaleit M, van der Heijde D, Landewé R, et al. The Assessment of SpondyloArthritis International Society classification criteria for peripheral spondyloarthritis and for spondyloarthritis in general. Ann Rheum Dis 2011;70(1):25–31.

---

it is composed of 2 different main compartments: a cartilaginous C-shaped or L-shaped portion that lies inferiorly and anteriorly and a ligamentous part that lies superiorly and posteriorly.[34,36–38] The anterocaudal portion has the anatomic characteristic of a cartilaginous articulation, resembling a symphysis with only the lower one-third lined by synovium (diarthrosis); the posterocephalad part is a syndesmosis and contains the strong interosseous ligament.[34,36–39] There are 2 different types of cartilage in the SIJs, hyaline cartilage covering the sacral surface and fibrocartilage covering the iliac surface. The sacral hyaline cartilage is 3 times to 5 times thicker than the fibrocartilage in the iliac aspect, which is why radiographic changes of sacroiliitis usually start and are more evident on the iliac side.[39] On the supine AP projection a significant overlap between the ilium and the sacrum is present, due to the oblique orientation of the joint from a medial to lateral direction, thus the evaluation of the entire SIJ in a 2-D projection can be challenging.[40,41] To improve the visualization of the joint space, more specific views, such as anteroposterior (AP) oblique Ferguson projections or AP views with cranial angulation, can be obtained; however, in most cases, these specialized views do not contribute additional information to the standard radiographic examination and cause an increase in a patient's radiation dose.[9,40]

Box 3

Modified New York criteria for ankylosing spondylitis

Clinical criteria

1. Low back pain and stiffness >3 months, improves with exercise, not relieved by rest

2. Limitation of motion of the lumbar spine in both sagittal and frontal planes

3. Limitation of chest expansion relative to normal values corrected for age and gender

Radiologic criterion

Sacroiliitis grade ≥2 bilaterally or grade 3 to 4 unilaterally

Definite AS: radiologic criterion + 1 clinical criterion

Data from van der Linden S, Valkenburg HA, Cats A. Evaluation of diagnostic criteria for ankylosing spondylitis. A proposal for modification of the New York criteria. Arthritis Rheum 1984;27(4):361–8.

Table 2 Grading of radiologic sacroiliitis	
Grade 0	Normal
Grade 1	Suspicious changes
Grade 2	Minimal abnormality Small localized areas with erosion or sclerosis, without alteration in joint width
Grade 3	Unequivocal abnormality Moderate or advanced sacroiliitis with 1 or more of the following: • Erosions • Evidence of sclerosis • Widening • Narrowing • Partial ankylosis
Grade 4	Severe abnormality–total ankylosis

Data from Bennett DL, Ohashi K, El-Khoury GY. Spondyloarthropathies: ankylosing spondylitis and psoriatic arthritis. Radiol Clin North Am 2004;42(1):121–34.

increasing role of MR imaging in the identification of sacroiliitis, however, conventional radiography remains the first line of imaging investigation in patients suspected of having inflammatory arthritis of all kinds.[10,40]

MR imaging is not generally recommended for initial diagnosis of axSpA, but it can be used as second-line examination in cases of high clinical suspicion but no radiographic evidence of sacroiliitis and as alternative first imaging method in young patients and in patients with short symptom duration (**Fig. 1**).[33]

Plain radiography is both sensitive and specific for diagnosis of established disease: in established and long-standing AS, more than 95% of patients show radiographic changes in the SIJ whereas approximately 50% to 70% of patients show spinal involvement with syndesmophytes and/or ankylosis of small vertebral joints.[3,6]

Conventional radiography should be used in long-term monitoring of established structural changes (in particular new bone formation) at SIJ and/or spine in patients with axSpA and it was shown superior to MR imaging in the detection of spinal syndesmophytes at cervical and lumbar spine, which are predicting of outcome/severity in patients with AS (**Fig. 2**).[4,33] It is also recommended in the follow-up protocol of to monitor structural changes in pSpA.

Finally, conventional radiography is the first-line imaging examination also if a vertebral fracture is suspected in patients with diagnosed axSpA.[33]

RADIOLOGIC MANIFESTATIONS

Although many imaging modalities are currently available, plain radiography remains the first line and the mainstay of radiologic investigation of these diseases.[10,40]

Changes related to axSpA and pSpA can be differentiated in active inflammation (SpA and spondylodiscitis, in cases of the spine), structural osteodestructive changes (erosions), and

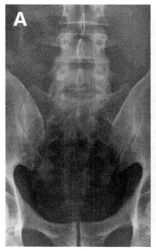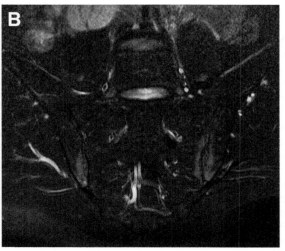

Fig. 1. Young patient with inflammatory back pain and HLA-B27 antigen positive. (*A*) Conventional radiography does not show any obvious abnormality of the SIJs. (*B*) Coronal T2 fast relaxation fast spin-echo fat saturated sequence from MR imaging study of the same patient, showing the presence of bone marrow edema in the SIJs, with irregularity of joint surfaces and presence of small erosions. Initial distribution typically involves the caudal portion of the joint.

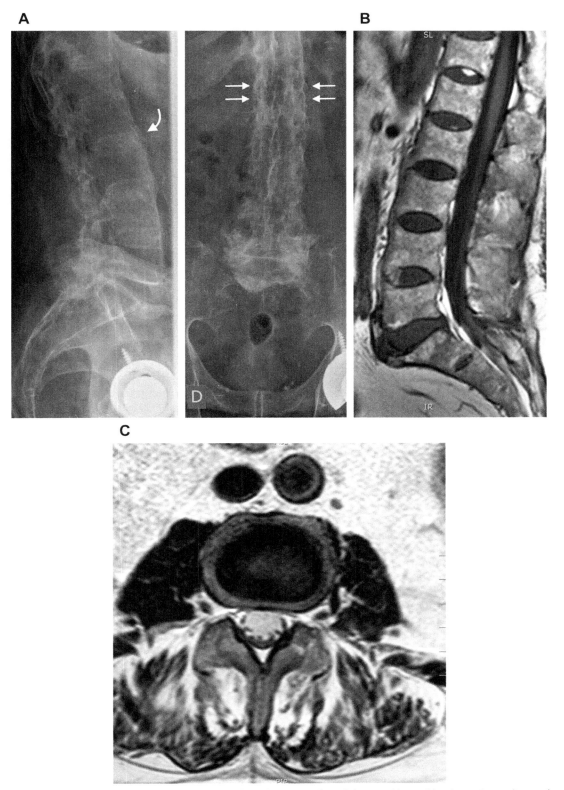

Fig. 2. A 73-year-old male patient with longstanding diagnosis of AS. (*A*) AP and lateral lumbar spine radiographs demonstrate progressive growth of syndesmophytes, extending anteriorly along the deep layer of the anterior

structural hyperproliferative changes (entheso-phytes, vertebral squaring, disk calcifications, spondylophytes, syndesmophytes, bony bridging, and vertebral ankylosis, in cases of the spine)[49–51]; conventional radiography cannot detect early signs of inflammation at the spine and other sites but seems superior to MR imaging in assessment and quantification of structural changes.[39]

In particular, radiography is the first-line imaging modality in detecting structural changes, such as spinal syndesmophytes at cervical and lumbar spine, which are predicting of outcome/severity in patients with AS.[4,33]

Axial Involvement

Sacroiliac joints

Sacroiliitis represents the most characteristic feature of these disorders; in absence of sacroilii-tis, the involvement of other sites of both axial and appendicular skeleton is unusual.

Pelvis AP (standard) and Ferguson (tube is angled 30°–35° in cephalad rotation and central beam directed toward the midportion of the pelvis, resulting in a tangential view of the SIJs, and sacral bone) are the standard views for the assessment of the SIJ. Five stages of radiographic changes in the SIJ can be identified,[45] which are described in the modified New York criteria (see **Box 3**).

The first changes in sacroiliitis consist of changes with poor definition of the joint outlines, in part due to the presence of erosions and in part due to the formation of new bone bridges (**Fig. 3**).

Erosions appear as scalloped–dentate contours in the caudal portion of the joint. If the process of erosion is marked, then there is the impression of pseudowidening of the joint space.

Eventually, sclerosis develops, typically involving the caudal portion of the joint, extending into the middle portion. This is normally broad and is predominant in the iliac side (**Fig. 4**).

Partial ankylosis and finally total ankylosis are the result of the progression of these lesions, particularly the bone bridging. Sometimes partial ankylosis is difficult to detect, mainly due to pro-jectional facts that may not allow assessing the joint space in its entirety and is only evident in

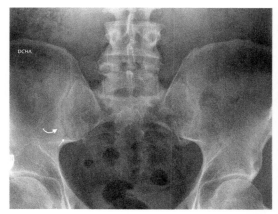

Fig. 3. A 26-year-old male patient with a year history of low back pain and positive HLA-B27 antigen. Initial changes in sacroiliitis consist of changes with poor defi-nition of the joint outlines (*curved arrow*), in part due to the presence of erosions and in part due to the for-mation of new bone. Erosions appear as scalloped–den-tate contours in the caudal portion of the joint (*straight arrow*). Eventually, sclerosis develops.

comparison with previous examinations. In total ankylosis, the whole of the normal outline of the joint is lost.

AS represents the prototype of axSpA: the involvement of the SIJ is usually bilateral and sym-metric and gradually progressive over years. The disease typically starts in the SIJ with tiny serrated erosions that resemble the appearance of the edge of a postage stamp, which start on the iliac side of the joint. As the disease progresses, defini-tion of the joint is lost and proliferative changes became predominant, with areas of subchondral sclerosis and superimposition of new bone forma-tion with narrowing and complete fusion of the joint in the final stages.[9,52]

In PsA, incidence of sacroiliitis is high, and this can be bilateral and symmetric, bilateral and asymmetric, or unilateral. Most typically this is uni-lateral (**Fig. 5**).

In ReA, the pattern tends to be asymmetric and bilateral. In early stages it can be unilateral; however, if inflammatory change progresses, involvement of both SIJs may become symmetric.

---

intervertebral ligament and involving the paravertebral soft tissue bridges the intervertebral space causing anky-losis (*curved arrow*). The extensive bone formation produces a smooth, undulating spinal contour, called the bamboo spine. There is extensive ossification over the dorsolateral aspect of the column, recognizable on the lateral projection, seen as what is called the tramlines sign on the AP projection, consisting of 2 parallel bands of sclerosis projected over the apophyseal joints (*straight arrows*). (*B*) Sagittal T1 turbo spin-echo from MR imag-ing study on the same patient. Note syndesmophytes and bone bridging are significantly less evident. (*C*) Axial T2 turbo spin-echo demonstrates ankylosis of the interapophyseal joints.

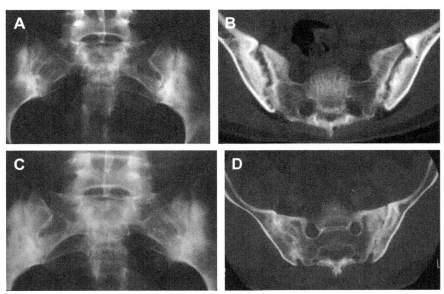

Fig. 4. Progression of changes in the SIJs. (A) AP sacroiliac (SI) joint radiograph demonstrates poor definition of the joint outlines, in part due to the presence of erosions, and in part due to the formation of new bone, with extensive sclerosis that extends mainly through the iliac aspect. (B) Axial CT images demonstrate erosions that appear as scalloped–dentate contours of the joint. If the process of erosion is marked, then there is the impression of pseudowidening of the joint space. (C) AP SI joint radiograph on the same patient 2.5 years later. Eventually, sclerosis progresses, and the joint line cannot be defined in some segments, features that are in keeping with ankylosis. (D) Axial CT image on the same patient shows almost complete loss of the outline of the left SIJ due to ankylosis.

In enteropathic arthritis, the pattern of distribution of inflammatory change in the SIJs is symmetric, similar to that of AS.

Spine

Regarding the spine, AP and lateral radiographs of cervical, thoracic, and lumbar spine should be obtained depending on the level of a patient's clinical

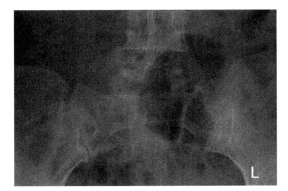

Fig. 5. A 55-year-old woman with PsA. AP radiograph of the sacroiliac joints shows unilateral asymmetric (left) sacroiliitis. In PsA, incidence of sacroiliitis is high, and this can be bilateral and symmetric, bilateral and asymmetric, or unilateral. Most typically this is unilateral.

symptoms.[20] Oblique views of the spine may be of some value, allowing further evaluation of the facet joints.

The involvement of the spine presents in approximately 50% of AS patients. The earliest changes, generally occur in the thoracolumbar and in the lumbosacral regions; as the disease progresses, the midlumbar, midthoracic, and cervical regions are affected. The cervical spine is rarely affected alone. This orderly progression in spine involvement represents a peculiar feature of AS, whereas in the other SpAs, the involvement of the spine tends to be more random.

In AS, the earliest changes in the spine appear as a result of enthesitis at the edges of the discovertebral joints. Three types were described by Cawley and colleagues.[53]

Type I lesions are localized central lesions in the vertebral endplate (Andersson type A lesions). These tend to be mild and focal and can be unchanged for months or years, unlike what happens with infectious discitis. They usually occur in the thoracolumbar spine (Fig. 6). Type I lesions are typically found in the first decade of the disease and demonstrate radiographically as endplate erosions. These lesions are in most cases asymptomatic and, therefore, are undetected.

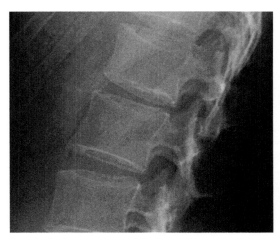

Fig. 6. Andersson type A lesions. These tend to be mild, focal erosions and can be unchanged for months or years, unlike what happens with infectious discitis, which is the main differential. They usually occur in the thoracolumbar spine.

MR imaging potentially is sensitive to this type of lesion (Fig. 7).

Type II lesions consist of localized peripheral erosive lesions (Romanus lesions) with reactive sclerosis (the shiny corner) (Fig. 8) at the anterior corner of vertebral endplates, mainly in the lumbar region. The same findings in the posterior vertebral corners are referred to as SpA marginalis.

These early changes can be short lived or long lived and generally difficult to detect on plain films unless there is a strong clinical suspicion.

Romanus lesions tend to resolve and lead to the formation of syndesmophytes that represent the ossification of the outer fibers of the annulus fibrosus, where Sharpey fibers attach to the vertebral bodies. Moreover, periosteal proliferation and new bone formation at the anterosuperior and anteroinferior vertebral margins result in squaring of vertebral borders (Fig. 9); this evidence is much easier to recognize in the lumbar spine, where vertebrae are normally concave in comparison with the more variable profile of cervical and thoracic vertebrae.[9,52] These syndesmophytes are thin and symmetric (Fig. 10).

The progressive growth of syndesmophytes, extending anteriorly along the deep layer of the anterior intervertebral ligament (prediscal type) and involving the paravertebral soft tissue, bridges the intervertebral space causing ankylosis, and the extensive bone formation produces a smooth, undulating spinal contour called the bamboo

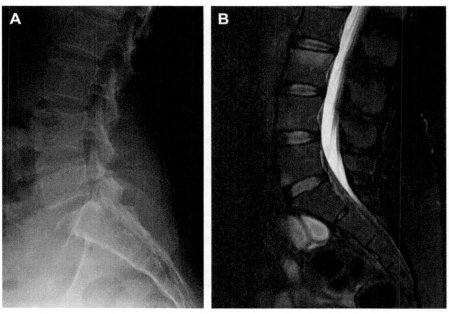

Fig. 7. A 27-year-old woman, with nonspecific back pain. (A) Lateral view of the lumbar spine was reported as normal. (B) On persistence of pain, MR imaging was performed 5 weeks later. There is increased signal intensity in the superior endplate of L3 as well as subtle foci of increased signal intensity in the anterior aspect of the inferior endplate of L4 and L5. MR imaging has high sensitivity to detect this type of lesions, not evident on radiographs. These lesions are in most cases asymptomatic and therefore go undetected. In this case symptoms were attributed to them, in absence of any other cause for pain. The patient had been diagnosed with ulcerative colitis and had a positive HLA-B27 antigen.

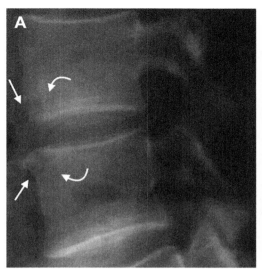
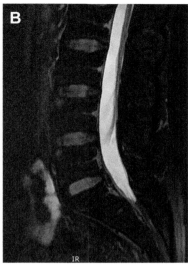

Fig. 8. Type II Cawley lesions consist of localized peripheral erosive lesions, also called the Romanus lesion. (A) Detail of a lateral lumbar spine radiograph with demonstration of the typical radiographic features of erosion at the anterior corner of vertebral endplates (*straight arrows*) with reactive sclerosis, also called the shiny corner (*curved arrows*). (B) Sagittal short tau inversion recovery from MR imaging of a different patient, showing the appearances of these lesions. Note the presence of high signal intensity in keeping with bone marrow edema in the anterior aspects of the superior endplates of L4 and L5.

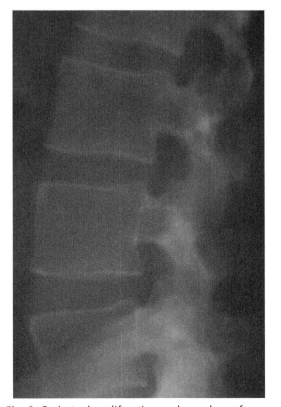

Fig. 9. Periosteal proliferation and new bone formation at the anterosuperior and anteroinferior vertebral margins results in squaring of vertebral. This evidence is much more easier to recognize in the lumbar spine, where vertebrae are normally concave in comparison with the more variable profile of cervical and thoracic vertebrae.

spine. The disk space is generally preserved (**Fig. 11**).[49–52]

This is not to be mistaken with diffuse idiopathic skeletal hyperostosis (DISH) syndrome, which is characterized by marginal ossifications

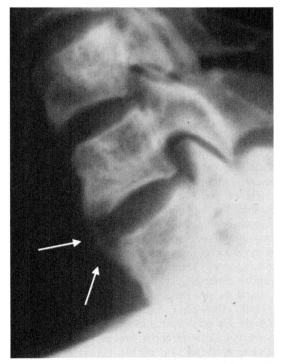

Fig. 10. Detail of a lateral cervical spine radiograph. Example of the typical thin and symmetric syndesmophytes on AS (*white arrows*).

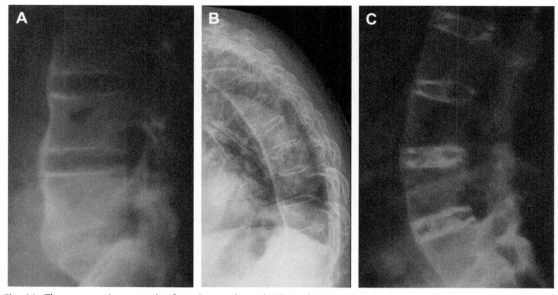

Fig. 11. The progressive growth of syndesmophytes bridges the intervertebral space, causing ankylosis, and the extensive bone formation produces a smooth, undulating spinal contour called the bamboo spine. The disk space is generally preserved. (*A*) Lateral lumbar spine view. (*B*) Thoracic spine lateral view. DISH syndrome can appear similar but is characterized by marginal ossifications that typically grow more laterally and in a horizontal direction. This vertical rather than horizontal orientation of the bony excrescences also establishes a difference with degenerative disease. (*C*) Lateral view of the lumbar spine demonstrates ossification of the intervertebral disks.

that typically grow more laterally and in a horizontal direction.[54] This vertical rather than horizontal orientation of the bony excrescences also establishes a difference with degenerative disease.

Square or barrel-shaped vertebrae are the result of inflammatory and osteoproliferative events in the ventral aspect of the vertebrae.

Type III, or Andersson type B, lesions consist of extensive central and peripheral lesions.[55] Classically they were described associated with the Andersson type A lesions. They represent a malunion or nonunion of an insufficiency fracture through the intervertebral disk, in the context of multisegmental ankylosis. They are typical of late stages of the disease and rare. When found, it is paramount to drive attention toward them given their severity. They usually occur in the thoracolumbar region (**Fig. 12**).

Patients normally report pain and improved mobility. They can be difficult to detect, especially if there are no previous radiographs. Risk factors are osteoporosis, trauma, and increased thoracolumbar kyphosis. Transverse lamina fractures in AP projection or dehiscence of the spinous processes in the lateral projection are characteristic features. Sometimes there is intense vertebral

endplate destruction, which is the result of resorption, and surrounding sclerosis, resembling in a pseudoarthrosis.

Inflammatory changes also develop in the posterior elements of the spine. Changes in the apophyseal joints are mixed result of arthritis and enthesitis. At early stages, this is difficult to detect on radiographs. In late stages, there is extensive ossification over the dorsolateral aspect of the column, recognizable on the lateral projection (**Fig. 13**), seen as what is called the tramlines sign on the AP projection, consisting of 2 parallel bands of sclerosis projected over the apophyseal joints.

Ligament ossifications are typical of late stages, and they involve the interspinal ligaments (dagger sign) and the iliolumbar ligaments.

Involvement of the craniocervical junction is uncommon. This point actually remains as the mobile point of cervical mobility if ankylosis affects the remainder of the cervical spine. In rare cases, the atlantoaxial ligament can be affected and in those cases there can be ventral subluxation of the atlas.[56]

In cases of PsA, features of involvement are similar, with destructive discovertebral lesions that resemble those of AS. Syndesmophytes

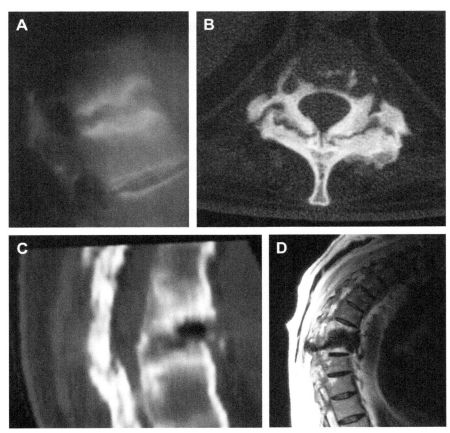

Fig. 12. Type III, or Andersson type B, lesions consist of extensive central and peripheral lesions. They represent a malunion or nonunion of an insufficiency fracture through the intervertebral disk, in the context of multisegmental ankylosis. They are typical of late stages of the disease and rare. When found, it is paramount to drive attention toward them given their severity. They usually occur in the thoracolumbar region. (*A*) Detail of a lateral view of the thoracic spine on a 76-year-old patient with known AS. Note the intense vertebral endplate destruction, which is the result of resorption, and surrounding sclerosis, resembling a pseudoarthrosis. (*B*) Axial CT images showing the fracture line and surrounding resoption and sclerosis. (*C*) Sagittal CT reconstruction. (*D*) Sagittal T2 spin-echo sequence on MR imaging shows intense sclerosis and loss of height of the vertebral bodies due to resorption. A hypointense transverse line of insufficiency fracture through the posterior columns is evident. (*Courtesy of* Dr Aparisi Rodriguez, Valencia, Spain.)

tend to be bulkier than those in AS and nonmarginal. Segmental involvement is more common in the upper lumbar spine (**Fig. 14**).[57]

In ReA, findings are again similar to those of AS. Romanus lesions and shiny corners can be seen but are rare. Asymmetric nonmarginal syndesmophytes are the most common (identical to the PsA ones). They tend to be bulky.[58]

The lower thoracic and upper lumbar segments are the commonly involved locations.

In cases of enteropathic arthritis, features and involvement are indistinguishable from AS.

Nonaxial Sites and Signs

Ankylosing spondylitis
The extra-axial manifestations of AS mainly involve the lower extremities in an asymmetric way.

The hips and knees are typically involved but also the shoulders.

Typical radiographic signs are periarticular demineralization, joint effusion, and diffuse joint narrowing. Erosions as such are seldom seen. In many patients, the only detectable changes are osteoarthritic changes due to premature degenerative disease resulting from the damage to the joint. Joint space narrowing combined with prominent osteophytosis is characteristic for hip disease on AS (**Fig. 15**).[59] Sometimes destruction can be prominent and at end stages ankylosis can also be found.

Involvement of small joints, in the hands and feet, is less common. Distribution tends to be asymmetric. Findings are typical for arthritis–demineralization, joint space narrowing, erosions, destruction, and soft tissue swelling. Ankylosis may appear soon after onset.

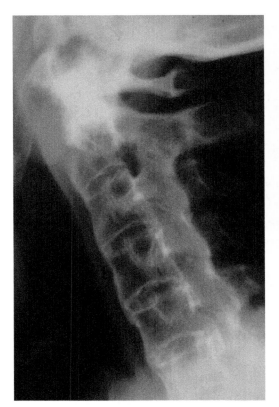

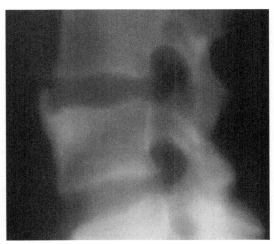

Fig. 14. In cases of PsA, features of involvement of the spine are similar to AS, with destructive discovertebral lesions. Syndesmophytes tend to be bulkier than the ones in AS and nonmarginal, as depicted in this detail of a lateral view of a lumbar spine. Segmental involvement is more common in the upper lumbar spine.

Fig. 13. Lateral view of the cervical spine. Changes in the apophyseal joints are mixed result of arthritis and enthesitis. In late stages there is extensive ossification over the dorsolateral aspect of the column, recognizable on the lateral projection. Note as well the typical characteristics of a bamboo spine in the anterior aspect of the vertebral bodies.

Enthesitis is the most characteristic sign of seronegative arthropathies. This consists of inflammatory affection of the ligamentous, tendinous, and capsular insertions.

Typically involved sites are the ischiatic tuberosities, trochanter, plantar calcaneal surface, triceps insertion, and patella but eventually any insertion could be affected.

Radiographically, an erosion with ill-defined margins is demonstrated, which forms a small groove. Subsequently, there is formation of new bone in the groove and surroundings. Eventually, this process relapses and there is a combination of erosion and proliferation of bone at the same time.

Other locations for inflammatory change are the symphysis pubis and manubriosternal sinchondrosis, with erosions, sclerosis, and soft tissue swelling.

Bursitis is another manifestation, anterior to the Achilles tendon insertion or at the trochanteric and ilipsoas bursae; for example, pressure erosions of

the bone, inflammatory destruction, and new bone formation can be seen associated with it.

Finally, but not less important, the incidence of osteoporosis in patients with AS is high.[60,61] Prevalence increases with age and duration of the disease and vertebral and peripheral involvement, mainly involving the spine, and predisposing to

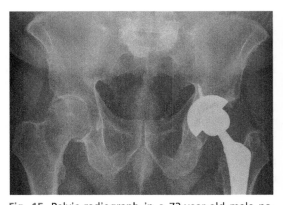

Fig. 15. Pelvic radiograph in a 73-year-old male patient with known AS, complaining of progression of right hip pain. Typical radiographic signs for AS involvement of the hip are periarticular demineralization, joint effusion, and diffuse joint narrowing. Erosions as such are only seldom seen. In many patients, the only detectable changes are osteoarthritic changes due to premature degenerative disease resulting from the damage to the joint. Joint space narrowing combined with prominent osteophytosis is characteristic for hip disease on AS. Note the complete ankylosis of the sacroiliac joints.

vertebral compression fractures and transdiscal insufficiency fractures. Bone mineral density should be monitored in these patients.

Psoriatic arthritis

Involvement of peripheral skeleton joints in PsA normally affects the distal interphalangeal joints of the hands and feet. Lesions tend to be asymmetric with an oligoarticular distribution, progressing to polyarticular distribution. There is a slight predilection for the great toe.

Vertical or horizontal patterns of affectation can be described in the digits; vertical involves all joints in 1 digit and horizontal translates affectation of all distal joints in a hand or foot (Fig. 16).

Large joints are involved in fewer than 10% of cases.

In cases of suspicion of PsA, examinations should include views of both hands and feet and lower thoracic spine, lumbar spine (and eventually other symptomatic sites) in 2 projections.

Early changes, which are often difficult to detect, consist of speculated or woolly foci of epiphyseal ossification on the distal phalanges (in the tuft), acro-osteolysis, and layered periosteal ossifications on the shafts of the tubular bones.

These changes are followed by the typical bone destruction–bone proliferation sequence of the seronegative arthritis, with irregularity of the joint lines, erosions, destruction of bone, specular ossifications at joint margins (especially at the bases of the distal phalanges), and eventually ankylosis. Insufficiency stress fractures are also possible (Fig. 17).

Enthesitis is also a feature of PsA, as it is of all seronegative spondyloarthritides. In this respect, as a typical feature, massive soft tissue swelling of the extra-articular soft tissues of a digit is called dactylitis (also described as sausage digits).[13]

Reactive arthritis

Peripheral skeleton joint involvement in ReA typically involves the lower extremities, in an asymmetric pattern.

Changes on radiographs are typically found in seronegative arthropathies, with marginal erosions and fluffy periosteal reaction, new bone formation, narrowing of the joint space, joint effusions, and soft tissue swelling. Ankylosis is also seen in late stages.

The forefoot is a common location. In particular, the first metatarsophalangeal joint is frequently involved.

Ankylosis may occur but is less common than it is in the hand in PsA.

If the knee is affected, the most common manifestation is a joint effusion.

The involvement of the upper extremities is at all similar to that in PsA, with dactylitis a common feature as well.

Enthesitis is one of the most frequent manifestations of ReA. The calcaneus is a common site of involvement, with erosion and formation of plantar or posterosuperior calcaneal spurs related to the insertions of the plantar fascia and Achilles tendon (Fig. 18).

A **B**

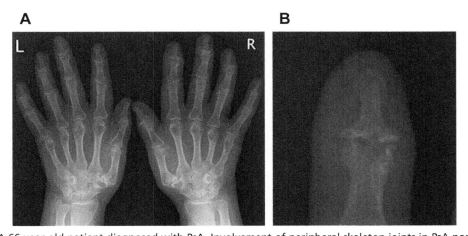

Fig. 16. A 66-year-old patient diagnosed with PsA. Involvement of peripheral skeleton joints in PsA normally affects the distal interphalangeal joints of the hands and feet. Lesions tend to be asymmetric with an oligoarticular distribution, progressing to polyarticular distribution (polyarticular involvement in this case). (A) Hands AP projection. Note the irregularity of the joint lines, erosions, destruction of bone, and specular ossifications at joint margins, especially at the bases of the distal phalanges, in this case seen more prominently in the distal interphalangeal joint (DIP) of the index finger of the right hand and fourth and fifth fingers of the left hand. (B) Detail of the DIP of the second finger of the right hand. Osteoarthritic changes are present in the trapezo-metacarpal joints bilaterally as well as in the proximal interphalangeal joint of the left index.

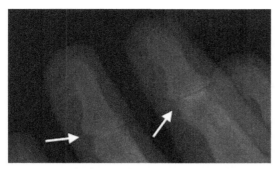

Fig. 17. Detail of early changes on PsA, with peripheral erosions, especially at the bases of the distal phalanges (*white arrows*).

Enteropathic arthritis

Typically arthritis involves lower extremities in asymmetric pattern.

Enthesitis is less common and dactylitis infrequent.

FROM QUALITATIVE DIAGNOSIS TO QUANTITATIVE EVALUATION
Axial Spondyloarthritis

Diagnosis of axSpA is based on the ASAS classification criteria (see **Box 1**).

Imaging is a key component of the criteria, in part due to the lack of specific clinical symptoms

as well as the variation of the disease activity over time.[33] Radiographic sacroiliitis is a crucial part of the modified New York criteria for diagnosis of AS (see **Box 3**).

As discussed previously, plain radiography is the recommended method for diagnosis and classification of SpA. Radiographic changes are a late development, however, and, therefore, sensitivity is limited in early stages of the disease.

Different methods have been described for scoring abnormalities in the spine.

Bath Ankylosing Spondylitis Radiology Index

The Bath Ankylosing Spondylitis Radiology Index (BASRI) consists of a global grading of the lateral cervical spine, the AP and lateral lumbar spine combined, and the SIJs.

Each site can be scored from 0 (normal) to 4 (severe disease in cases of SI, fusion involving at least 3 vertebrae in cases of the spine). The sum of sites gives the BASRI–Spine, which ranges from 0 to 12.[62]

A similar 0 to 4 grading is described for the hips.[63] This is added to the spine score to result in the BASRI total score, with a maximum score of 16 (scores are summarized in **Table 3**).

The system presents the problem of ceiling effects (changes cannot be measured above a certain level) and poor reproducibility and poor sensitivity to change with only 20% of cases demonstrating change over a period of 2 years.[64]

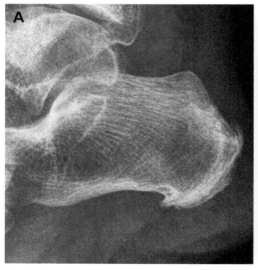
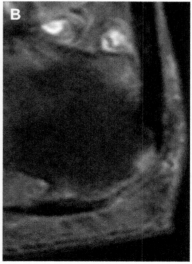

Fig. 18. Enthesitis is one of the most frequent manifestations of ReA. The calcaneus is a common site of involvement, with erosion and formation of plantar or posterosuperior calcaneal spurs related to the insertions of the plantar fascia and Achilles tendon. (*A*) Detail of a lateral radiograph of the left foot of a 47-year-old male patient diagnosed with ReA. Note the secondary spurs in the insertions of the plantar fascia and Achilles tendon. (*B*) Detail of sagittal proton density–weighted spectral attenuated inversion recovery of the MR imaging from the same patient. Note the increased signal intensity in the insertion of the Achilles tendon and plantar fascia, in keeping with bone marrow edema. There is also a small pre-Achilles bursitis.

Table 3
Bath Akylosing Spondylitis Radiology Index

Score	Grade	Lumbar and Cervical Spine Changes
0	Normal	No change
1	Suspicious	No definite change
2	Mild	Any number of erosions, squaring or sclerosis ± syndesmophytes on ≤2 vertebrae
3	Moderate	Syndesmophytes on ≥3 vertebrae ± fusion involving 2 vertebrae
4	Severe	Fusion involving ≥3 vertebrae

Score	Sacroiliac Joint Changes
0	No disease
1	Suspicious for disease
2	Minimal disease
3	Moderate disease
4	Severe disease

Score	Hip Changes
0	No disease
1	Suspicious for disease
2	Minimal disease
3	Moderate disease
4	Severe disease

Data from MacKay K, Mack C, Brophy S, et al. The Bath Ankylosing Spondylitis Radiology Index (BASRI): a new, validated approach to disease assessment. Arthritis Rheum 1998;41(12):2263–70.

Stoke Ankylosing Spondylitis Spine Score

The Stoke Ankylosing Spondylitis Spine Score (SASSS) is obtained on lateral views of the lumbar spine (from the inferior endplate of T12 to superior endplate of S1 inclusive), to assess abnormalities in the anterior and posterior corners of each vertebra. This scoring system does not include the cervical or the thoracic spine.[65]

Each corner is scored for the presence of no abnormality (0), squaring (1), sclerosis (1), erosions (1), syndesmophytes (2), and bridging syndesmophytes (3).

This scoring system also has low sensitivity to change.[64]

Modified Stoke Ankylosing Spondylitis Spine Score

In the Modified SASSS (mSASSS) scoring method, the cervical spine is also assessed, (from inferior endplate of C2 to superior endplate of T1 inclusive) in combination with the lumbar spine (lateral views). The total of sites assessed is 24.[66]

The thoracic spine is not assessed, even though it is frequently affected, due to the frequent superimposition of structures in the lateral view.

The scoring system is the same as the one used on SASSS.

Each total number of particular scores is multiplied by 1, 2, or 3, respectively, and the results added, for a grand total that ranges between 0 and 72.

Progression is defined as "change greater than 0" in a 2-year interval follow-up.[67]

Berlin X-Ray score

The Berlin X-ray score method is based on AP and lateral views, in this case including the cervical, thoracic, and lumbar segments, and focuses on changes in the vertebral units, defined as the region between 2 virtual lines drawn through the middle of each vertebra. The method was developed in analogy to the T1-weighted MR imaging score, the Ankylosing Spondylitis Spine MRI score for chronic changes (ASspiMRI-c).[68]

A total of 21 vertebral units are scored by a value between 0 and 6, with grade 0 normal, 1 suspicious, 2 minor erosion and or squared vertebrae, grade 3 small single syndesmophytes and or more severe erosions, grade 4 two or more syndesmophytes or SpA/spondylodiscitis, and grade 5 vertebral bridging and 6 fusion.

The total score is 126. This scoring system has the particularity of its analogy with the

ASspiMRI-c scoring system, which makes findings in both scoring systems easily comparable.

Radiographic ankylosing spondylitis spine score

The radiographic AS spine score (RASSS) method is similar to the mSASSS, with the addition of assessment of the thoracic spine in lateral views.[69]

In the recent EULAR recommendations for the use of imaging in the diagnosis and management of SpA in clinical practice,[33] a comprehensive review of 6 different studies[67–72] comparing these 5 radiographic scoring methods was carried out. Of these 6 studies reviewed, 2 reported mSASSS superior to BASRI and SASSS.[67,72] RASSS was reported as superior to mSASSS in 1 study,[69] whereas another did not find advantage of 1 over another.[71]

Currently, mSASSS seems to be the most widely used system of scoring in clinical trials.

Peripheral Spondyloarthritis

When pSpA is suspected, ultrasound (US) or MR imaging is recommended for initial assessment of enthesitis, arthritis, tenosynovitis, or bursitis.[33] The role of radiography in this case is mainly focused on follow-up of structural changes, with the possibility of obtaining additional information from US or MR imaging if needed.

Several scoring methods have been described to monitor structural changes in PsA, all of them having their basis in scoring methods for rheumatoid arthritis.

Modified Steinbrocker Method

The modified Steinbrocker method scores according to the worst joint. Each joint is scored on a scale of 0 to 4: 0 representing normal, 1 juxta-articular osteopenia or soft tissue swelling, 2 presence of erosions, 3 presence of erosion and joint space narrowing, and 4 total destruction (osteolysis, ankylosis). This scoring system includes all the joints of the hand (considering the wrist as 1 joint), the metatarsophalangeal joints, and the interphalangeal joint of the great toe (40 joints in total). The score range is 0 to 160.[73]

Psoriatic arthritis Ratingen score

The PsA Ratingen score method also includes 40 joints of the hands and feet. Each joint is scored separately for destruction and proliferation. Destruction score ranges from 0 to 5 and proliferation score ranges from 0 to 4. The total destruction score ranges from 0 to 200 and the proliferation score from 0 to 160. Both are added to give a total score[74] (Table 4).

Psoriatic arthritis scoring method based on Sharp scoring method for rheumatoid arthritis

The PsA scoring method based on Sharp scoring method for rheumatoid arthritis scale assesses erosion and joint space narrowing separately. Assessment for erosion is applied to 21 joints in each hand (total score ranging from 0 to 210) and 6 on joints on each foot (total score ranging 0–60) and narrowing of the joint space to 20 joints in each hand (range 0–160) and 5 joints in each foot (range 0–40). The scale was expanded to include the scores of 6 and 7 in

Table 4
Psoriatic arthritis Ratingen score

Psoriatic Arthritis Ratingen Score Scale	Destruction	Proliferation
0	Normal	Normal
1	≥1 definite erosions with interruption of the cortical plate >1 mm but <10% of joint surface destroyed	Proliferation of 1–2 mm measured from original bone surface not exceeding 25% or the original diameter
2	Destruction of 11%–25% of joint surface	Proliferation of 2–3 mm or bone growth of 25%–50%
3	Destruction of 25%–50% joint surface	Proliferation of >3 mm or bone growth of >50%
4	Destruction of 51%–75% joint surface	Ankylosis
5	Destruction >75% joint surface	—

Data from Wassenberg S, Fischer-Kahle V, Herborn G, et al. A method to score radiographic change in psoriatic arthritis. Z Rheumatol 2001;60(3):156–66.

bone erosion/destruction, given the more extensive bone destruction that can be seen in PsA, and the score of 5 in joint space narrowing, which actually consists of widening due to extensive osteolysis. These added scores are not added directly but noted separately (**Table 5**).[75]

Sharp–van der Heijde–Modified Scoring Method for Psoriatic Arthritis

The Sharp–van der Heijde (SVH)–Modified Scoring Method for Psoriatic Arthritis is similar to the system described for rheumatoid arthritis. The same joints are assessed for erosions and joint space narrowing, with the addition of the 8 distal interphalangeal joints of the hands for both variables and the interphalangeal of the thumbs for the assessment of joints space narrowing. The grand total, given more joints are assessed, is, therefore, higher than in this same method used for rheumatoid arthritis. Again, gross osteolysis is scored separately. This method, applied to rheumatoid arthritis, has proved of great precision and sensitivity to change and is the most widely used in clinical trials (**Table 6**).[64,75]

RADIOLOGIC FINDINGS IN PARALLEL AND FUTURE PERSPECTIVES

Imaging modalities other than conventional radiology are not generally recommended in the initial diagnosis of ax SpA.

MR imaging can be used as second-line examination in cases of high clinical suspicion but no radiographic evidence of sacroiliitis and as an alternative first imaging method in young patients and in patients with short symptom duration.[33]

MR imaging is a highly sensitive method to detect bone marrow edema, which is a nonspecific sign on itself but associated with the presence of inflammatory change. On this basis, it is recommended as a tool to monitor disease activity in axSpA, in combination with clinical and biochemical assessments. Conventional radiography should still be used in long-term monitoring of established structural changes (in particular new bone formation) at SIJ and/or spine in patients with axSpA, given it has been shown superior to MR imaging in the detection of spinal syndesmophytes at cervical and lumbar spine (which are predictive of outcome/severity in patients with AS[4,33]).

The prediction of good response to anti–TNF-α treatment in axSpA, particularly in patients with AS, is based on the extension of inflammatory change on MR imaging. In this respect, MR imaging can be used as well as a tool to help in the decision of initiation of treatment, in addiction to clinical and biochemical findings.

MR imaging is also a first-line imaging method in the diagnosis of pSpA, able to demonstrate enthesitis (most common manifestation) arthritis, tenosynovitis, or bursitis. In this regard, the strength of the recommendation based on EULAR criteria equals that of the use of ultrasound; both techniques allow for good assessment of the soft tissues.

Table 5
Psoriatic arthritis scoring method based on the Sharp scoring method for rheumatoid arthritis

Sharp Psoriatic Arthritis Scale	Erosion	Joint Space Narrowing
0	No erosion	Normal
1	1 discrete erosion or <21% joint area affected	Asymmetric and/or minimal
2	2 discrete erosions or 21%–40% joint area affected	Definite narrowing with loss up to 50% of joint space
3	3 discrete erosions or 41%–60% joint area affected	Definite narrowing with loss 51%–99% of joint space or subluxation
4	4 discrete erosions or 61%–80% joint area affected	Absence of joint space ankylosis
5	Extensive destruction involving >80% of the joint	Widening of the joint due to extensive osteolysis
6–7	Extensive destruction, such as ostelysis or pencil-in-cup	—

Data from van der Heijde D. Quantification of radiological damage in inflammatory arthritis: rheumatoid arthritis, psoriatic arthritis and ankylosing spondylitis. Best Pract Res Clin Rheumatol 2004;18(6):847–60.

Table 6
Sharp–van der Heijde–Modified Scoring Method for Psoriatic Arthritis

Sharp–van der Heijde Scale for Psoriatic Arthritis	Erosion	Joint Space Narrowing
0	Normal	Normal
1	Discrete erosion	Asymmetric or minimal narrowing up to 25% of the joint space
2	Large erosion not passing midline	Definite narrowing with loss of up to 50% of the joint space
3	Large erosion passing midline	Definite narrowing with loss of 50%–99% of the joint space or subluxation
4	—	Absence of joint space (ankylosis or complete subluxation)

Data from van der Heijde D. Quantification of radiological damage in inflammatory arthritis: rheumatoid arthritis, psoriatic arthritis and ankylosing spondylitis. Best Pract Res Clin Rheumatol 2004;18(6):847–60.

MR imaging and US indistinctly are also first-line methods for the follow-up of disease activity, in conjunction with clinical and biochemical markers. Normally, the follow-up periods are tailored to clinical circumstances. US with high frequency color or power Doppler is sufficient to detect inflammation and widely used as an activity monitorization tool. When it comes to structural changes in pSpA, conventional radiography is still the method of choice, with eventual consideration of US as a complementary assessment.

The use of CT as a first-line tool for diagnosis is rare, given the wide availability of MR imaging. CT has an excellent spatial resolution and allows for complete assessment of the SIJ, implying that structural damage in the SIJ could be probably best recognized with CT; however, sensitivity of conventional radiography and the added information on inflammatory activity that MR imaging provides, added to the high dose of ionizing radiation, make this technique unsuitable as a first-line diagnosis method or a method to evaluate progression of the disease over time.[46] CT may be able to provide additional information if conventional radiography is negative and MR imaging cannot be performed.

CT is, however, invaluable in the assessment of vertebral fractures. If a vertebral fracture is suspected and conventional radiography is negative, CT should be performed.[33] CT allows for 3-D reconstruction, making it extremely useful for surgical planning (**Fig. 19**).

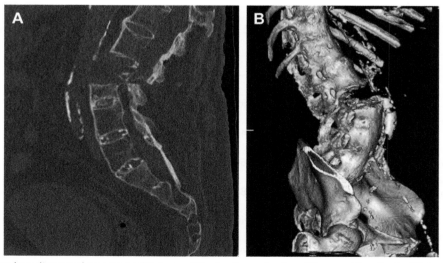

Fig. 19. Complete distracted transverse fracture of the lumbar spine in a 63-year-old patient with known AS. (*A*) Sagittal CT reconstructions, demonstrating small bone fragments in the neural canal. (*B*) 3-D reconstruction. (*Courtesy of* Dr Aparisi Rodriguez, Valencia, Spain.)

Nuclear medicine studies, such as scintigraphy, were frequently used in the past decades. The specificity of a positive test for early arthritis in patients with HLA-B27 and inflammatory back pain was considered acceptable.[56] Progressively, the use of CT and MR imaging have relegated the use of nuclear medicine studies. MR imaging is as sensitive and more specific.

The scintigraphic technique has developed as well into single-photon emission CT, and this is useful in revealing inflammatory foci in the spine; however, in clinical practice, MR imaging is more widely available. Nuclear medicine techniques are still useful to show inflammatory foci and direct more-specific studies.

Incidence of osteoporosis in patients with axSpA is high.[60,61] Regular assessment should be performed with hip and AP spine dual-energy X-ray absorptiometry (DXA); however, sometimes these patients present a challenge for spine DXA assessment, due to the presence of syndesmophytes, sclerosis, and the added involvement of the apophyseal joints. Alternatives if this is the case are the use of DXA in the hip and extrapolation (useful if there is no significant involvement of the hip) supplemented by either spine DXA in the lateral projection or quantitative CT, especially in cases of severe vertebral and hip involvement present.

SUMMARY

Changes related to ax-SpA and pSpA can be differentiated into active inflammation, structural osteodestructive changes (erosions), and structural hyperproliferative changes, such as enthesophytes, vertebral squaring, disk calcifications, spondylophytes, syndesmophytes, bony bridging, and finally ankylosis.

Sacroiliitis represents the most characteristic feature of spondyloarthritides; in the absence of sacroiliitis, the involvement of other sites of both axial and appendicular skeleton is unusual. Diagnosis of sacroiliitis is, therefore, a key criterion in the diagnosis of these diseases.

Although many imaging modalities are currently available, plain radiography remains the first line and the mainstay of radiologic investigation of SpA, playing a first-line role in the diagnosis, according to the ASAS and EULAR recommendations. Plain radiography is both sensitive and specific for diagnosis of established disease, able to detect structural changes that are the consequences of the inflammatory process.

Early sacroiliitis is often difficult to identify and, because the progression of radiographic damage is generally slow, there can be a significant delay between the onset of the first symptoms and the diagnosis. The identification of early sacroiliitis has improved dramatically with the use of MR imaging technique that is able to detect the inflammatory changes that precede osteodestructive changes in patients that show no evidence of abnormalities on conventional radiography.

To cover the entire spectrum of the disease, the new concept of nr-axSpA was introduced in 2009. This group includes patients without signs of sacroiliitis on conventional radiographs but who satisfy clinical criteria for diagnosis for axSpA as well as patients with active inflammation in the SIJ detected by MR imaging. Nr-axSpA can be considered an early stage of axSpA, with progression reported in approximately 10% of cases over 2 years. It is still unclear, however, what the predisposing factors are of the subgroup of patients who end up developing radiographic signs of sacroiliitis.

Radiography has been shown superior to MR imaging in the detection of spinal syndesmophytes at cervical and lumbar spine, which are predictive of outcome/severity in patients with AS. Conventional radiography remains the first line of imaging investigation to monitor structural changes once a diagnosis of axSpA or pSpA has been achieved.

Multiple scoring systems based on radiographic assessment are available for axial and peripheral structural changes.

The most widely used scoring system in clinical trials for axSpA is the mSASSS, and the most widely used scoring system for pSpA is the SvH–Modified Scoring Method for Psoriatic Arthritis.

Conventional radiography remains as well as the first-line imaging examination if a vertebral fracture is suspected in patients with diagnosed axSpA.

The adequate training of a radiologist in the recognition of early changes, grading of lesions, and evaluation of progress of structural changes has a clear impact on the management of the condition and, therefore, influences the outcome of the disease in these patients.

REFERENCES

1. Dougados M, van der Linden S, Juhlin R, et al. The European Spondylarthropathy Study Group preliminary criteria for the classification of spondylarthropathy. Arthritis Rheum 1991;34(10):1218–27.
2. van Tubergen A, Weber U. Diagnosis and classification in spondyloarthritis: identifying a chameleon. Nat Rev Rheumatol 2012;8(5):253–61.
3. Rudwaleit M. New approaches to diagnosis and classification of axial and peripheral spondyloarthritis. Curr Opin Rheumatol 2010;22(4):375–80.
4. Eshed I, Hermann KG. Novel imaging modalities in spondyloarthritis. Curr Opin Rheumatol 2015;27(4): 333–42.

5. Rudwaleit M, Sieper J. Referral strategies for early diagnosis of axial spondyloarthritis. Nat Rev Rheumatol 2012;8(5):262–8.

6. Braun J, Sieper J. Early diagnosis of spondyloarthritis. Nat Clin Pract Rheumatol 2006;2(10):536–45.

7. Braun J, Sieper J. Ankylosing spondylitis. Lancet 2007;369(9570):1379–90.

8. Van der Linden S, van der Heijde D. Ankylosing spondylitis. Clinical features. Rheum Dis Clin North Am 1998;24(4):663–76, vii.

9. Amrami KK. Imaging of the seronegative spondyloarthopathies. Radiol Clin North Am 2012;50(4): 841–54.

10. Mielants H, Veys EM, Goemaere S, et al. A prospective study of patients with spondyloarthropathy with special reference to HLA-B27 and to gut histology. J Rheumatol 1993;20(8):1353–8.

11. Khan MA. Immunogenetics of ankylosing spondylitis: clinically oriented aspects. Clin Exp Rheumatol 1987;5(Suppl 1):S49–52.

12. Anandarajah AP, Ritchlin CT. Pathogenesis of psoriatic arthritis. Curr Opin Rheumatol 2004;16(4): 338–43.

13. Olivieri I, Barozzi L, Favaro L, et al. Dactylitis in patients with seronegative spondylarthropathy. Assessment by ultrasonography and magnetic resonance imaging. Arthritis Rheum 1996;39(9):1524–8.

14. Jablonka K, Freyschmidt J. Psoriatic arthritis and psoriatic spondyloarthritis. In: Pope TL, Bloem HL, Beltran J, et al, editors. Imaging of the musculoskeletal system. Philadelphia: Saunders Elsevier; 2008. p. 1113–9.

15. Amor B. Reiter's syndrome. Diagnosis and clinical features. Rheum Dis Clin North Am 1998;24(4): 677–95.

16. Nissman D, Pope TL. Reactive arthritis. In: Pope TL, Bloem HL, Beltran J, et al, editors. Imaging of the musculoskeletal system. Philadelphia: Saunders Elsevier; 2008. p. 1120–30.

17. Kataria RK, Brent LH. Spondyloarthrotpathies. Am Fam Physician 2004;69(12):2853–60.

18. De Keyser F, Elewaut D, De Vos M, et al. Bowel inflammation and the spondyloarthropathies. Rheum Dis Clin North Am 1998;24(4):785–813. ix-x.

19. Fianyo E, Wendling D, Poulain C, et al. Non-radiographic axial spondyloarthritis: what is it? Clin Exp Rheumatol 2014;32(1):1–4.

20. Sieper J, Rudwaleit M, Baraliakos X, et al. The Assessment of SpondyloArthritis international Society (ASAS) handbook: a guide to assess spondyloarthritis. Ann Rheum Dis 2009;68(Suppl 2):ii1–44.

21. Rudwaleit M, Landewe R, van der Heijde D, et al. The development of Assessment of SpondyloArthritis international Society classification criteria for axial spondyloarthritis (part I): classification of paper patients by expert opinion including uncertainty appraisal. Ann Rheum Dis 2009;68(6):770–6.

22. Rudwaleit M, van der Heijde D, Landewe R, et al. The development of Assessment of SpondyloArthritis international Society classification criteria for axial spondyloarthritis (part II): validation and final selection. Ann Rheum Dis 2009;68(6):777–83.

23. Boonen A, Sieper J, van der Heijde D, et al. The burden of non-radiographic axial spondyloarthritis. Semin Arthritis Rheum 2015;44(5):556–62.

24. Baraliakos X, Braun J. Non-radiographic axial spondyloarthritis and ankylosing spondylitis: what are the similarities and differences? RMD open 2015; 1(Suppl 1):e000053.

25. Rudwaleit M, Haibel H, Baraliakos X, et al. The early disease stage in axial spondylarthritis: results from the German Spondyloarthritis Inception Cohort. Arthritis Rheum 2009;60(3):717–27.

26. Sampaio-Barros PD, Bortoluzzo AB, Conde RA, et al. Undifferentiated spondyloarthritis: a longterm followup. J Rheumatol 2010;37(6):1195–9.

27. Poddubnyy D, Rudwaleit M, Haibel H, et al. Rates and predictors of radiographic sacroiliitis progression over 2 years in patients with axial spondyloarthritis. Ann Rheum Dis 2011;70(8):1369–74.

28. Molto A, Paternotte S, van der Heijde D, et al. Evaluation of the validity of the different arms of the ASAS set of criteria for axial spondyloarthritis and description of the different imaging abnormalities suggestive of spondyloarthritis: data from the DESIR cohort. Ann Rheum Dis 2015;74(4):746–51.

29. Sieper J, van der Heijde D. Review: Nonradiographic axial spondyloarthritis: new definition of an old disease? Arthritis Rheum 2013;65(3):543–51.

30. Kiltz U, Baraliakos X, Karakostas P, et al. Do patients with non-radiographic axial spondylarthritis differ from patients with ankylosing spondylitis? Arthritis Care Res 2012;64(9):1415–22.

31. Sieper J, Rao SA, Chen N, et al. FRI0286 Burden of the disease in axial spondyloarthritis. Ann Rheum Dis 2013;71(Suppl 3):410–1.

32. Ciurea A, Scherer A, Exer P, et al. Tumor necrosis factor alpha inhibition in radiographic and nonradiographic axial spondyloarthritis: results from a large observational cohort. Arthritis Rheum 2013;65(12): 3096–106.

33. Mandl P, Navarro-Compan V, Terslev L, et al. EULAR recommendations for the use of imaging in the diagnosis and management of spondyloarthritis in clinical practice. Ann Rheum Dis 2015;74(7): 1327–39.

34. Navallas M, Ares J, Beltran B, et al. Sacroiliitis associated with axial spondyloarthropathy: new concepts and latest trends. Radiographics 2013;33(4): 933–56.

35. Klauser A, Bollow M, Calin A, et al. Workshop report: clinical diagnosis and imaging of sacroiliitis, Innsbruck, Austria, October 9, 2003. J Rheumatol 2004;31(10):2041–7.

36. Puhakka KB, Melsen F, Jurik AG, et al. MR imaging of the normal sacroiliac joint with correlation to histology. Skeletal Radiol 2004;33(1):15–28.
37. Vleeming A, Schuenke MD, Masi AT, et al. The sacroiliac joint: an overview of its anatomy, function and potential clinical implications. J Anat 2012; 221(6):537–67.
38. Egund N, Jurik AG. Anatomy and histology of the sacroiliac joints. Semin Musculoskelet Radiol 2014; 18(3):332–9.
39. Hermann KG, Althoff CE, Schneider U, et al. Spinal changes in patients with spondyloarthritis: comparison of MR imaging and radiographic appearances. Radiographics 2005;25(3):559–69 [discussion: 69–70].
40. Luong AA, Salonen DC. Imaging of the seronegative spondyloarthropathies. Curr Rheumatol Rep 2000; 2(4):288–96.
41. McLauchlan GJ, Gardner DL. Sacral and iliac articular cartilage thickness and cellularity: relationship to subchondral bone end-plate thickness and cancellous bone density. Rheumatology (Oxford) 2002;41(4):375–80.
42. Doran MF, Brophy S, MacKay K, et al. Predictors of longterm outcome in ankylosing spondylitis. J Rheumatol 2003;30(2):316–20.
43. Brophy S, Mackay K, Al-Saidi A, et al. The natural history of ankylosing spondylitis as defined by radiological progression. J Rheumatol 2002;29(6): 1236–43.
44. Jang JH, Ward MM, Rucker AN, et al. Ankylosing spondylitis: patterns of radiographic involvement–a re-examination of accepted principles in a cohort of 769 patients. Radiology 2011;258(1):192–8.
45. van der Linden S, Valkenburg HA, Cats A. Evaluation of diagnostic criteria for ankylosing spondylitis. A proposal for modification of the New York criteria. Arthritis Rheum 1984;27(4):361–8.
46. Poddubnyy D, Sieper J. Radiographic progression in ankylosing spondylitis/axial spondyloarthritis: how fast and how clinically meaningful? Curr Opin Rheumatol 2012;24(4):363–9.
47. Feldtkeller E, Khan MA, van der Heijde D, et al. Age at disease onset and diagnosis delay in HLA-B27 negative vs. positive patients with ankylosing spondylitis. Rheumatol Int 2003;23(2):61–6.
48. Braun J, Bollow M, Eggens U, et al. Use of dynamic magnetic resonance imaging with fast imaging in the detection of early and advanced sacroiliitis in spondylarthropathy patients. Arthritis Rheum 1994; 37(7):1039–45.
49. Gaucher AA, Pere PG, Gillet PM. From ankylosing spondylitis to Forestier's disease: ossifying enthesopathy, a unifying concept. J Rheumatol 1990; 17(6):854–6.
50. Calin A. Radiology and spondylarthritis. Baillieres Clin Rheumatol 1996;10(3):455–76.
51. Dihlmann W. Current radiodiagnostic concept of ankylosing spondylitis. Skeletal Radiol 1979;4(4): 179–88.
52. Ostergaard M, Lambert RG. Imaging in ankylosing spondylitis. Ther Adv Musculoskelet Dis 2012;4(4): 301–11.
53. Cawley MI, Chalmers TM, Kellgren JH, et al. Destructive lesions of vertebral bodies in ankylosing spondylitis. Ann Rheum Dis 1972;31(5):345–58.
54. Cammisa M, De Serio A, Guglielmi G. Diffuse idiopathic skeletal hyperostosis. Eur J Radiol 1998; 27(Suppl 1):S7–11.
55. Bron JL, de Vries MK, Snieders MN, et al. Discovertebral (Andersson) lesions of the spine in ankylosing spondylitis revisited. Clin Rheumatol 2009;28(8): 883–92.
56. Schorn C, Lingg G. Ankylosing spondylitis. In: Pope TL, Bloem HL, Beltran J, et al, editors. Imaging of the musculoskeletal system. Philadelphia: Saunders Elsevier; 2008. p. 1120–30.
57. Gladman DD. Current concepts in psoriatic arthritis. Curr Opin Rheumatol 2002;14(4):361–6.
58. Gladman D. Spondyloarthropaties. In: Lahita R, Weinstein A, editors. Educational review manual on rheumatology. 2nd edition. New York: Castle Conolly Graduate Medica; 2002. p. 1–26. Review.
59. Resnick D, Niwayama G. Ankylosing spondylitis. In: Resnick D, Niwayama G, editors. Diagnosis of joint and bone disorders. 2nd edition. Philadelphia: WB Saunders; 1988. p. 1103–70.
60. Mitra D, Elvins DM, Speden DJ, et al. The prevalence of vertebral fractures in mild ankylosing spondylitis and their relationship to bone mineral density. Rheumatology (Oxford) 2000;39(1):85–9.
61. Bessant R, Keat A. How should clinicians manage osteoporosis in ankylosing spondylitis? J Rheumatol 2002;29(7):1511–9.
62. MacKay K, Mack C, Brophy S, et al. The Bath Ankylosing Spondylitis Radiology Index (BASRI): a new, validated approach to disease assessment. Arthritis Rheum 1998;41(12):2263–70.
63. MacKay K, Brophy S, Mack C, et al. The development and validation of a radiographic grading system for the hip in ankylosing spondylitis: the bath ankylosing spondylitis radiology hip index. J Rheumatol 2000;27(12):2866–72.
64. Carmona R. Appendix: imaging scoring methods in arthritis. In: O'Neill J, editor. Essential imaging in rheumatology. New York: Springer; 2014. p. 397–405.
65. Averns HL, Oxtoby J, Taylor HG, et al. Radiological outcome in ankylosing spondylitis: use of the Stoke Ankylosing Spondylitis Spine Score (SASSS). Br J Rheumatol 1996;35(4):373–6.
66. Creemers MC, Franssen MJ, van't Hof MA, et al. Assessment of outcome in ankylosing spondylitis: an extended radiographic scoring system. Ann Rheum Dis 2005;64(1):127–9.

67. Wanders AJ, Landewé RB, Spoorenberg A, et al. What is the most appropriate radiologic scoring method for ankylosing spondylitis? A comparison of the available methods based on the Outcome Measures in Rheumatology Clinical Trials filter. Arthritis Rheum 2004;50(8):2622–32.

68. Braun J, Baraliakos X, Golder W, et al. Analysing chronic spinal changes in ankylosing spondylitis: a systematic comparison of conventional x rays with magnetic resonance imaging using established and new scoring systems. Ann Rheum Dis 2004; 63(9):1046–55.

69. Baraliakos X, Listing J, Rudwaleit M, et al. Development of a radiographic scoring tool for ankylosing spondylitis only based on bone formation: addition of the thoracic spine improves sensitivity to change. Arthritis Rheum 2009;61(6):764–71.

70. Lubrano E, Marchesoni A, Olivieri I, et al. The radiological assessment of axial involvement in psoriatic arthritis: a validation study of the BASRI total and the modified SASSS scoring methods. Clin Exp Rheumatol 2009;27(6):977–80.

71. Ramiro S, van Tubergen A, Stolwijk C, et al. Scoring radiographic progression in ankylosing spondylitis: should we use the modified Stoke Ankylosing Spondylitis Spine Score (mSASSS) or the Radiographic Ankylosing Spondylitis Spinal Score (RASSS)? Arthritis Res Ther 2013;15(1):R14.

72. Salaffi F, Carotti M, Garofalo G, et al. Radiological scoring methods for ankylosing spondylitis: a comparison between the Bath Ankylosing Spondylitis Radiology Index and the modified Stoke Ankylosing Spondylitis Spine Score. Clin Exp Rheumatol 2007; 25(1):67–74.

73. Rahman P, Gladman DD, Cook RJ, et al. Radiological assessment in psoriatic arthritis. Br J Rheumatol 1998;37(7):760–5.

74. Wassenberg S, Fischer-Kahle V, Herborn G, et al. A method to score radiographic change in psoriatic arthritis. Z Rheumatol 2001;60(3):156–66.

75. van der Heijde D. Quantification of radiological damage in inflammatory arthritis: rheumatoid arthritis, psoriatic arthritis and ankylosing spondylitis. Best Pract Res Clin Rheumatol 2004;18(6):847–60.

Conventional Radiology in Crystal Arthritis
Gout, Calcium Pyrophosphate Deposition, and Basic Calcium Phosphate Crystals

Thibaut Jacques, MD, MSc[a,b,*], Paul Michelin, MD[c],
Sammy Badr, MD, MSc[a,b], Michelangelo Nasuto, MD[d],
Guillaume Lefebvre, MD[a,b], Neal Larkman, MD, MPH[e],
Anne Cotten, MD, PhD[a,b]

KEYWORDS

- Gout • Calcium pyrophosphate • CPPD • Crystal deposition • Crystal arthropathy
- Basic calcium phosphate • Hydroxyapatite

KEY POINTS

- Crystal deposition diseases are a common finding and their radiographic features should be known to help the referring physician in the differential.
- Classic features of gout are tophi, large para-articular erosions contrasting with articular-space sparing, and bone hyperostosis without bone rarefaction.
- CPPD arthropathy involves joints usually spared by osteoarthritis, with severe joint narrowing, marked subchondral osteosclerosis, with no or few osteophytes.
- Basic calcium phosphate deposits are usually amorphous and frequently asymptomatic.
- Their density and shape vary when resorbing or migrating into an adjacent structure during an acute and painful flare.

This article reviews the radiographic aspects of the 3 main crystal deposition diseases: monosodium urate (gout), calcium pyrophosphate (CPPD), and basic calcium phosphate (BCP).

GOUT
Introduction

Gout is a crystal-induced deposition disease caused by saturation and precipitation of monosodium urate (MSU) crystals. This common condition affects up to 1% of the general population. Its prevalence is increasing in both developed[1,2] and developing[3,4] countries, mostly because of the evolution of lifestyle and particularly eating habits.[5]

Men are affected 4 to 10 times more often than women,[6] gout being the most frequent cause of inflammatory arthritis in men older than 60 years.[7] In cases of early onset, secondary causes must be considered, because their diagnosis can change further patient care.

Disclosure Statement: The authors have nothing to disclose.
[a] Division of Radiology and Musculoskeletal Imaging, University Hospital of Lille, Rue du Professeur Emile Laine, Lille Cedex 59037, France; [b] University of Lille, 42, rue Paul Duez, Lille 59000, France; [c] Department of Radiology, CHRU de Rouen, 1 rue de Germont, Rouen Cedex 76031, France; [d] Department of Radiology, University of Foggia, Viale Luigi Pinto 1, Foggia 71100, Italy; [e] Department of Radiology, Leeds Teaching Hospital Trust, Chapeltown Road, Leeds, West Yorkshire LS7 4SA, UK
* Corresponding author. Division of Radiology and Musculoskeletal Imaging, University Hospital of Lille, Rue du Professeur Emile Laine, Lille Cedex 59037, France.
E-mail address: thib.jacques@gmail.com

Radiol Clin N Am 55 (2017) 967–984
http://dx.doi.org/10.1016/j.rcl.2017.04.004
0033-8389/17/© 2017 Elsevier Inc. All rights reserved.

Several factors are required for MSU crystals to form. The main underlying factor is hyperuricemia, which is a consequence of either excessive production of uric acid or a lack of its clearance.

Excessive production can be either exogenous, due to excessive intake of purines (eg, meat, seafood, alcohol),[6,8] or endogenous, especially in case of massive cell lysis (eg, chemotherapy or myeloproliferative disorders). Insufficient uric acid clearance can result from chronic kidney disease, drug interactions, or genetic predispositions. Familial diseases that directly affect enzymes involved in purine metabolism are less frequent, such as Lesch-Nyhan disease.

Several local factors can play a crucial role in MSU crystal formation, such as trauma or repetitive microtrauma, arthritis, infection, lack of tissue perfusion, lower blood pH, or lower tissue temperature.[9]

Clinically, gout is characterized by recurrent episodes of arthritis involving one or multiple joints. In the absence of care, the disease can evolve into chronic tophaceous gout. Ultimately, patients can suffer from visceral consequences, such as gouty nephropathy. However, hyperuricemia remains asymptomatic in 90% of patients.

Acute flares are either due to oversaturation of MSU crystals in synovial fluid or to their relapse from hyaline cartilage into the joint, triggering inflammation pathways and resulting in the production of cytokines such as tumor necrosis factor-α and interleukin (IL)-1β.[10] Secondary recruitment of neutrophils worsen local inflammation.[11]

Acute gouty arthritis is typically of sudden onset, involving one or few joints (less frequently polyarticular), with a preference for inferior limbs (in 85% of cases[12]), particularly for the first metatarsophalangeal space. Clinical and biological inflammatory patterns are frequently noted,[13] sometimes mimicking an infectious process, also leading to difficult differential diagnoses with inflammatory diseases, such as rheumatoid arthritis. The synovial fluid analysis would display an inflammatory fluid containing 2000 to 5000 white blood cells per mm^3 (sometimes more) and typical MSU crystals, elongated and birefringent under polarized light, but no germs on Gram staining.

These acute flares usually resolve spontaneously in 5 to 10 days, followed by an asymptomatic period lasting from months to years before recurring.[14] Chronic tophaceous gout is characterized by the presence of *tophi*, which are MSU deposits in either hypodermic soft tissues, articular and para-articular spaces, tendons, or bursae. It tends to occur years after the initial episode of gout and in the absence of adequate treatment (5 years for 30% of patients).[12] *Tophi* are related to the duration and levels of hyperuricemia, and tend to diminish under treatment.

Imaging Findings

In the event of an acute arthritis (if the patient has not yet reached the chronic tophaceous gout stage), plain radiographs are most of the time normal or display a nonspecific joint effusion and/or periarticular soft tissue edema (Fig. 1).

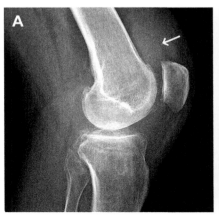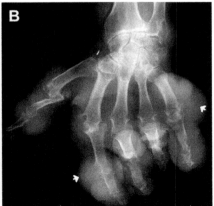

Fig. 1. (A) Acute knee arthritis with nonspecific intra-articular effusion (arrow); joint aspiration showed MSU crystals. (B) Severe chronic tophaceous gout with large subcutaneous tophi (arrowheads) and polyarticular involvement of the hand.

The following are the main radiographic features seen in chronic tophaceous gout:

- Polyarticular involvement, typically asymmetric and more frequently in the lower limbs.
- Subcutaneous *tophi*, of variable sizes, shapes, and topography, most of the time asymmetric. Although this can vary, their intermediate to high density is highly suggestive of gout (Fig. 2A). However, *tophi* rarely calcify in the absence of renal disease. *Tophi* can erode the underlying bone or even the skin in front of them, which can result in the presence of internal gas.
- Bone erosions, adjacent to a tophus, most of the time well circumscribed with overhanging sclerotic margins (Fig. 2B). These erosions are typically large and parallel to the long axis of the bone diaphysis (see Fig. 2B; Fig. 3A). Gout is strongly suspected whenever bone spicules are found at the edges of these erosions (Fig. 2C). Para-articular location, at a distance from the joint, is also highly suggestive of gout.
- Intraosseous *tophi* (Fig. 3B), less frequent, and not to be confused with bone erosions, although they share similar features, such as large size, sclerotic margins, and long-axis parallelism. These pseudo-cystic lesions are usually found around joints and can also mimic subchondral cysts (geodes) and even sometimes destroy the articular space and lead to ankylosis. They are typically seen in severe disorders and in association with the other typical radiographic features of gout.
- Exuberant bone hyperostosis in front of a tophus (with or without associated bone erosions). It can range from large and irregular bony formations (Fig. 2D), osteophytes, or enthesophytes, to regular periosteal apposition (Fig. 4A).
- Long period of articular-space sparing, which contrasts with the usual large size of the

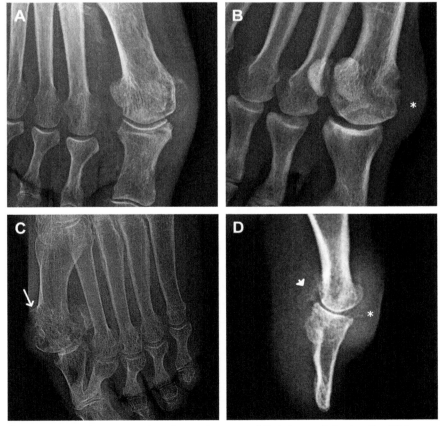

Fig. 2. (*A*) Subcutaneous tophus suggestive of gout because of its intermediate density. (*B*) Large erosion, well circumscribed with overhanging sclerotic margins, in front of a tophus of low density (*asterisk*). (*C*) Large erosion with proximal bone spicule (*arrow*). (*D*) Large bony formations (*arrowhead*) around an interphalangeal joint, adjacent to a tophus (*asterisk*).

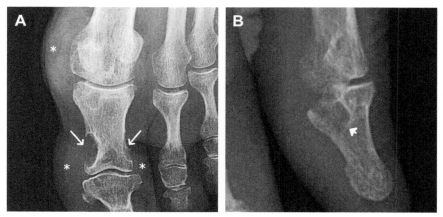

Fig. 3. (A) Two large and symmetric para-articular erosions (arrows) near subcutaneous tophi (asterisks). (B) Intraosseous tophus (arrowhead) mimicking a large subchondral cyst. Note the sparing of the joint-space width.

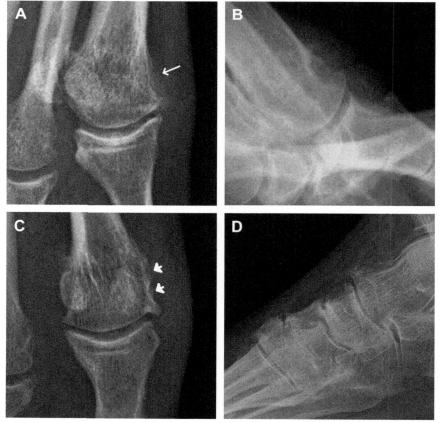

Fig. 4. (A) Subtle periosteal appositions in gout (arrow). (B) Large erosions contrasting with a preserved articular space. (C) Cortical irregularities in gout (arrowheads). (D) "Spiky-foot" aspect on lateral view.

erosions (as opposed to other rheumatisms) (**Figs. 4**B and **5**B).

- No rarefaction of the adjacent bone, which is a reliable tool to help differentiating gout from other inflammatory rheumatisms, when marginal bone erosions are seen.

Gout can affect any joint, but some are more common:

- In the foot, the first metatarsophalangeal space is the initial site in up to 50% of patients, followed in order of frequency by the interphalangeal spaces, then the tarsometatarsal joints.[15] It is first seen on the medial and dorsal sides of the first metatarsal head, and erosions can be seen only as cortical irregularities (**Fig. 4**C). Gout can also frequently affect sesamoid bones, sometimes mimicking a tumoral process. Bone overgrowth (osteophytes, enthesophytes) is frequently seen on the dorsal side of the foot, giving a "spikyfoot" aspect on lateral views (**Fig. 4**D).

- In the knee, the patella is frequently involved, mostly because of the existence of prepatellar *tophi* leading to anterior patellar erosions or reactional anterior bony formations (**Fig. 5**A). Large erosions of the lower femoral cortical bone also can be noted, especially in the intercondylar notch.
- Hands and wrists are involved in advanced gout (see **Fig. 5**B), especially when hyperuricemia is related to a diuretic treatment,[16] usually asymmetrically. Interphalangeal joints (see **Fig. 2**D) are more often affected than metacarpophalangeal or carpometacarpal joints (**Fig. 5**B). Carpal ankylosis can happen in very advanced stages.
- In the elbow, the most common site is the olecranon, with either an olecranon bursitis, erosions, or bony formations of the olecranon (see **Fig. 5**C, D).
- Other joints (eg, shoulder, hip, spine, sacroiliac, temporomandibular) can also be affected, but rarely with an isolated pattern.[17,18]

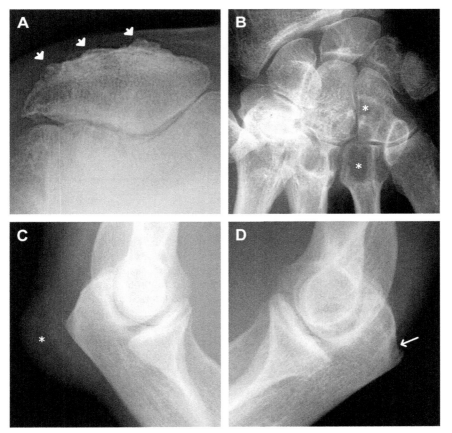

Fig. 5. (*A*) Anterior cortical irregularities of the patella in gout (*arrowheads*). (*B*) Large carpal and metacarpal erosions (*asterisks*) contrasting with the absence of joint narrowing and no subchondral bone rarefaction. (*C*) Large olecranon tophus (*asterisk*). (*D*) Olecranon erosion in gout (*arrow*).

Diagnostic criteria	
Acute arthritis	Nonspecific effusion and/or periarticular soft tissue edema
Chronic tophaceous gout: positive signs	Polyarticular and asymmetric involvement; usually lower limbs (especially first metatarsophalangeal space) Subcutaneous *tophi*: intermediate to high density Bone erosions: large, para-articular, well limited, parallel to the long axis of bone, frequent sclerotic margins Bony formations: spicules, osteophytes, enthesophytes, exuberant periosteal reaction Intraosseous *tophi* (pseudo-cystic) ± intra-articular rupture
Chronic tophaceous gout: negative signs	Articular-space sparing contrasting with large erosions No rarefaction of the adjacent bone

Differential diagnosis	
Septic arthritis	Main differential in the event of an acute arthritis If persistent doubt, joint aspiration required
Rheumatoid arthritis	No tophi Typically, symmetric and most common in hands and wrists Early articular-space narrowing Marginal erosions; no para-articular erosions No bony formations
Psoriatic arthritis	No tophi Early articular-space narrowing Small marginal erosions Frequent bony formations, usually irregular, blurry, and micro-spiculated
Osteoarthritis	No tophi No erosions (especially para-articular) Subchondral cysts (geodes) Articular-space narrowing
CPPD	No tophi No erosions (especially para-articular) Different joint involvement pattern

CALCIUM PYROPHOSPHATE DEPOSITION DISEASE
Introduction

CPPD is caused by the deposition of calcium pyrophosphate crystals in joints. This condition is frequent, affecting up to 1% to 2% of the general population between the ages of 60 and 70, 6% to 8% between 70 and 80, and 20% to 30% after the age of 80.[19,20]

Calcium pyrophosphate (CPP) crystals can lead to several clinical manifestations, such as acute arthritis, chronic arthritis, or destructive arthropathy.[21]

Chondrocalcinosis is defined by radiological or histologic articular cartilage calcification, either hyaline cartilage or fibrocartilage. Chondrocalcinosis is due in the clear majority of cases to CPP crystals, sometimes associated with calcium phosphate crystals or calcium oxalate crystals.[21] The diagnosis is theoretically proven only by the microscopic evidence of CPP crystals in either synovial fluid or a fragment from synovium or cartilage. These crystals have a small size (5–10 μm), and a rodlike shape. Recommendations for the positive diagnosis of CPPD[21] have been proposed, based on the following:

- Clinical features: symptoms usually develop quickly (from 6 to 24 hours) with an important inflammatory pattern (fever, local swelling). Topography is highly suggestive when involving knee, shoulders, or wrists, especially in patients older than 65.

- Biological features: fluctuant inflammatory syndrome.
- Radiographic and/or ultrasonographical features. The absence of chondrocalcinosis in conventional radiography does not exclude the diagnosis of CPPD, especially during an acute event.
- The absence of clinical findings consistent with another disease, especially rheumatoid arthritis or septic arthritis.

Acute CPPD flares ("pseudo-gout") are due to the relapse of CPP crystals (from cartilage, fibrocartilage, or synovium) into the synovial fluid. Crystals are then phagocyted by leukocytes, which triggers an inflammatory response, inducing cytokines and interleukin secretion, especially IL-1β.[22] Acute flares resolve spontaneously in 3 to 4 days, quicker under appropriated treatment.[23]

The exact mechanism leading to chronic CPP arthritis and its relation with osteoarthritis remains unclear.

Clinical features of CPPD are highly variable, being most of the time monoarticular or oligoarticular, polyarticular involvement happening in only 11% of cases. CPPD is frequently asymptomatic, discovered by incidental calcifications seen on conventional radiography.[23]

Sex ratio of chondrocalcinosis is 1:1, with degenerative arthropathy (osteoarthritis) being an important underlying factor for the development of sporadic CPPD. For example, patients suffering from knee osteoarthritis have 3 times more risk to develop chondrocalcinosis.[23]

Familial forms are rare and revealed by early polyarticular calcifications (20–40 years old), frequently followed by severe arthropathy.[24]

Secondary CPPD is the consequence of metabolic diseases, which are to be searched for, especially in young patients or when facing a diffuse and polyarticular disease.

The following are the most frequent metabolic causes:

- Hyperparathyroidism (primary or secondary). Eight percent to 57% of these patients will eventually suffer from CPPD.[25] Radiological calcifications do not resolve after parathyroidectomy.
- Hemochromatosis. The exact mechanism is yet unclear, but excessive iron concentration is thought to increase intra-articular CPP concentration. Thirty-eight percent of patients who are homozygotes for C282Y mutation will eventually have CPPD, whereas 21% of heterozygotes will.[26]

- Other metabolic causes are less frequent: hypomagnesemia (eg, in Gitelman syndrome), hypophosphatasia, or familial hypocalciuric hypocalcemia.[19,27,28]

Imaging Findings

On conventional radiography, CPPD is characterized by 2 main abnormalities: calcifications (articular or soft tissues) and arthropathy.

Calcifications tend to be symmetric and can involve the following[20]:

- Hyaline cartilages, delineating a thin linear opacity parallel to subchondral bone but separated from it by 1 to 2 mm (Fig. 6A). This opacity can be continuous or not, less frequently granular (Fig. 6B).
- Fibrocartilages, displaying thicker calcifications, frequently stratified or granular[29] (Fig. 6C).
- Synovial membranes (Fig. 6D) and bursae, displaying cloudy and blurry calcifications, particularly involving knees, wrists, and hands.
- Articular capsules, with thin, linear, and regular calcifications.
- Tendons, with linear and stratified calcifications, oriented toward the long axis of the tendon (as opposed to BCP deposition) (see Fig. 10A), and ligaments, especially in the wrist.
- Other tissues with a pseudotumoral form that can mimic gout or soft tissue sarcoma.[30]

The main specificities of CPPD arthropathy, when compared with osteoarthritis are as follows:

- The involvement of joints usually spared by osteoarthritis: radiocarpal (Fig. 7A), metacarpophalangeal, talo-calcaneo-navicular, or elbow for example.
- Severe joint narrowing, sometimes with crenated aspect of articular surfaces (Figs. 7B and 8), rapidly worsening with subchondral bone fragmentation and intra-articular foreign bodies (see Fig. 8).
- Marked subchondral and well-defined osteosclerosis (Fig. 7C).
- Sometimes absent or few osteophytes, contrasting with the severity of joint narrowing (see Fig. 7A, B).
- Numerous subchondral cysts (geodes), frequently displaying a microcystic pattern in subchondral bone (with sometimes larger cysts) (Fig. 7D).

The most frequently affected joint is the knee, where any kind of calcification can be seen.[31,32]

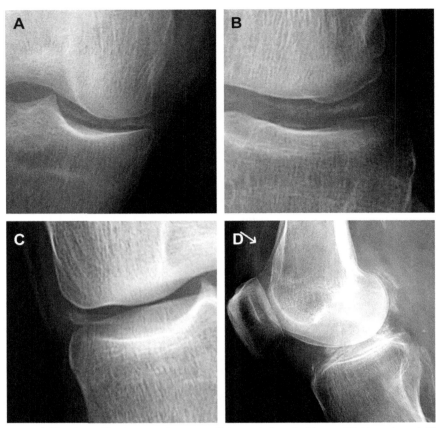

Fig. 6. (*A*) Linear calcification of hyaline cartilage, parallel to subchondral bone. (*B*) Granular calcification of hyaline cartilage. (*C*) Stratified calcifications of meniscus. (*D*) Cloudy synovial calcifications (*arrow*).

CPPD can affect either 1 or both femorotibial compartments at the same time, which is not frequent in osteoarthritis and helps in the differential. The femoropatellar joint also can be affected, and suggests CPPD when isolated and severe, sometimes with a crenated aspect (see **Figs.** 7B and 8).

In the wrist, an isolated scaphotrapezial joint involvement is typical, with features highly suggestive of CPPD: severe joint narrowing, dense and well-limited subchondral sclerosis, with no or few osteophytes[33] (see **Fig.** 7C; **Fig.** 9A). CPPD also can affect ligaments, especially the lunotriquetral ligament, scapholunate ligament, and the triangular fibrocartilage complex (TFCC) (**Fig.** 9B). Scapholunate ligament involvement and rupture can then lead to a scapholunate advanced collapse (SLAC-Wrist)[34] (see **Fig.** 9B). Other patterns can be seen less frequently, such as a distal radioulnar joint involvement. In the hand, metacarpophalangeal spaces are frequently affected (particularly the

second and third spaces), with cartilage calcifications, synovial calcifications, and/or joint-space narrowing (**Fig.** 9C, D). Interphalangeal spaces are rarely affected, as opposed to osteoarthritis, in which metacarpophalangeal spaces are spared.

In the hip and shoulder, CPPD can affect hyaline cartilage, periarticular tendons, articular capsule, or articular labrum (**Fig.** 10A). Ultimately, shoulder or hip osteoarthritis can be seen. Several features, such as bone fragmentation or microcystic subchondral geodes, can help differentiating from degenerative arthropathy, but these are not always present.

In the elbow, except for classic CPPD features, specific calcifications of the triceps tendon are important to recognize.

In the ankle and foot, the most commonly affected joints are the talo-calcaneonavicular and tarsometatarsal joints, where it may sometimes mimic neuropathic arthritis due to the extent of lesions.[35]

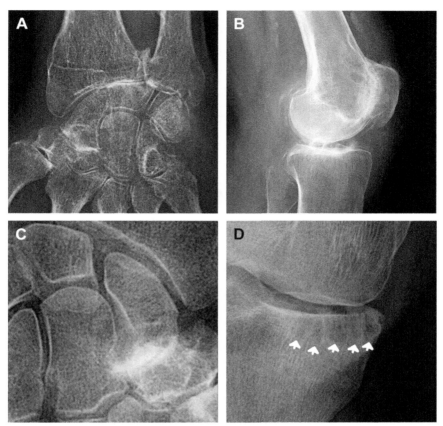

Fig. 7. (A) Radiocarpal CPPD arthropathy; severe joint narrowing contrasting with the relative absence of osteophytes. (B) Severe femoro-patellar joint narrowing without osteophytes. (C) Marked osteosclerosis, well defined, in the subchondral bone of a scaphotrapezial joint. (D) Microcystic pattern of subchondral bone in CPPD (arrowheads).

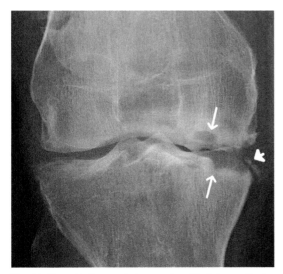

Fig. 8. Crenated aspect (arrows) with intra-articular fragments (arrowhead) of the medial femorotibial compartment in CPPD.

The main spinal lesions of CPPD are located as follows:

- In the discs, with subtle linear calcifications usually predominating in the peripheral part of the disc[36] (Fig. 10B). Degenerative discopathies are a common finding and suggest the diagnosis of CPPD when severe, multiple (more than 3 levels), and erosive, sometimes associated with an intradiscal vacuum.
- In the spinal ligaments, every single one of them can be affected. Ligamental involvement is frequent and peri-odontoid deposition is highly suggestive, depicting the classic "crowned-dens syndrome."[37]
- In the facet joints or interspinous bursae.

Many more joints can be affected, such as sternoclavicular, acromioclavicular, sacroiliac and temporomandibular joints, or pubic symphysis.[38,39]

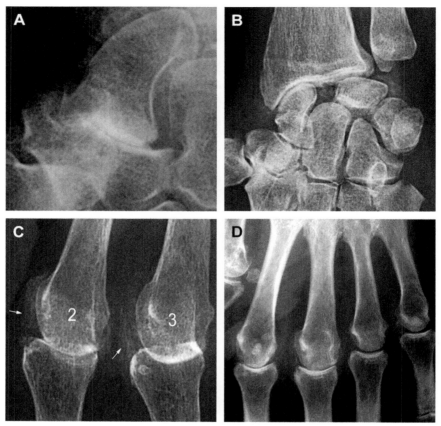

Fig. 9. (A) Scaphotrapezial arthropathy with severe joint narrowing and well-limited marked subchondral osteo-sclerosis, highly suggestive of CPPD. (B) SLAC-wrist with scapholunate diastasis and calcifications of both scapho-lunate ligament and TFCC. (C, D) Joint narrowing of the second and third metacarpophalangeal spaces, suggestive of CPPD (arrows = capsulo-synovial calcifications).

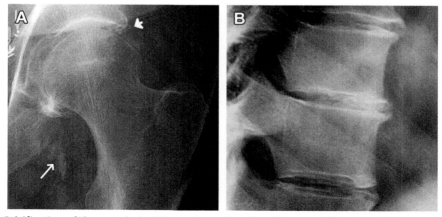

Fig. 10. (A) Calcification of the acetabular labrum (arrowhead) and linear calcifications of the hamstring tendons (arrow) in CPPD. (B) CPPD discal involvement with subtle linear calcifications located on the peripheral part of the discs.

Diagnostic criteria	
Calcifications	Hyaline cartilage (thin, linear, less frequently granular) Fibrocartilage (thick, stratified, or granular) Synovium (cloudy and blurry) Articular capsule (thin, linear, regular) Ligaments and tendons (stratified, parallel to long) Soft tissue: pseudotumoral form
Arthropathy	Affecting joints usually spared by osteoarthritis (metacarpophalangeal, wrist, tarsus, elbow) Severity of joint narrowing (crenated, subchondral bone fragmentation) Marked subchondral osteosclerosis (well defined) Absent or few osteophytes, contrasting with the severity of joint narrowing Numerous subchondral cysts (microcystic)

Differential diagnosis	
BCP calcifications	Amorphous deposits, of higher density Not stratified
Osteoarthritis	Different joint topography Frequent osteophytes
Hemochromatosis	Hooklike osteophytes Frequent arthropathy of second and third metacarpophalangeal space (fourth and fifth also can be involved) Less frequent than CPPD
Septic arthritis	Main differential in the event of an acute arthritis If persistent doubt, joint aspiration required

BASIC CALCIUM PHOSPHATE DEPOSITION DISEASE
Introduction

BCP crystal deposition disease is characterized by the presence of BCP crystals, mostly hydroxyapatite but also tricalcium phosphate and octacalcium phosphate, in either the periarticular soft tissues (tendons and bursae) or in the intraarticular space, where it can lead to acute arthritis or destructive arthropathy (eg, Milwaukee shoulder).[40,41]

The most frequent topography for this crystal deposition disease is the shoulder, accounting for 60% of cases, followed in order of frequency by hip, knee, elbow, wrist, and hand, but any joint can theoretically be affected.

Although its etiology is still unclear,[42] and only a few familial forms have been reported,[43] no systemic factors are found in most cases. Interestingly, periarticular depositions, especially in tendons, tend to not be related to physical activity or professional activity, and happen mostly on previously intact tendons.[44,45]

Most calcifications are asymptomatic and incidental findings; reports on shoulder calcifications showed that only approximately 30% of calcifications would eventually become symptomatic.[46] They can resorb locally or extrude in adjacent bursa, joint, or bone. This extrusion can be chronic (no symptoms or chronic pain) or acute, and associated with excruciating pain (acute tendinobursitis).[47]

When intra-articular, BCP crystals are rarely proven microscopically because they are too small to be reliably detected even under polarized light. They can result from either periarticular calcification resorption into the joint, or from primary intra-articular deposit.[48] Consequences are either acute arthritis, mimicking septic arthritis because of the frequent fever and swelling, or destructive arthropathy, especially in the shoulder (Milwaukee shoulder), knee, and hip. BCP-related destructive arthropathy is more frequent in women between the ages of 50 and 90, bilateral in 65% of cases, with coexistent trauma or excessive use found in 25% of cases.[40]

Imaging Findings

BCP crystal deposition disease diagnosis is based primarily on conventional radiography.

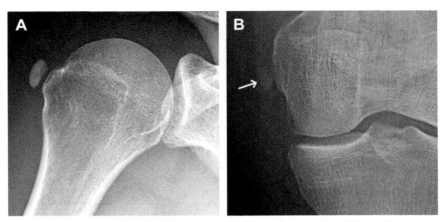

Fig. 11. (A) Internal rotation of shoulder displaying an amorphous, dense, and well-limited quiescent calcification of the infraspinatus tendon. (B) Cloudy, ill-defined calcification of the medial collateral ligament, of lesser density, in a patient with acute knee pain, typical of acute resorption (*arrow*).

Periarticular calcifications are typically amorphous, dense, round or oval-shaped, with well-limited borders while quiescent (**Fig. 11**A). They locate on insertion sites of tendons, especially zones of relative hypoxia (eg, in the supraspinatus tendon) but also in tendon sheets and bursae.

When calcifications resorb, they tend to become cloudy, less dense with an ill-defined shape (**Fig. 11**B), and can migrate into adjacent structures: bursae, joints, or bones (leading to cortical erosions) (**Fig. 12**). It is important to notice that in the event of an acute resorption, calcification may not be seen in conventional radiography, thus leading to misdiagnosis[49] (see **Fig. 12**). When calcification is seen in such a situation around cortical erosion, it frequently displays a "comet-tail" shape, better seen on computed tomography (CT).

Intra-articular BCP crystal deposition disease can lead to destructive arthropathy, such as "Milwaukee shoulder," which combines glenohumeral space narrowing, humeral head ascent, moderate subchondral bone sclerosis, and subtle or absent osteophytosis. Ultimately, subchondral bone fragmentation and even neoarticulations are seen[40] (**Fig. 13**). Destructive arthropathy with bone fragmentation also can be seen; for example, in the knee and spine (erosive spondylodiscitis).

In the shoulder, rotator cuff calcifications are well known, frequent, and sometimes multiple. They can be bilateral in up to 46% of cases and affect by order of frequency the *supraspinatus* (80%) (**Fig. 14**A), *infraspinatus* (15%) (see **Fig. 11**A), and *subscapularis* (5%) tendons.[46] On

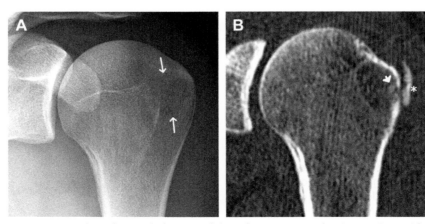

Fig. 12. Intraosseous resorption of BCP calcification of the infraspinatus tendon in a patient with acute shoulder pain. On conventional radiography (A), the calcification is not seen but there is a focal zone of bone lucency (*arrows*). (B) On CT (performed the same day), the calcification is better seen (*asterisk*) with a focal zone of cortical bone interruption in front of it, and an intraosseous resorption (*arrowhead*).

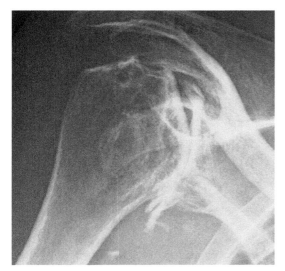

Fig. 13. Milwaukee shoulder due to intra-articular BCP. Gleno-humeral space narrowing, moderate sub-chondral bone sclerosis, and or few osteophytes.

anteroposterior views, the use of 3 routine shoulder positions (external rotation, neutral, and internal rotation) help in discriminating which tendon is affected.[50] Calcifications involving the *biceps brachii* affect more often the proximal aspect of its long head's tendon (**Fig. 14**B) rather than its short head.[51]

Numerous structures can be affected in the elbow, among which epicondyle tendons, collateral ligaments, olecranon bursa, tendon of *biceps brachii* near its radial insertion, or *triceps brachii* near the olecranon.[52]

Any flexor or extensor tendon can be affected in the wrist or hand, although the most frequently affected is *flexor carpi ulnaris*, in front and above pisiform bone (**Fig. 14**C), frequently linked with repetitive microtrauma.[42,50] These calcifications are better seen on profile views. Periarticular deposits are often seen around metacarpophalangeal and proximal interphalangeal joints.[42] Interestingly, the myotendinous

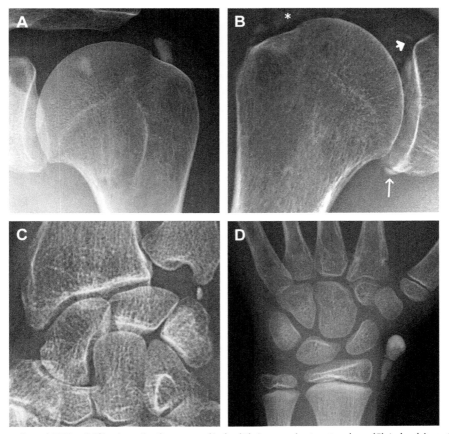

Fig. 14. Examples of BCP calcifications in the upper limb. (*A*) Supraspinatus tendon. (*B*) Labral insertion of the long head of *biceps brachii* (*arrowhead*), labral insertion of *triceps brachii* (*arrow*), and subacromial-subdeltoid bursa (*asterisk*). (*C*) *Flexor carpi ulnaris* above the pisiform bone. (*D*) Periarticular deposit in front of the radiocarpal space.

junction of lumbrical and interosseous muscles also can be calcified.

The most frequent calcification site around the hip is the insertion of the gluteal muscles onto the greater trochanter (**Fig. 15**A) and adjacent bursae. Cortical erosions can be associated.[50,53,54] Nearly any tendon can be affected in the pelvic region, thus leading to frequent misdiagnoses.

Around the knee, calcifications can involve collateral ligaments (less frequently cruciate ligaments), bursae, or tendons, especially *biceps femoris* above the fibular head, mimicking sciatica when resorbing (**Fig. 15**B) or quadriceps tendon and/or patellar ligament.[50,55]

The most frequent site for BCP calcifications around the ankle and foot are tendons of *flexor hallucis longus, flexor hallucis brevis,* and fibular tendons[50] (**Fig. 15**C, D). Soft tissues around metatarsophalangeal spaces also can be involved. When affecting the hallux, the diagnosis may often be misinterpreted as gout, thus probably underestimating the real incidence of BCP in this region.

In the spine, BCP crystal deposition disease appears as dense and amorphous calcifications, in a central position inside the intervertebral discs, affecting one or several discs, especially in the lower thoracic spine[56] (**Fig. 16**A), but the cervical spine also can be involved, particularly in children. They can usually be easily distinguished from CPPD, which displays linear calcifications in the peripheral part of the disc. Their size and shape can vary over time and resorb during an acute episode of pain, mimicking spondylodiscitis, and/or migrate in the adjacent environment (epidural space, vertebral plates). Another classic location for BCP crystal deposition disease is the *longus colli* muscle, especially its superior and oblique fibers that are projecting on lateral view under the anterior body of C1 (**Fig. 16**B) (less frequently its vertical fibers, seen from C4 to C6).[57] Its acute resorption is responsible for acute cervicalgia and/or dysphagia, mimicking meningitis, spondylodiscitis or cervical tumor. In addition to the visible calcification, a frequent prevertebral

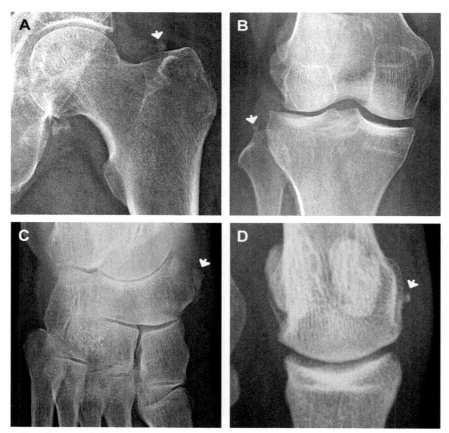

Fig. 15. Examples of BCP calcifications in the lower limb (*arrowheads*). (*A*) Gluteal tendons near the greater trochanter. (*B*) Resorbing calcification in the tendon of *biceps femoris* above the fibular head, in a patient with acute sciatica. (*C*) *Tibialis posterior* tendon. (*D*) *Flexor hallucis brevis* tendon.

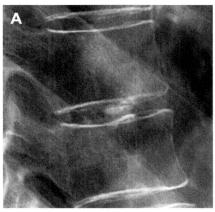
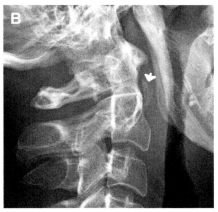

Fig. 16. (A) Amorphous calcification in a central position inside a thoracic intervertebral disc, highly suggestive of BCP. (B) Typical appearance of *longus colli* calcification (*arrowhead*), projecting under the anterior body of C1, in a patient with acute cervicalgia.

soft tissue enlargement in the upper cervical region can be seen on conventional radiography during acute resorption. An anterior accessory bone of C1 can be mistaken for a *longus colli* calcification.

Numerous other structures can be calcified in the spine, especially bursae, apophyseal joints, or ligaments. One special feature is the "crowned-dens syndrome," due to calcification above and around the odontoid, better seen on CT. This syndrome also can be seen in CPPD with overlapping radiological findings, none being specific on conventional radiography.[58,59] Both can lead to acute resorption and acute cervical symptoms.

Careful analysis of the structure of BCP deposits shows only calcified matter, without cortical or trabecular bone organization, therefore distinguishing it from intervertebral ossifications (degenerative or spondyloarthropathy-related).

Diagnostic criteria	
Periarticular BCP crystal deposition disease	Calcifications: amorphous, dense, round or oval; cloudy aspect while resorbing Bursal space: can present as an opaque and sloping collection Bone erosions: marginal when close to a joint (mimicking arthritis) or cortical when distant from a joint (mimicking tumoral or infectious process)

Differential diagnosis	
If calcification is not seen	If calcification is seen
Septic arthritis or bursitis Aspiration needed if suspected	CPPD Main differential diagnosis Frequently multifocal and/or symmetric Thin, linear, and/or stratified calcifications Frequent intra-articular calcifications
Gout *Tophi* are less dense than BCP calcifications Look for large bone erosions, bony spicules, or intraosseous *tophi*	*Tumoral* calcifications (sarcoma, venous malformation) *Infectious* calcifications (cysticercosis) *Posttraumatic* calcifications

PEARLS, PITFALLS, VARIANTS

- Septic arthritis should never be ruled out solely based on radiographic features
- Erosions in gout are para-articular and their large size contrasts with the relative absence of joint-space narrowing
- Most *tophi* are of intermediate density (not calcified except if renal disease)
- Know the main locations of osteoarthritis and those that are suggestive of CPPD, such as scaphotrapezial, radiocarpal, or metacarpophalangeal joints
- Joint narrowing in CPPD arthropathy and marked subchondral osteosclerosis contrast with the relative absence of osteophytes
- BCP calcifications are asymptomatic and incidental findings in most cases, but their resorption can cause excruciating pain
- Accessory bones can be misdiagnosed for BCP calcifications
- Different crystal diseases can coexist and the diagnosis can be challenging

WHAT THE REFERRING PHYSICIAN NEEDS TO KNOW

- Which deposition disease is the most likely considering the radiographic features?
- If not initially suspected, what are the elements in favor of a crystal-related arthropathy instead of differentials (eg, osteoarthritis or inflammatory rheumatism)?
- Which structures are involved, and what are the anatomic locations of the deposits?
- Are the findings incidental, or can they be related to the symptoms of the patient?
- Is further imaging needed (ultrasound, CT, MR imaging)?

SUMMARY

This article reviews the radiographic characteristics of the main crystal-related deposition diseases: gout, calcium pyrophosphate, and BCP. Their radiographic semiology should be known to help the referring physician in the differential between them, or between a crystal arthropathy and another articular disease, especially inflammatory rheumatism and osteoarthritis. Even though certain features are highly suggestive, it is sometimes impossible to identify or differentiate crystal deposition diseases based on conventional radiology, and advanced imaging (CT, MR imaging) may be needed.

REFERENCES

1. Annemans L, Spaepen E, Gaskin M, et al. Gout in the UK and Germany: prevalence, comorbidities and management in general practice 2000-2005. Ann Rheum Dis 2008;67(7):960–6.
2. Lawrence RC, Felson DT, Helmick CG, et al. Estimates of the prevalence of arthritis and other rheumatic conditions in the United States. Part II. Arthritis Rheum 2008;58(1):26–35.
3. Chuang SY, Lee SC, Hsieh YT, et al. Trends in hyperuricemia and gout prevalence: nutrition and health survey in Taiwan from 1993-1996 to 2005-2008. Asia Pac J Clin Nutr 2011;20(2):301–8.
4. Xiang YJ, Dai SM. Prevalence of rheumatic diseases and disability in China. Rheumatol Int 2009;29(5):481–90.
5. Bolzetta F, Veronese N, Manzato E, et al. Tophaceous gout in the elderly: a clinical case review. Clin Rheumatol 2012;31(7):1127–32.
6. Cea Soriano L, Rothenbacher D, Choi HK, et al. Contemporary epidemiology of gout in the UK general population. Arthritis Res Ther 2011; 13(2):R39.
7. Zhang W, Doherty M, Pascual E, et al. EULAR evidence based recommendations for gout. Part I: diagnosis. Report of a task force of the standing committee for international clinical studies including therapeutics (ESCISIT). Ann Rheum Dis 2006; 65(10):1301–11.
8. Choi HK, Atkinson K, Karlson EW, et al. Purine-rich foods, dairy and protein intake, and the risk of gout in men. N Engl J Med 2004;350(11):1093–103.
9. Roddy E, Doherty M. Epidemiology of gout. Arthritis Res Ther 2010;12(6):223.
10. Martinon F. Mechanisms of uric acid crystal-mediated autoinflammation. Immunol Rev 2010; 233(1):218–32.
11. Popa-Nita O, Naccache PH. Crystal-induced neutrophil activation. Immunol Cell Biol 2010;88(1):32–40.
12. Richette P, Bardin T. Gout. Lancet 2010;375(9711):318–28.
13. Rousseau I, Cardinal EE, Raymond-Tremblay D, et al. Gout: radiographic findings mimicking infection. Skeletal Radiol 2001;30(10):565–9.
14. Lioté F, Lancrenon S, Lanz S, et al. GOSPEL: prospective survey of gout in France. Part I: design and patient characteristics (n = 1003). Joint Bone Spine 2012;79(5):464–70.
15. Dhanda S, Jagmohan P, Quek ST, et al. A re-look at an old disease: a multimodality review on gout. Clin Radiol 2011;66(10):984–92.
16. Andracco R, Zampogna G, Parodi M, et al. Risk factors for gouty dactylitis. Clin Exp Rheumatol 2009; 27(6):993–5.

17. King JC, Nicholas C. Gouty arthropathy of the lumbar spine: a case report and review of the literature. Spine 1997;22(19):2309–12.

18. Bhattacharyya I, Chehal H, Gremillion H, et al. Gout of the temporomandibular joint: a review of the literature. J Am Dent Assoc 2010;141(8):979–85.

19. Richette P, Bardin T, Doherty M. An update on the epidemiology of calcium pyrophosphate dihydrate crystal deposition disease. Rheumatol Oxf Engl 2009;48(7):711–5.

20. Neame RL, Carr AJ, Muir K, et al. UK community prevalence of knee chondrocalcinosis: evidence that correlation with osteoarthritis is through a shared association with osteophyte. Ann Rheum Dis 2003;62(6):513–8.

21. Zhang W, Doherty M, Bardin T, et al. European league against rheumatism recommendations for calcium pyrophosphate deposition. Part I: terminology and diagnosis. Ann Rheum Dis 2011;70(4):563–70.

22. Moltó A, Ea HK, Richette P, et al. Efficacy of anakinra for refractory acute calcium pyrophosphate crystal arthritis. Jt Bone Spine Rev Rhum 2012;79(6):621–3.

23. Zhang W, Doherty M, Pascual E, et al. EULAR recommendations for calcium pyrophosphate deposition. Part II: management. Ann Rheum Dis 2011;70(4):571–5.

24. Gruber BL, Couto AR, Armas JB, et al. Novel ANKH amino terminus mutation (Pro5Ser) associated with early-onset calcium pyrophosphate disease with associated phosphaturia. J Clin Rheumatol 2012;18(4):192–5.

25. Huaux JP, Geubel A, Koch MC, et al. The arthritis of hemochromatosis. A review of 25 cases with special reference to chondrocalcinosis, and a comparison with patients with primary hyperparathyroidism and controls. Clin Rheumatol 1986;5(3):317–24.

26. Pawlotsky Y, Le Dantec P, Moirand R, et al. Elevated parathyroid hormone 44-68 and osteoarticular changes in patients with genetic hemochromatosis. Arthritis Rheum 1999;42(4):799–806.

27. Volpe A, Guerriero A, Marchetta A, et al. Familial hypocalciuric hypercalcemia revealed by chondrocalcinosis. Jt Bone Spine Rev Rhum 2009;76(6):708–10.

28. Alix L, Guggenbuhl P. Familial hypocalciuric hypercalcemia associated with crystal deposition disease. Jt Bone Spine Rev Rhum 2015;82(1):60–2.

29. Steinbach LS. Calcium pyrophosphate dihydrate and calcium hydroxyapatite crystal deposition diseases: imaging perspectives. Radiol Clin North Am 2004;42(1):185–205, vii.

30. Yamazaki H, Uchiyama S, Kato H. Median nerve and ulnar nerve palsy caused by calcium pyrophosphate dihydrate crystal deposition disease: case report. J Hand Surg 2008;33(8):1325–8.

31. Yang BY, Sartoris DJ, Resnick D, et al. Calcium pyrophosphate dihydrate crystal deposition disease: frequency of tendon calcification about the knee. J Rheumatol 1996;23(5):883–8.

32. Misra D, Guermazi A, Sieren JP, et al. CT imaging for evaluation of calcium crystal deposition in the knee: initial experience from the multicenter osteoarthritis (MOST) study. Osteoarthritis Cartilage 2015;23(2):244–8.

33. Donich AS, Lektrakul N, Liu CC, et al. Calcium pyrophosphate dihydrate crystal deposition disease of the wrist: trapezioscaphoid joint abnormality. J Rheumatol 2000;27(11):2628–34.

34. Kahloune M, Libouton X, Omoumi P, et al. Osteoarthritis and scapholunate instability in chondrocalcinosis. Diagn Interv Imaging 2015;96(1):115–9.

35. Lomax A, Ferrero A, Cullen N, et al. Destructive pseudo-neuroarthropathy associated with calcium pyrophosphate deposition. Foot Ankle Int 2015;36(4):383–90.

36. Lefebvre G, Pansini V, Dodre E, et al. Maladie des dépôts de cristaux de phosphate de calcium basique (rhumatisme apatitique). EMC Radiol Imag Médicale Musculosquelettique Neurol Maxillofac 2015;10(4):1–10.

37. Chang EY, Lim WY, Wolfson T, et al. Frequency of atlantoaxial calcium pyrophosphate dihydrate deposition at CT. Radiology 2013;269(2):519–24.

38. Hanai S, Sato T, Nagatani K, et al. Pseudogout of the sternoclavicular joints. Intern Med 2014;53(5):521–2.

39. Kenzaka T, Wakabayashi T, Morita Y. Acute crystal deposition arthritis of the pubic symphysis. BMJ Case Rep 2013;2013 [pii: bcr2013009239].

40. McCarty DJ, Swanson AB, Ehrhart RH. Hemorrhagic rupture of the shoulder. J Rheumatol 1994;21(6):1134–7.

41. Gerster JC. Intraarticular apatite crystal deposition as a predictor of erosive osteoarthritis of the fingers. J Rheumatol 1994;21(11):2164–5.

42. Doumas C, Vazirani RM, Clifford PD, et al. Acute calcific periarthritis of the hand and wrist: a series and review of the literature. Emerg Radiol 2007;14(4):199–203.

43. Hajiroussou VJ, Webley M. Familial calcific periarthritis. Ann Rheum Dis 1983;42(4):469–70.

44. Serafini G, Sconfienza LM, Lacelli F, et al. Rotator cuff calcific tendonitis: short-term and 10-year outcomes after two-needle US-guided percutaneous treatment–nonrandomized controlled trial. Radiology 2009;252(1):157–64.

45. Uhthoff HK, Loehr JW. Calcific tendinopathy of the rotator cuff: pathogenesis, diagnosis, and management. J Am Acad Orthop Surg 1997;5(4):183–91.

46. Clavert P, Sirveaux F, Société française d'arthroscopie. Shoulder calcifying tendinitis. Rev Chir Orthop

Reparatrice Appar Mot 2008;94(8 Suppl):336–55 [in French].

47. Pascual E, Bardin T, Richette P. Crystal arthropathies. In: Bijlsma JWJ, editor. EULAR texbook on rheumatic diseases. UK: BMJ Group; 2012. p. 301–12.

48. Gerster JC, Fournier D. Acute apatite arthritis of the shoulder in a young woman. Clin Rheumatol 1995; 14(1):95–9.

49. Kraemer EJ, El-Khoury GY. Atypical calcific tendinitis with cortical erosions. Skeletal Radiol 2000; 29(12):690–6.

50. Holt PD, Keats TE. Calcific tendinitis: a review of the usual and unusual. Skeletal Radiol 1993;22(1):1–9.

51. Kim KC, Rhee KJ, Shin HD, et al. A SLAP lesion associated with calcific tendinitis of the long head of the biceps brachii at its origin. Knee Surg Sports Traumatol Arthrosc 2007;15(12):1478–81.

52. Park JY, Gupta A, Park HK. Calcific tendinitis at the radial insertion of the biceps brachii: a case report. J Shoulder Elbow Surg 2008;17(6):e19–21.

53. Fritz P, Bardin T, Laredo JD, et al. Paradiaphyseal calcific tendinitis with cortical bone erosion. Arthritis Rheum 1994;37(5):718–23.

54. Sakai T, Shimaoka Y, Sugimoto M, et al. Acute calcific tendinitis of the gluteus medius: a case report with serial magnetic resonance imaging findings. J Orthop Sci 2004;9(4):404–7.

55. Varghese B, Radcliffe GS, Groves C. Calcific tendonitis of the quadriceps. Br J Sports Med 2006;40(7):652–4 [discussion: 654].

56. Chanchairujira K, Chung CB, Kim JY, et al. Intervertebral disk calcification of the spine in an elderly population: radiographic prevalence, location, and distribution and correlation with spinal degeneration. Radiology 2004;230(2):499–503.

57. Park SY, Jin W, Lee SH, et al. Acute retropharyngeal calcific tendinitis: a case report with unusual location of calcification. Skeletal Radiol 2010;39(8):817–20.

58. Malca SA, Roche PH, Pellet W, et al. Crowned dens syndrome: a manifestation of hydroxy-apatite rheumatism. Acta Neurochir (Wien) 1995;135(3–4): 126–30.

59. Wu DW, Reginato AJ, Torriani M, et al. The crowned dens syndrome as a cause of neck pain: report of two new cases and review of the literature. Arthritis Rheum 2005;53(1):133–7.

Ultrasound in Arthritis

Iwona Sudoł-Szopińska, MD, PhD[a,b,]*,
Claudia Schueller-Weidekamm, MD, MBA[c], Athena Plagou, MD, PhD[d],
James Teh, MD, MBBS, MRCP, FRCR[e]

KEYWORDS

• Ultrasound • Imaging • Arthritis • Rheumatoid arthritis • Spondyloarthritis
• Connective tissue diseases

KEY POINTS

- Ultrasound is one of the most commonly used methods in the diagnosis of arthritis; to make an initial diagnosis, monitor treatment, and define remission.
- The most frequent findings in ultrasound in arthritis are synovitis, tenosynovitis, bursitis, enthesopathy, and erosions.
- Ultrasound is an excellent tool to guide diagnostic and therapeutic procedures.
- Quantitative methods of inflammation assessment, as well as criteria for differential diagnosis of arthropathies and remission, still remain to be elaborated.

INTRODUCTION

Conventional radiography remains an important diagnostic tool for the diagnosis and monitoring of treatment in arthritis. The importance of early diagnosis and the necessity for accurate monitoring of modern treatment in patients with rheumatic diseases are the main reasons ultrasound and MR imaging are being performed more and more often,[1–4] because they can both visualize early inflammatory lesions within the soft tissues. MR imaging can also visualize subchondral bone marrow edema.

SPECTRUM OF PATHOLOGIES SEEN ON ULTRASOUND IN ARTHRITIS

In patients with rheumatological conditions, ultrasound is conducted mainly for the diagnosis of inflammatory lesions in peripheral joints, tendon sheaths, bursae, and entheses. The following abnormalities in rheumatologic diseases can be seen on ultrasound[2,4–10]:

- Effusions, synovitis, and bursitis
- Tendon pathology (also referred to as tendinopathy), including tendinosis, tenosynovitis, and tendon tears
- Cartilaginous, osseous, or osteochondral lesions (cartilage damage, cysts, erosions, fractures)
- Enthesopathy, encompassing pathologic changes at tendon, ligament, fascia, or joint capsule attachments
- Compression neuropathy
- Postoperative complications

The advantages of ultrasound include the following:

- Assessment of inflammation activity by detecting and measuring vascularity (eg, of the synovium or enthesis)

Disclosure Statement: The authors declare no financial or commercial conflicts of interest nor any funding sources.
[a] Department of Radiology, National Institute of Geriatrics, Rheumatology, and Rehabilitation, Street Spartanska 1, Warsaw 02-637, Poland; [b] Department of Diagnostic Imaging, Warsaw Medical University, St. Żwirki i Wigury 61, Warsaw 02-091, Poland; [c] Division of Neuroradiology and Musculoskeletal Radiology, Department of Biomedical Imaging and Image-guided Therapy, Vienna General Hospital, Medical University of Vienna, Waehringer Guertel 18-20, Vienna 1090, Austria; [d] Ultrasound Private Institution, 15 Ionias Street, Athens 14671, Greece; [e] Nuffield Orthopaedic Centre, Oxford University Hospitals NHS Trust, Windmill Road, Oxford, OX3 7LD, UK
* Corresponding author.
E-mail address: sudolszopinska@gmail.com

radiologic.theclinics.com

- Comparison of the target joint with the asymptomatic contralateral side
- Assessment of the tendons, joints by dynamic ultrasound
- Presentation of the pathologies to patients to increase their compliance
- Noninvasive character
- Invasive procedures guidance

The disadvantages of ultrasound include the following:

- Low specificity, because several arthropathies exhibit the same spectrum of features. This includes, among others, undifferentiated arthritis, in which neither imaging nor immunologic nor laboratory tests allow diagnosis
- Inability to assess the bone marrow
- Limited field of view
- Considerable dependence on the examiner's experience and equipment quality
- Steep learning curve

Inflammatory Features in the Peripheral Joints

Synovitis

Synovitis is the early sign of rheumatic diseases both inflammatory, such as connective tissue diseases and spondyloarthritides, and noninflammatory arthropathies, such as osteoarthritis and crystallopathies. It is visible as synovial thickening of various degrees in a joint capsule, tendon sheath, or bursa resulting from hyperplasia of the intima layer of the synovium and edema of the underlying subintima caused by its inflammatory infiltrates.[11] Inflamed synovium is of low echogenicity, similar to that of an effusion, which usually accompanies synovial pathology (Fig. 1).[4,8–10,12] The

differentiation between these 2 pathologies is possible by applying pressure with a transducer, which causes slight compression of the thickened synovium and movement or swirling of low-pressure effusions.[2,4,8–10] Active synovitis is characterized by neoangiogenesis, and results in increased vascularity. As the disease progresses, Doppler ultrasound reveals blood flow in the synovium, the intensity of which (the number of vessels) correlates with the severity of inflammation (Fig. 2).[2,13–15] In chronic conditions, synovial hypertrophy is observed and echogenicity of the synovium increases. This hypertrophied synovium assumes varied forms that may undergo fragmentation, which results in the appearance of so-called "rice bodies."

Erosions, cartilage loss, and inflammatory cysts

Erosions, resulting from the destructive activity of the pannus, initially develop between the border of an articular surface covered with cartilage and the joint capsule attachment (the so-called *bare area* and the so-called *marginal erosions*). Subsequently, erosions develop in the subchondral bone of a joint, which is preceded by cartilage damage (so-called *subchondral erosions*). Erosions are visible on ultrasound as cortical bone defects of various sizes in 2 perpendicular planes, filled with the synovial membrane that is inactive or demonstrates features of blood flow (Fig. 3).[2,4,8–10,12,16]

An analogous destructive process can occur in the bone marrow, where certain cytokines promote osteoclasts that destroy trabeculae. The result of this destructive process is the formation of inflammatory cysts, which become erosions when the cortical bone is disrupted[11,14,17,18] (Fig. 4). The progressive erosional-destructive process leads to the destruction of joint surfaces, with subluxation of the joint. As on radiographs, an ultrasound examination does not enable the assessment of all joint surfaces. This is a potential disadvantage of ultrasound when compared with MR imaging.[4,8]

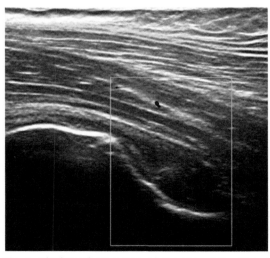

Fig. 1. Thickened synovium of the hip joint without increased vascularization.

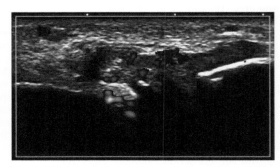

Fig. 2. Thickened, hyperemic synovium of the MTP 1 joint.

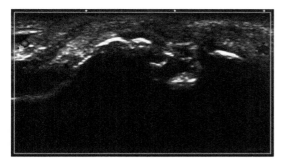

Fig. 3. Erosions in the MTP 5 joint.

Tenosynovitis and Tendinopathy

Tenosynovitis is manifest by thickened synovium in the tendon sheath, and is frequently associated with hypervascularization and accompanying effusions (Fig. 5).[4,9,12]

Inflammatory vessels originating in a tendon sheath may, later in the course of the disease, infiltrate the tendon. The inflammatory process causes tendon weakness and predisposes to tendon damage that is seen initially as a partial tear, and, subsequently, as a complete tear (Fig. 6).[14] A spontaneous tear is a typical feature of rheumatoid arthritis. Before surgery for a full-thickness tendon tear, the quality of the remaining tendon, the level of damage, the distance between tendon stumps, and the distance between unaltered fragments should be assessed.[4] A dynamic examination reveals splitting stumps. Ultrasound dynamic examination helps also reveal an abnormal shift of a tendon (eg, extensor carpi ulnaris) caused by stretching or tearing of its retinaculum. Moreover, in the case of adhesions between a tendon and a sheath (postsurgical, postinflammatory), the mobility of the tendon in relation to the sheath is restricted. The same concerns a tendon sheath/retinaculum conflict.

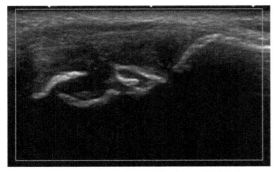

Fig. 4. Erosion and small cysts in the MCP 2 joint.

Enthesopathy

Enthesitis affecting tendons, ligaments, joint capsules and fasciae is considered the typical feature of peripheral spondylarthritis (SpA). The clinical examination for enthesitis is sometimes equivocal and ultrasound is helpful to identify an abnormal enthesis. However, to date, there are no known morphologic features in either histopathological or imaging studies that would enable the differentiation between inflammation and chronic overuse, microinjury, and degeneration of the entheses.[19,20] What is more, there are several hypotheses regarding the etiology of enthesitis, including mechanical, inflammatory, autoimmune, and genetic causes.[21] McGonagle and colleagues[22] proposed an enthesitis-based model for the pathogenesis of spondyloarthritis when interactions between biomechanical factors and the innate immune response (eg, to bacterial products) may lead to disease. Recent studies have shown that mechanical strain plays an important role in enthesitis and bone formation in SpA, and underscored the importance of stromal cells.[23] Regardless of the pathogenesis, an ultrasound image usually demonstrates a thickened and inhomogeneous attachment due to its inflammatory edema, structural intratendinous tears, and scars. Vessels of the inflammatory-repair process can be observed, as well as cysts and erosions in the bony attachment[2,8] (Fig. 7). However, according to the study by Feydy and colleagues,[24] neither power doppler ultrasound nor MR imaging can discriminate between patients with SpA and without SpA and the differential diagnosis includes enthesopathy due to overuse and traumatic lesions.

Bursitis

Bursitis is manifest by thickening and increased blood flow in the synovium of the bursa, and effusions.[9] A bursa that is filled with fluid and hypertrophied synovium can rupture (usually the gastrocnemius-semimembranosus bursa) or may compress adjacent nerves (femoral nerve by iliopsoas bursa, median nerve by bicipitoradialis bursa). The ongoing inflammatory process within bursae can lead to the development of erosions in its bony wall or inflammation in the surrounding soft tissues (Fig. 8).

Inflammation of the Intra-articular and Extra-articular Fat Tissue

The fat tissue, both intra-articular as well as extra-articular, next to the synovium and subchondral bone tissue, is another site for inflammatory processes.[25,26] Ultrasound signs that indicate

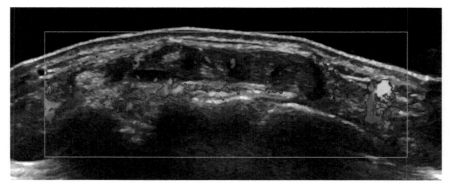

Fig. 5. Tenosynovitis of the fourth compartment of extensor tendons in a 32-year-old woman.

fat-tissue inflammation are its increased echogenicity and hyperemia (**Fig. 9**).[26]

Peripheral Neuropathies

In patients with arthritides, ultrasound enables the determination of the level and cause of nerve compression by inflammatory lesions, hematomas, metal devices, or nerve entrapment in scars. Also, it can help to differentiate of the origin of various symptoms (eg, Wartenberg syndrome from de Quervain tenosynovitis or from trapeziometacarpal joint synovitis).[7,27] The most commonly encountered neuropathies in arthritis are the following:

- Median nerve compression (mainly at the level of the wrist as a result of carpal tunnel narrowing due to tenosynovitis of the flexor digitorum tendons, so-called carpal tunnel syndrome) (**Fig. 10**)
- Ulnar nerve impingement (mainly at the level of the elbow joint as a result of nerve compression by inflammatory lesions in the posterior joint recess, proliferative degenerative changes, or ganglia)
- Tibial nerve compression (at the level of the tarsal tunnel by inflammatory lesions in the

joint recess or effusions in the tendon sheaths of the flexor digitorum and hallucis longus)
- Interdigital perineural fibrosis (so-called Morton neuroma, which may result from compression of the neurovascular bundle by intermetatarsophalangeal bursa inflammation)
- Femoral nerve compression (irritation by the iliopsoas bursitis or hematomas after endoprosthesoplasty)
- Sciatic nerve neuropathy (direct damage during endoprosthesoplasty, or impingement by a hematoma)

ROLE OF ULTRASOUND IN THE DIAGNOSIS AND MONITORING OF SPECIFIC ARTHRITIDES
Connective Tissue Disorders

Rheumatoid arthritis
Rheumatoid arthritis (RA) has a typical appearance, which is usually characterized by symmetric involvement of multiple synovial joints in both the upper and lower limbs. Involvement is typically seen in the wrist, MCP (metacarpophalangeal), MTP (metatarsophalangeal), and PIP (proximal interphalangeal) joints of the hands and feet. Two characteristic sites for foot RA include the interphalangeal joint of the big toe

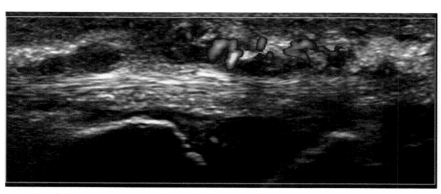

Fig. 6. Tenosynovitis of the extensor carpi ulnaris tendon sheath.

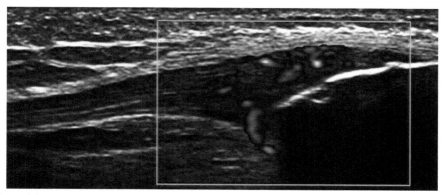

Fig. 7. Thickened, hyperemic proximal enthesis of the patellar tendon in a 17-year-old girl with JIA, with a small cyst in an attachment; enthesitis.

and MTP 5 joint. Tendon sheaths and bursae are involved as well (Fig. 11). Significantly, tenosynovitis can be the only manifestation of RA. Other lesions include rheumatoid nodules, which are the most common cutaneous manifestation of active RA.[10] Ultrasound can visualize the early stages of inflammation within the soft tissues.[2,9,28,29]

Typical for chronic RA are tendon tears, both in small joints (typical spontaneous tearings of tendons of the hand) and large joints (eg, rotator cuff tears).[28]

In RA, ultrasound

- Helps identify synovial pathologies in joint cavities, tendon sheaths, and bursae, their location and activity (vascularization)
- Enables a diagnosis of destructive lesions that result from the activity of pannus (cysts, bony erosions, articular cartilage destruction, and tendon injuries)
- Is conducted to monitor the efficacy of treatment, guide drug administration or joint decompression, and to confirm remission

Juvenile idiopathic arthritis

Juvenile idiopathic arthritis (JIA) is the most common chronic, systemic autoimmune disease of the connective tissue that affects both children and adolescents.[30] The disease most frequently affects the knees (frequently with a monoarticular onset), hands and wrists, and hip, ankle, and tarsal joints. Ultrasound findings are similar to the features in RA.[31]

In JIA, ultrasound[32–36]

- Can evaluate the activity of the inflammation (persistent activity is a risk factor for subsequent destructive disease)
- Has higher sensitivity than clinical assessment in monitoring treatment effects
- Can diagnose subclinical JIA, which can result in reclassification of the type of JIA, mainly from oligoarthritis to polyarthritis

Adult-onset Still disease

Still disease shares characteristics of RA and is considered an adult form of JIA. At the ultrasound examination, signs of arthritis are sought, as in RA and JIA.

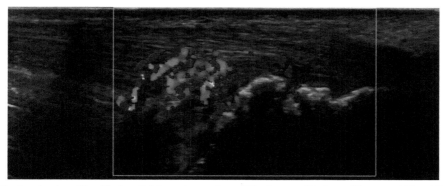

Fig. 8. Achilles tendon bursitis: effusion, thickened synovium of the bursa with signs of increased blood flow; erosions in the calcaneal wall of the bursa; inflammatory vessels of the bursa infiltrating the Achilles tendon leading to tears.

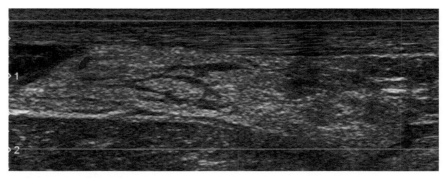

Fig. 9. Edema of the Kager fat pad tissue.

Systemic lupus erythematosus

One of the most common manifestations of systemic lupus erythematosus (SLE) is lupus arthritis, which can affect any joint. The disease typically involves numerous joints symmetrically, usually in the hand (wrist, MCP, and PIP), and sometimes in the foot.

Periarticular tissue inflammation is typical and may lead to joint subluxation and contracture, called Jaccoud arthropathy. Spontaneous tendon tears may be concomitant. Hand deformity in SLE is named "lupus hand." The form of the disease with deformities and erosions is referred to as *rhupus*.

Ultrasound is used to diagnose the following:

- Tenosynovitis, tendinitis, and tendon damage
- Arthritis
- Erosions in patients with deformities

Scleroderma, systemic sclerosis, progressive systemic sclerosis

The disease involves the skin, subcutaneous tissue, muscles, bones, and joints. The following lesions may be seen: soft tissue atrophy usually occurring in the fingers, calcifications in the soft tissues, and bone resorption, which can affect various anatomic regions (**Fig. 12**).[37,38]

Ultrasound is used to diagnose the following:

- Skin and subcutaneous involvement in systemic sclerosis (SSc) as a progressive thickening and increased echogenicity due to fibrosis, also referred to as morphea
- Calcifications in soft tissues (calcinosis), including incipient digital calcifications that may inflame or ulcerate in more than a negligible proportion of cases
- Synovitis, tenosynovitis, myositis, bone changes (erosions, acroosteolysis)
- Overlap conditions, consisting of SSc and RA, or SSc and myositis (also called scleromyositis), which requires the early initiation of adequate therapy.

Polymyositis, dermatomyositis

Polymyositis (PM) is a chronic inflammation of striated muscles, and dermatomyositis (DM) is a form of PM with accompanying dermatitis.

Ultrasound can

- Differentiate the cause of improper position of fingers (contracture, tendon tear, or articular surface damage)
- Identify the signs of myositis

Sjögren syndrome

Within the musculoskeletal system, the spectrum of inflammatory changes seen in patients with

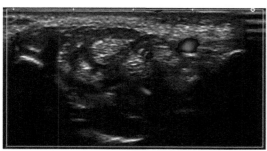

Fig. 10. Medial nerve compression by the flexor digitorum tendon tenosynovitis.

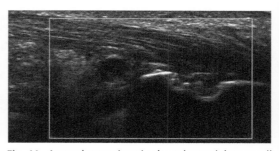

Fig. 11. Avascular erosions in the calcaneal, bony wall of the Achilles tendon bursa, typical of chronic RA.

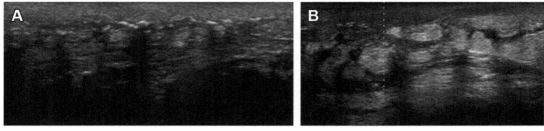

Fig. 12. Scleroderma, numerous small calcifications (*A*), edema and increased echogenicity of subcutaneous tissues (*B*).

Sjögren syndrome is identical to that in RA: synovial pathologies; effusions, erosions, and cysts.

Mixed connective tissue disease

Mixed connective tissue disease is a chronic systemic inflammatory disease with clinical and radiological features of more than one connective tissue disorder, such as SLE, SSc, PM (or DM), RA, or psoriatic arthritis (PsA).

At ultrasound, signs of arthritis, cysts, erosions, and periarticular calcifications may be seen.

Spondyloarthritis

The most frequently affected joints in SpA are the hip and glenohumeral joint,[39] followed by knee, ankle, and foot. Ultrasound is used to diagnose a spectrum of pathology in the peripheral SpA, presenting with symptoms of enthesitis, arthritis, and dactylitis.

Ultrasound is used to diagnose the following:

- Inflammatory lesions in the peripheral joints, sheaths, and bursae, similar to those seen in RA
- Enthesopathy, mainly at the calcaneal tuberosity, clinically diagnosed as enthesis, which

radiographically does not differ from those seen in degenerative, overload enthesopathy
- Features of PsA,[8,40–42] such as dactylitis (**Fig. 13**), extracapsular inflammation, PIP, and especially distal interphalangeal joint involvement that differentiates PsA from RA
- Juvenile SpA (JSpA), in which the disease usually begins with inflammation in a single joint or several or multiple large lower-limb joints; depending on the type of JSpA, one of the first involved joints can be the sternoclavicular joints (**Fig. 14**), or first MTP and interphalangeal joints, and, sometimes (mainly reactive and juvenile enteropathic arthritis), sausage toes are seen

Osteoarthritis

Articular cartilage breakdown, osteophyte formation, subchondral sclerosis, and bone marrow lesions are best seen on conventional radiographs, CT,[28] and MR imaging. Ultrasound is used to diagnose synovitis, and can visualize proliferative changes and cartilage loss in areas that are assessible with ultrasound. In patients with RA, secondary osteoarthritis (OA) may develop, which complicates the diagnosis due

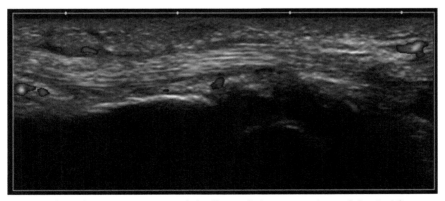

Fig. 13. Dactylitis resulting from tenosynovitis of the flexor digitorum tendons of the 2nd finger.

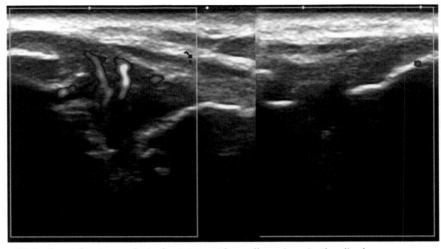

Fig. 14. Synovitis in the right sterno-clavicular joint, with small erosions in the diaphyses.

to overlap syndromes. The same is true for enthesitis, which is considered to initiate OA in some patients, whereas, so far, being specific for SpA only.[19]

Crystal Diseases

The most common diseases caused by crystals are gout, pyrophosphate arthropathy, and hydroxyapatite arthropathy.[25,28,39,42]

Gout

Usually, the first involved joints are the MTP and interphalangeal joints of the great toe.

In an acute arthritis (gout attack), ultrasound shows the following:

- Thickening and hypervascularization of the synovium in joint capsules, tendon sheaths (particularly of flexors and extensors of the hand), and bursae (particularly the prepatellar and olecranon bursa). As the disease progresses, the synovium becomes rich in hyperechoic foci (a snowstorm sign: starry sky)
- Effusions: anechoic in the first gout attack, and subsequently with single hyperechoic echoes, tiny or clustered, representing sodium urate crystals
- The incrustation of the superficial layer of the hyaline cartilage, the so-called *double contour image* resulting from the presence of a hyperechoic bone contour and a parallel layer of sodium urate deposition, divided by a layer of hypoechoic cartilage (**Fig. 15**)

Chronic gout (crystal deposits in joints and soft tissues) in ultrasound presents with the same spectrum as in the acute phase and additionally the following:

- Hyperechoic, hypoechoic, or isoechoic solid gouty nodules (tophi) localized in the periarticular subcutaneous tissue, usually on the ulnar side of the hands and the extensor side of the knees and elbows; they are initially homogeneous and later heterogeneous, sometimes with acoustic posterior shadowing or hypoechoic halo around the tophi, a sign of inflammation of the adjacent tissues (**Fig. 16**)
- Tendon and ligament heterogeneity, thickening, including entheseal inflammatory and

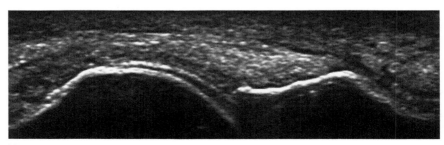

Fig. 15. Double contour sign at the MTP 1 joint.

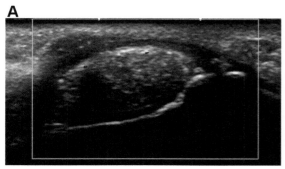
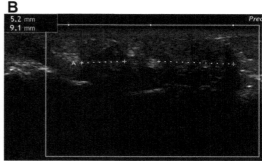

Fig. 16. Hyperechoic, avascular tophus with calcifications, localized in the soft tissues at the PIP 3 joint level (A), and 2 hypoechoic tophi at the ulnar side of the wrist (B).

postinflammatory lesions secondary to the presence of gouty nodules
• Bony lesions: cysts, characteristic erosions, and proliferative reactions

Calcium pyrophosphate dihydrate deposition disease, chondrocalcinosis
On ultrasound, the following features can be seen:

• Calcification in the layer of the hyaline cartilage, usually of the femoral condyle and the head of the humerus, first scattered and later linear and parallel to the bone and cartilage outline
• Calcification within tendon and ligament attachments, mostly within the Achilles tendon
• Calcification in the triangular fibrocartilage complex or within the meniscus

Ultrasound enables the collection of synovial fluid for microscopic analysis.

Hydroxyapatite deposition disease, calcium hydroxyapatite, crystal deposition disease, basic calcium phosphate crystal deposition disease
Ultrasound shows the following:

• Synovial pathologies (thickening, hyperemia) and effusions in joints and bursae
• Calcifications in tendons and bursae with or without a subsequent posterior acoustic shadow, including calcium deposits, usually localized between the layer of the upper humeral capsule and the supraspinatus tendon
• Partial or complete tendon tears, including "Milwaukee shoulder"

MONITORING OF ARTHRITIS AND ESTABLISHING REMISSION

Ultrasound is used to diagnose and follow-up treatment results. The assessment of inflammatory lesions in a ultrasound examination, both at the initial stage and during follow-up, is usually qualitative. Power Doppler (PD) or color Doppler signal also can be assessed either semiquantitatively or using quantification methods, after placing a region of interest in the area of interest or calculating a resistive index from spectral Doppler measurements of flow (Fig. 17).[8] PD scores correlate well both with clinical disease activity and serum biomarkers.[4,8,43,44] Nevertheless, semiquantitative and quantificative measures are rarely used in clinical practice. This is also true of microbubble sonographic contrast agents.

In patients following joint replacement, ultrasound is used to diagnose and monitor postoperative complications, which include abnormal fluid collections in the region of an endoprosthesis, hematomas at various stages of resorption and organization, abscesses, tendon injuries, neuropathies, for example, peroneal nerve palsy following knee joint replacement, or sciatic nerve damage during hip joint replacement.

In case of remission, in a substantial number of cases, residual disease cannot be differentiated from chronic arthritis. For example, a definitive answer of whether or not avascular synovium is inactive or represents a chronic stage of disease

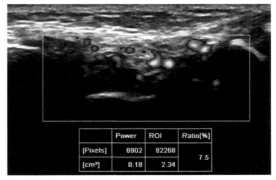

	Power	ROI	Ratio[%]
[Pixels]	6902	92268	7.5
[cm²]	0.18	2.34	

Fig. 17. Quantification of radio-carpal and midcarpal joint synovitis.

is impossible. The criteria for remission in ultrasound examination, both in adults and in children with JIA, have not yet been established.[45–48]

ULTRASOUND-GUIDED INTERVENTIONS IN PATIENTS WITH ARTHRITIS

Flexibility, availability, and low cost make ultrasound the best tool to guide interventional therapeutic procedures.[49,50] These procedures can be divided into diagnostic and therapeutic interventions, and include[49–52] the following:

- Biopsy for diagnostic purposes
- Arthrocentesis for diagnostic purposes
- Joint and soft tissue injections (corticosteroids, hyaluronic acid)
- Drainage (bursitis, hematomas)
- Treatment of cystic lesions (ganglia, popliteal cysts)
- Percutaneous lavage (barbotage) and debridement for crystal arthropathies
- Monitoring of radioisotope administration during radioisotope synovectomy

SUMMARY

Ultrasound is currently an integrated part of the workup in patients with rheumatic diseases, for both adults and children. Ultrasound has several advantages, which have been listed in many articles, including a consensus paper of the European Society of Musculoskeletal Radiology experts.[53] Among the limitations of the method, low specificity is the most important one. New developments in ultrasound have opened perspectives for a more precise diagnosis. These include more sensitive Doppler techniques and tools for quantification of inflammation, elastography, fusion techniques, and 3-dimensional ultrasound. However, at present, evidence suggests these techniques do not provide any revolution in terms of quantification of synovitis or improved specificity.[4,8,54] A further disadvantage of ultrasound is that it provides no information about the intramedullary bone structure. Marrow edema-like lesions detected on MR imaging are known to be an important prognostic factor and are considered biomarkers for disease progression.[4]

The most urgent research priorities for ultrasound include the following[2,10,47]:

1. Identification of more sensitive and specific ultrasound features that will provide early diagnosis and identification of high-risk patients
2. Clarification of definitive outcome measurements, including quantification to provide increased accuracy in monitoring disease
3. Establishing remission criteria

REFERENCES

1. Narvaez JA, Narvaez J, De Lama E, et al. MR imaging of early rheumatoid arthritis. Radiographics 2010;30:143–63.
2. Boutry N, Morel M, Flipo RM, et al. Early rheumatoid arthritis: a review of MRI and sonographic findings. AJR Am J Roentgenol 2007;189:1502–9.
3. Freeston JE, Bird P, Conaghan G. The role of MRI in rheumatoid arthritis: research and clinical issues. Curr Opin Rheumatol 2009;21:95–101.
4. Grainger AJ, Rawbotham EL. Rheumatoid arthritis. Semin Musculoskelet Radiol 2013;1(17):69–73.
5. Teh J. Ultrasound of soft tissue masses of the hand. J Ultrason 2012;12:381–401.
6. Tan AL, McGonagle D. Psoriatic arthritis: correlation between imaging and pathology. Joint Bone Spine 2010;77:206–11.
7. Wilson D, Allen GM. Imaging of the carpal tunnel. Semin Musculoskelet Radiol 2012;2(16):137–73.
8. Rowbotham EL, Wakefield RJ, Grainger AJ. The technique and application of ultrasound in the diagnosis and management of inflammatory arthritis. Semin Musculoskelet Radiol 2012;5(16):360–6.
9. Boutry N, Moraes do Carmo CC, Flipo R-M, et al. Early rheumatoid arthritis and its differentiation from other joint abnormalities. Eur J Radiol 2009;71:217–24.
10. Rowbotham EL, Grainger AJ. Rheumatoid arthritis: ultrasound versus MRI. AJR Am J Roentgenol 2011;197:541–6.
11. Sudoł-Szopińska I, Kontny E, Maśliński W, et al. The pathogenesis of rheumatoid arthritis in radiological studies. Part I: Formation of inflammatory infiltrates within the synovial membrane. J Ultrason 2012;12(49):202–21.
12. Wakefield RJ, Balint PV, Szkudlarek M, et al. Musculoskeletal ultrasound including definitions for ultrasonographic pathology. J Rheumatol 2005;32:2485–7.
13. Ellegard K, Torp-Pedersen S, Terslev L, et al. Ultrasound colour Doppler measurements in a single joint as measure of disease activity in patients with rheumatoid arthritis–assessment of concurrent validity. Rheumatology 2009;48:254–7.
14. Bliddal H, Boesen M, Christensen R, et al. Imaging as a follow-up tool in clinical trials and clinical practice. Best Pract Res Clin Rheumatol 2008;22:1109–26.
15. Gullick NJ, Evans HG, Church LD, et al. Linking power Doppler ultrasound to the presence of Th17 cells in the rheumatoid arthritis joint. PLoS One 2010;5:e125160.
16. Grainger AJ, McGonagle D. Imaging in rheumatology. Imaging 2007;19:310–23.
17. Bugatti S, Caporali R, Manzo A, et al. Involvement of subchondral bone marrow in rheumatoid arthritis: lymphoid neogenesis and in situ relationship to

subchondral bone marrow osteoclast recruitment. Arthritis Rheum 2005;52:3448–59.

18. Jimenez-Boy E, Redlich K, Türk B, et al. Interaction between synovial inflammatory tissue and bone marrow in rheumatoid arthritis. J Immunol 2005; 175:2579–88.

19. McGonagle D, Hermann K-GA, Tan AL. Differentiation between osteoarthritis and psoriatic arthritis: implications for pathogenesis and treatment in the biologic therapy era. Rheumatology 2015;54: 29–38.

20. Sudoł-Szopińska I, Kwiatkowska B, Prochorec-Sobieszek M, et al. Enthesopathies and enthesitis. Part 2: Imaging studies. J Ultrason 2015;15:196–207.

21. Sudoł-Szopińska I, Kwiatkowska B, Prochorec-Sobeszek M, et al. Enthesopathies and enthesitis. Part 1. Etiopathogenesis. J Ultrason 2015;15(60): 72–84.

22. McGonagle D, Stockwin L, Isaacs J, et al. An enthesitis based model for the pathogenesis of spondyloarthropathy additive effects of microbial adjuvant and biomechanical factors at diseases sites. J Rheumatol 2001;28:2155–9.

23. Jacques P, Lambrecht S, Verheugen E, et al. Proof of concept: enthesitis and new bone formation in SpA are driven by mechanical strain and stromal cells. Ann Rheum Dis 2014;73:437–45.

24. Feydy A, Lavie-Bryon MC, Gossec L, et al. Comparative study of MRI and power Doppler ultrasonography of the heel in patients with spondyloarthritis with and without heel pain and in controls. Ann Rheum Dis 2012;71:498–503.

25. Kontny E, Plebanczyk M, Lisowska B, et al. Comparison of rheumatoid articular adipose and synovial tissue reactivity to proinflammatory stimuli: contribution to adipocytokine network. Ann Rheum Dis 2012; 71:262–7.

26. Sudoł-Szopińska I, Kontny E, Zaniewicz-Kaniewska K, et al. Role of inflammatory factors and adipose tissue in pathogenesis of rheumatoid arthritis and osteoarthritis. Part I: rheumatoid adipose tissue. J Ultrason 2013;13:192–201.

27. Tagliafico A, Cadoni A, Fisci E, et al. Nerves of the hand beyond the carpal tunnel. Semin Musculoskelet Radiol 2012;2(16):129–36.

28. Sankaye P, Ostlere S. Arthritis at the shoulder joint. Semin Musculoskelet Radiol 2015;3(19):307–17.

29. Boutry N, Khalil C, Jaspart M, et al. Imaging of the hip in patients with rheumatic disorders. Eur J Radiol 2007;63:49–58.

30. Ravelli A, Martini A. Juvenile idiopathic arthritis. Lancet 2007;369:767–78.

31. Malattia C, Damasio MB, Magnaguagno F, et al. Magnetic resonance imaging, ultrasonography, and conventional radiography in the assessment of bone erosions in juvenile idiopathic arthritis. Arthritis Rheum 2008;59(12):1764–72.

32. Sparchez M, Fodor D, Miu N. The role of power Doppler ultrasonography in comparison with biological markers in evaluation of disease activity in juvenile idiopathic arthritis. Med Ultrason 2010;12(2): 97–103.

33. Kakati P, Sodhi KS, Sandhu MS, et al. Clinical and ultrasound assessment of the knee in children with juvenile rheumatoid arthritis. Indian J Pediatr 2007; 74(9):831–6.

34. Wakefield RJ, Green MJ, Marzo-Ortega H, et al. Should oligoarthritis be reclassified? Ultrasound reveals a high prevalence of subclinical disease. Ann Rheum Dis 2004;63:382–5.

35. Magni-Manzoni S, Epis O, Ravelli A, et al. Comparison of clinical versus ultrasound-determined synovitis in juvenile idiopathic arthritis. Arthritis Rheum 2009;61(11):1497–504.

36. Breton S, Jousse-Joulin S, Cangemi C, et al. Comparison of clinical and ultrasonographic evaluations for peripheral synovitis in juvenile idiopathic arthritis. Semin Arthritis Rheum 2011;41:272–8.

37. Pracoń G, Płaza M, Walntowska-Janowicz M, et al. The value of ultrasound in the diagnosis of limited scleroderma–a case report. J Ultrason 2015;15: 326–31.

38. Boutry N, Hachulla E, Zanetti-Musielak C, et al. Imaging features of musculoskeletal involvement in systemic sclerosis. Eur Radiol 2007;17:1172–80.

39. Resnick D. Diagnosis of bone and joint disorders. 4th edition. Philadelphia: WB Saunders; 2002. p. 1023–54, 1082–1089.

40. Coates LC, Hodgson R, Conaghan PG, et al. MRI and ultrasonography for diagnosis and monitoring of psoriatic arthritis. Best Pract Res Clin Rheumatol 2012;26:805–22.

41. Fournie B, Margarit-Coll N, Champetier de Ribes TL, et al. Extrasynovial ultrasound abnormalities in the psoriatic finger. Prospective comparative power-Doppler study versus rheumatoid arthritis. Joint Bone Spine 2006;73(5):527–31.

42. O'Connor P. Cristal deposition disease and psoriatic arthritis. Semin Musculoskelet Radiol 2013;1(17): 74–9.

43. Ribbens C, Andre B, Marcelis S, et al. Rheumatoid hand joint synovitis: gray-scale and power Doppler US quantifications following anti-tumor necrosis factor-alpha treatment: pilot study. Radiology 2003; 229:562–9.

44. Weidekamm C, Köller M, Weber M, et al. Diagnostic value of high-resolution B-mode and Doppler sonography for imaging of hand and finger joints in rheumatoid arthritis. Arthritis Rheum 2003;48(2): 325–33.

45. Breton S, Jousse-Joulin S, Finel E, et al. Imaging approaches for evaluating peripheral joint abnormalities in juvenile idiopathic arthritis. Semin Arthritis Rheum 2011;41(5):698–711.

46. Karmazyn B, Bowyer L, Schmidt KM, et al. US findings of metacarpophalangeal joints in children with idiopathic juvenile arthritis. Pediatr Radiol 2007;37: 475–82.

47. Cellerini M, Salti S, Trapani S, et al. Correlation between clinical and ultrasound assessment of the knee in children with mono-articular or pauci-articular juvenile idiopathic arthritis. Pediatr Radiol 1999;29:117–23.

48. Gylys VM, Graham TB, Blebea JS, et al. Knee in early juvenile rheumatoid arthritis: MR imaging findings. Radiology 2001;220:696–706.

49. Davidson J, Jayaraman S. Guided interventions in musculoskeletal ultrasound: what's the evidence? Clin Radiol 2011;66:140e152.

50. del Cura JL. Ultrasound-guided therapeutic procedures in the musculoskeletal system. Curr Probl Diagn Radiol 2008;37:203–18.

51. Kowalska B. Ultrasound-guided joint and soft tissue interventions. J Ultrason 2014;14:163–70.

52. Ćwikła JB, Zbikowski P, Kwiatkowska B, et al. Radiosynovectomy in rheumatic diseases. J Ultrason 2014;14:241–51.

53. Klauser A, Tagliafico A, Allen GM, et al. Clinical indications for musculoskeletal ultrasound: a Delphi-based consensus paper of the European Society of Musculoskeletal Radiology. Eur Radiol 2012;22: 1140–8.

54. Drakonaki E. Ultrasound elastography for imaging tendons and muscles. J Ultrason 2012;12(49):214–25.

Computed Tomography and MR Imaging in Rheumatoid Arthritis

Antonio Barile, MD[a],*, Francesco Arrigoni, MD[a],
Federico Bruno, MD[a], Giuseppe Guglielmi, MD[b],
Marcello Zappia, MD[c], Alfonso Reginelli, MD[d],
Piero Ruscitti, MD[e], Paola Cipriani, MD[e],
Roberto Giacomelli, MD[e], Luca Brunese, MD[c],
Carlo Masciocchi, MD[a]

KEYWORDS

- Rheumatoid arthritis imaging • MR imaging • CT • Rheumatology imaging

KEY POINTS

- Rheumatoid arthritis (RA) is one of the most prevalent chronic inflammatory diseases that primarily affects joints.
- Clinical diagnosis of RA is supported by imaging findings, especially using CT and MR imaging; knowledge of the different imaging sequences and study protocols is important to obtain the best diagnostic information.
- Early diagnosis and prompt initiation of treatment, also guided by the imaging findings, are important to reduce structural damage and disability in patients with RA.

INTRODUCTION

Rheumatoid arthritis (RA) is one of the most prevalent chronic inflammatory diseases that primarily affects joints, but it has been shown to be associated with extra-articular manifestations and systemic comorbidities.[1] Its prevalence is approximately 1% to 2% of the world's population and is more common in the female population between 30 and 50 years of age. Articular and periarticular manifestations of these patients include joint swelling and tenderness, with morning stiffness and severe motion impairment in the involved joints. The clinical presentation of RA varies, but an insidious onset of pain with symmetric swelling of small joints is the most frequent finding. Although RA may affect any joint, it is typically found in metacarpophalangeal (MCP), proximal interphalangeal, and metatarsophalangeal joints, as well as in the wrists and knee.[2]

Joint swelling in RA reflects synovial membrane inflammation consequent to immune activation,

Disclosure Statement: The authors have nothing to disclose.
[a] Diagnostic and Interventional Radiology, Department of Biotechnological and Applied Clinical Sciences, University of L'Aquila, Via Vetoio 1, L'Aquila, Coppito 67100, Italy; [b] Department of Radiology, Scientific Institute Hospital "Casa Sollievo della Sofferenza" S. Giovanni Rotondo, University of Foggia, v.le Cappuccini 1, San Giovanni Rotondo, Foggia 71013, Italy; [c] Department of Medicine and Health Science "V. Tiberio", University of Molise, Via F. De Santis, Campobasso 86100, Italy; [d] Department of Internal and Experimental Medicine, Magrassi-Lanzara, Institute of Radiology, Second University of Naples, Via Pansini 6, Naples 80131, Italy; [e] Department of Biotechnological and Applied Clinical Sciences, Rheumatology Clinic, University of L'Aquila, Via Vetoio 1, L'Aquila, Coppito 67100, Italy
* Corresponding author.
E-mail addresses: antonio.barile@cc.univaq.it; abarile63@gmail.com

Radiol Clin N Am 55 (2017) 997–1007
http://dx.doi.org/10.1016/j.rcl.2017.04.006

and it is characterized by leukocyte infiltration into the synovial compartment. A strong tissue response mediated by different cells occurs in the affected joints. Synovial fibroblasts assume an aggressive inflammatory, matrix regulatory, and invasive phenotype, together with enhanced chondrocyte catabolism and synovial osteoclastogenesis. This mechanism results in cartilage degradation and bone erosion, thus leading to articular destruction.[1,2]

RA clinical diagnosis is supported by imaging findings. In the American College of Rheumatology (ACR)/European League Against Rheumatism (EULAR) 2010 criteria for RA classification, RA is based on the presence of clinical synovitis (swelling at clinical examination) in 1 or more joints with the absence of an alternative diagnosis that better explains the synovitis.[3,4] Because MR imaging has proven its value in imaging joint pathology,[5–15] its role is also established in the evaluation of joint involvement in RA.[16,17]

Early diagnosis and target therapy can stop or, at least, slow the disease progression. The disappearance of the rheumatoid inflammatory process is the major therapeutic target; if inflammation is reduced, physical function may be strongly improved without further structural damage of the affected joints.

IMAGING TECHNIQUE

Imaging techniques have played an important role in assessing disease progression and response to treatment in RA for many years. Conventional radiology (CR) has played an essential role in diagnosing and measuring progression of RA.

More recently, MR imaging, directly visualizing bone and soft tissues and measuring inflammatory activity, has gained the most important role in the management of this pathology.

MR imaging is increasingly being used because of its superiority over CR in detecting bone erosion, osteitis, and synovitis and for its high rate of reproducibility. Ultrasound, despite being a very diffuse and handy technique,[18,19] is highly operator-dependent and lacks a standardized method of measurement reproducibility. An example is represented by controversy in measuring the synovial thickness that is one of the most important findings identified with ultrasound.[20]

MR Imaging Scanners

High-field MR imaging is the most used modality to image joints affected by RA in both clinical and research settings. Since the introduction of extremity-dedicated low-field magnets (<0.5 T), there has been interest in comparing the diagnostic performance of these patient-friendly scanners to high-field (>1.0 T) scanners.[21] High-field MR imaging scanners generate images of higher resolution and better signal-to-noise ratio (SNR). This, however, does not necessarily translate into a greater diagnostic power, especially in patients with RA. Imaging hands and wrists in whole-body high-field scanners may also be complicated by uncomfortable positioning of the patient ("Superman" position). This problem can be solved using dedicated low-field (0.2–0.4 T) and high-field (1.0 T) extremity scanners, the newly developed "mid-field" open scanners (0.6–1.0 T), or the newest whole-body high-field (1.5–3.0 T) scanners allowing off-center imaging with the hand along the side of the body. Extremity low-field magnets often require less physical space and shielding and use low-field magnets. Cost is also significantly reduced and the machine can be located conveniently in a simple room.[22] Patient comfort is enhanced by the design of the magnet. In addition to all these advantages, however, there are also some drawbacks. Lower magnet strengths result in reduced SNRs and fields of view.[23] In addition, low-field MR imaging presents a limited number of image acquisition techniques, with no possibility to obtain frequency-selective fat-saturation (FS) sequences (which are the optimum for detecting bone edema). The low-field systems use a short-tau inversion-recovery (STIR) sequence, providing fat-suppression images, which are, however, impaired by reduced SNR and limited spatial resolution. Despite all these limitations, it appears that low-field MR imaging is equivalent to high-field MR imaging for the assessment of erosions, although it is less sensitive for edema and requires contrast to adequately identify synovitis.[22] Comparing high-field and low-field MR imaging using the RA MR imaging scoring system (RAMRIS) has also shown good interobserver and intraobserver reproducibility with reference to synovitis, bone marrow edema, and erosions in most studies.[21] The Outcome Measures in Rheumatology Clinical Trials (OMERACT) MR imaging group has also confirmed these findings demonstrating equivalent scores for images obtained in patients with RA using high-field and low-field systems.

Three-Tesla MR imaging can visualize musculoskeletal structures more clearly than 1.5-T MR imaging because of enhanced SNR and higher spatial resolution.[24,25] In addition, the conspicuity of contrast enhancement is likely to be increased compared with lower field scanners due to the relatively stronger shortening of increased T1 relaxation times by gadolinium.[24] With recent advances in MR imaging hardware, 3-T scanners have decreased scan times.[25]

Imaging Protocols and Sequences

To obtain the best possible spatial and contrast resolution, it is crucial to choose proper imaging sequences and study protocols.

We report in **Box 1** the imaging protocols recommended by OMERACT.[26]

Three-dimensional isotropic T1-weighted gradient-echo sequences

A 3-dimensional (3D) isotropic T1-weighted gradient-echo sequence or a T1-weighted spin-echo sequence in the coronal and axial planes is acquired before and after gadolinium injection for detection of erosions and synovitis. The isotropic 3D acquisition offers the advantage of subsequent reconstruction in the orthogonal plane, allowing performance of fewer scan planes and saving patient time in the scanner. Another advantage of the 3D gradient-echo sequence is the smaller voxel size, reducing the partial volume artifact, which can be a problem when dealing with small erosions on the 2D spin-echo sequences with a slice thickness of 2 to 5 mm.[21]

Selective fat suppression or water excitation are important for increasing T1 contrast between cartilage and adjacent joint fluid or subchondral bone (marrow fat) and for eliminating chemical shift effects,[27] which distort cartilage-bone interfaces and can simulate cartilage thinning and joint space narrowing (JSN). Fat-suppressed, T1-weighted, 3D gradient-echo pulse sequences are the most commonly used for evaluating bone erosion in multicenter randomized controlled trials of RA.[27]

Short-time inversion-recovery sequences

Short-time inversion-recovery (STIR) sequences are based on the rapid T1 recovery of fat and are not substantially impaired by field inhomogeneity. However, STIR images have inherently less signal and are not adequate for the detection of contrast medium enhancement because STIR suppresses all short T1 species, including tissues that have absorbed gadolinium.[28]

Iterative decomposition of water and fat with echo asymmetry and least-squares estimation sequences

FS is commonly used in clinical imaging to improve tissue contrast and lesion characterization.[28] However, acquisition of high-quality MR images of the hand and finger with uniform FS is challenging because of the complex magnetic environments commonly encountered during clinical MR imaging.[29] Although higher-field MR imaging can visualize musculoskeletal structures more clearly due to the enhanced SNR and the higher spatial resolution, the tendency to fail to select suppression pulses in chemical shift selective method is increased by higher magnetic inhomogeneity. Adequate fat suppression is critical in identifying and quantifying bone marrow edema (BME) in bone marrow. Factors including field inhomogeneity and motion can cause failure of fat suppression using conventional FS methods.[30]

Iterative decomposition of water and fat with echo asymmetry and least-squares estimation (IDEAL) imaging is a new method that can steadily separate fat and water by using 3 asymmetric echo times and the 3-point Dixon method.[29,30] IDEAL sequences provide images with high SNR and uniform water and fat separation. IDEAL sequences, especially with multifrequency fat reconstruction, are robust to provide uniform water and fat suppression.[30] In addition, IDEAL sequences can provide water, fat, in-phase, out-of-phase, and field map simultaneously, which provide

---

Box 1

Imaging protocols recommended by the rheumatology clinical trials (Outcome Measures in Rheumatology Clinical Trials [OMERACT])

- Coronal and axial T2-weighted iterative decomposition of water and fat with echo asymmetry and least-squares estimation (IDEAL) fast spin-echo (FSE) images (repetition time (TR)/echo time (TE) 1/4 3500/50 ms, in plane resolution 1/4 0.2 mm, slice thickness 1/4 2 mm)

- Coronal T1-weighted IDEAL FSE images (TR/TE 1/4 600/9.9 ms, in plane resolution 1/4 0.4 mm, slice thickness 1/4 2 mm)

- Coronal T1-weighted IDEAL spoiled gradient-echo (SPGR) images (TR/TE 1/4 15.3/2.9 ms, in plane resolution 1/4 0.2 mm, slice thickness 1/4 1 mm)

- Coronal 3-dimensional dynamic contrast-enhanced (DCE) SPGR images acquired during gadolinium-diethylenetriaminopentaacetic (Gd-DTPA) injection (TR/TE 1/4 6.4/2.1 ms, in plane resolution 1/4 0.4 mm, slice thickness 1/4 3 mm, temporal resolution 12 s, 32 time points, agent injection delay 1/4 45 s)

- Postcontrast coronal T1-weighted IDEAL FSE images (using the same parameters as precontrast T1-weighted IDEAL FSE images)

multiple images with different contrast among tissues and may facilitate further image analysis (such as registration between dynamic contrast-enhanced [DCE]-MR imaging and IDEAL fast spin-echo [FSE] images).

Dynamic contrast-enhanced MR imaging sequences

Intravenous contrast is necessary to estimate the degree of synovial inflammation and to differentiate the enhancing synovium from the surrounding tissues.[1,25] Synovitis tends to be overestimated if it is scored based on the STIR or T2 FS images, partly because joint effusion cannot be differentiated from synovitis using the latter sequences.

DCE-MR imaging involves the acquisition of sequential images in rapid succession during and after the intravenous administration of contrast agent,[28,31,32] allowing the time-course of the synovial enhancement to be analyzed. Measurements made from the enhancement curve are sensitive to various parameters, including synovial perfusion and capillary permeability. Consequently, they are expected to be good markers for inflammation. Contrast is usually administered as a rapid, intravenous, bolus injection. A contrast dose of 0.1 mmol/kg gadolinium is usually given, but 0.05 to 0.3 mmol/kg has been used. Injection rate directly affects the DCE-MR imaging measurements, hence consistency is important and a power injector may be helpful.[32] The conflicting demands of joint coverage, temporal resolution, and spatial resolution are particularly important in DCE-MR imaging.[28] Inflamed synovitis enhances rapidly over the first 20 to 30 seconds after a bolus of intravenous contrast and a temporal resolution of less than 10 seconds is advantageous to accurately characterize the initial enhancement phase. The small size of the wrist and MCP joints means that a spatial resolution of at least 1 mm is helpful. Three-dimensional sequences with high resolution in all 3 planes improve reproducibility in serial studies. Typically, images of the wrist from 3-mm slices acquired in less than 30 seconds are adequate, although a wide range of imaging protocols have been used in different studies with temporal resolutions of 2.6 to 70 seconds and slice thicknesses from 1 to 7 mm. Imaging is usually carried out at 1.5 T, although field strengths between 0.2 and 3 T have been used.[32] In general, increased signal at higher field strengths allows better spatial and/or temporal resolution. In addition to high temporal and spatial resolution, the imaging protocol must provide strongly T1-weighted images that are sensitive to the gadolinium. Most studies have therefore used rapid T1-weighted gradient-echo sequences with relatively short echo times and repetition times. The region of interest of inflamed synovium from which the enhancement curve is determined may be chosen in different ways. The entire enhancing synovium should be included. Because of the time involved in manually outlining all the inflamed synovium, several investigators have used automated or semiautomated methods.[33] Parameters that can be measured from the enhancement curve include the early enhancement rate, the maximum enhancement, and the late or static enhancement. The relative early enhancement rate is often used in preference to the absolute early enhancement rate, as it is independent of the units of signal intensity and is proportional to the gadolinium concentration in the synovium.

IMAGING FINDINGS: MR IMAGING

The main MR imaging findings are synovitis, BME, also defined as osteitis, and bone erosion. MR imaging allows standardization in the evaluation of the degree of disease. For this purpose, RAMRIS was presented in 2002 by 2 groups that evaluated MR imaging signs of RA in the wrist and in the hand (OMERACT and EULAR).

Bone erosions, synovitis, and BME were classified with semiquantitative scoring of MR images of hands and wrists (**Box 2**). The groups also have produced a reference image atlas for scoring synovitis, BME, and erosions in RA wrist and MCP joints.[3,4]

Box 2
Rheumatoid arthritis MR imaging scoring system (RAMRIS) according to OMERACT and European League Against Rheumatism (EULAR)

OMERACT RAMRIS

Edema

  0 = no edema

  1 = 1%–33% of the bone edematous

  2 = 34%–66% of the bone edematous

  3 = 67%–100% of the bone edematous

Synovitis

  0 = normal

  1 = mild

  2 = moderate

  3 = severe

Bone erosion

  From 0 to 10 with intervals of 10% volume involvement

Bone Marrow Edema

BME is a unique MR imaging feature that represents inflammatory infiltrates in trabecular bone (also called osteitis). It shows high signal intensity on STIR or T2-weighted fat-suppressed images and low signal intensity on T1-weighted images (**Fig. 1**).

Recently, a shorter protocol has been identified[34] based on evaluation of BME using T1-weighted images. It was demonstrated that T1 sequences with Gadolinuim (T1Gd) and T2 images are equally suitable for scoring BME in early arthritis and advanced RA.

According to McQueen,[35] BME consists of infiltration by leukocytes and an increased number of osteoclasts. BME has been shown to be a strong independent predictor of progressive joint damage and can therefore be used for prognostication of the disease course.[36–41] Nieuwenhuis and colleagues[42] demonstrated that, when BME was present at first clinical presentation, it frequently persisted at subsequent measurements during the first year and it frequently evolved in erosive progression.

Lisbona and colleagues[43] demonstrated high values of BME in patients with progressive erosions after sustained remission. Subclinical inflammation and, consequently, high scores of BME may explain the structural progression reported on MR imaging in patients with RA despite clinical remission. The aim of this study was to define the critical cutoff of BME for the development of erosions or erosion progression in RA. According to the OMERACT scoring system, BME is considered as "a lesion within the trabecular bone, with ill-defined margins and signal characteristics consistent with increased water content."[3,4]

Synovitis

Synovitis is defined as a thickness area in the synovial compartment with abnormal enhancement after intravenous administration of contrast agent. It is observed on postcontrast agent T1-weighted images. It can be more easily identified in 3 areas: radio-ulnar, radiocarpal, and intracarpal-carpometacarpal areas (**Fig. 2**).

On MR imaging, synovitis has been shown to relate to the histologic degree of synovial inflammation.

Chew and colleagues,[44] comparing the total sum scores of the right hand and wrist joints with the left hand and wrist joints of individual patients, suggested that there was positive correlation in all 3 parameters (synovitis, BME, erosion), with high mean sum score for both the sides; however, as to synovitis alone, there was a side prevalence on the left side, with higher values compared

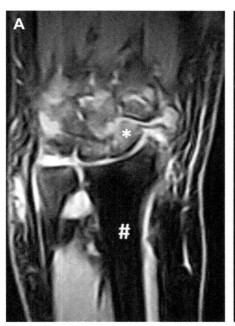
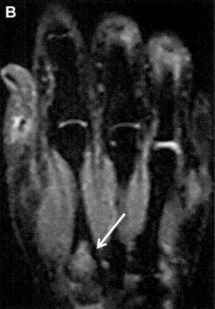

Fig. 1. Bone edema MR imaging. (*A*) Coronal T2-weighted FS image of the wrist: note the difference in signal intensity between the scaphoid bone (*asterisk*) (affected by bone edema) and the radius (*hash*) with normal spongious signal. (*B*) Coronal T2-weighted FS image of the hand: bone edema of the proximal epiphysis of the second metacarpal bone (*arrow*).

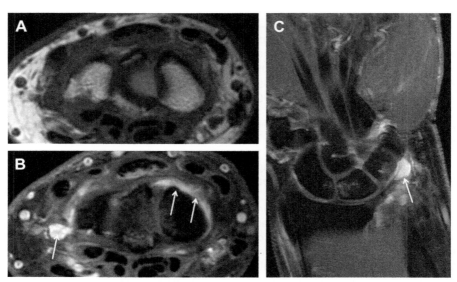

Fig. 2. Synovitis MR imaging. (*A*) T1-weighted axial MR image of the wrist. (*B, C*) T1-weighted FS contrast-enhanced axial (*B*) and coronal (*C*) images of the wrist: thickened synovium with contrast enhancement (*arrows*).

with the right one. There is no evidence about prognostic value of tenosynovitis. In fact, in a cross-sectional analysis, Nieuwenhuis and colleagues[42] did not find higher tenosynovitis scores in anti-citrullinated protein antibodies (ACPA)-positive patients with RA, a group that is characterized by more severe joint destruction.

Synovitis is defined by the OMERACT as an "area in the synovial compartment that shows above normal post-gadolinium enhancement of a thickness greater than the width of the normal synovium."[3]

Bone Erosion

Bone erosion is a juxta-articular marginated lesion, a cortical break. On T1-weighted images, it shows loss of normal low signal intensity of the cortical bone and loss of high signal intensity of the trabecular component of the bone (**Fig. 3**). A primarily common finding is the cartilage damage caused by proteases. Increased serum levels of cartilage matrix proteins are predictable of radiographic joint damage.

In 2012, a single study was conducted to prove the role of T2* to reflect cartilage hydration and collagen integrity,[45] but the results have low diagnostic value.

The natural evolution of cartilage damage is bone erosion. MR imaging erosion scores aim to study the effects of new therapies on structural joint damage progression in RA. Koevoets and colleagues[46] demonstrated that erosions in the wrist are the only independent predictors of functional disability.

Bone erosion is defined as "a sharply marginated bone lesion with correct juxta-articular localization visible in 2 planes and showing a cortical break in at least one plane,"[3] sometimes with pannus or enhancing synovium inside the erosion.

IMAGING FINDINGS: COMPUTED TOMOGRAPHY

CT is more advantageous than MR imaging for the study of bones and can detect more subtle alterations of the bone cortex, in particular compared with CR. However, CT is unable to detect inflammation processes such as synovitis, tenosynovitis, or BME. CT has the ability to detect bone erosions more accurately than other techniques.[47,48] CT allows a careful evaluation of bone damage. The latest CT scanners may detect even minimal bone changes. Thus, they may be considered the gold standard for bone erosions, even though exposure to ionizing radiation represents a strong limitation to its daily use.[49]

A novel, sensitive imaging technique is high-resolution peripheral quantitative CT (HR-pQCT).[50] HR-pQCT allows analysis of the cortical and trabecular microarchitecture of peripheral bones with an isotropic resolution of 82 μm. This technique is now also applied for 3D assessment of the bone microarchitecture in the hand joints.[50,51] A study by Stach and colleagues[50] demonstrated that HR-pQCT is more sensitive than CR in detecting cortical breaks in the hand joints in RA and also in healthy controls. However, the resolution of the HR-pQCT images can be of

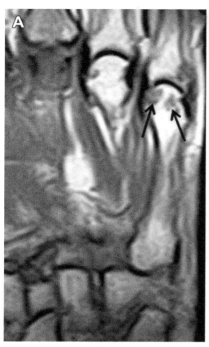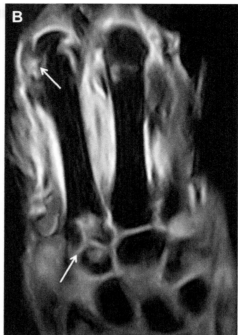

Fig. 3. Bone erosion MR imaging. (*A*) Coronal spin echo (SE) T1-weighted image and (*B*) coronal T2-weighted FS image of the hand and wrist: typical bone erosion of the metacarpal and carpal bone (*arrows*).

the same order as the thickness of the cortical bone in finger joints. Due to partial-volume effects, it is possible that thin cortices are falsely identified as breaks. Therefore, in particular with thin cortices, the reliability, sensitivity, and specificity of the measurements might be impaired and depend on the reader's perception.

It is important to understand some specific characteristics of MR imaging and CT. Although CT scanners provide optimal visualization of bone and other calcified tissues, MR imaging signal depends on the presence of mobile protons in the tissue and the technique is less suitable for the direct detection of erosion; sclerotic lesions can lead to an overestimation of the erosion dimension in MR imaging, whereas soft tissue infiltration can result in underestimation of the erosion dimension.[47]

For these reasons, according to Lee and colleagues,[52] MR imaging is less sensitive and accurate than HR-pQCT for the detection of bony erosions (Fig. 4).

The most important limiting factor in applying CT in routine clinical practice is the radiation exposure, but HR-pQCT has a very low radiation dose. The total effective dose for the MCP and wrist scans in this study was approximately 25 μSv per visit.

Quantification of bone erosion in RA has been divided into stages. Stage 1 (inflammation): BME without erosion; stage 2: low-degree erosion detectable only by HR-pQCT; stage 3: progress of disease, with large erosion areas detectable by both HR-pQCT and MR imaging; and in the last stage (stage 4), the erosion areas are large enough to be detected by all 3 modalities (CR, HR-pQCT, and MR imaging).[52]

Regensburger and colleagues[53] do not believe in MR imaging as a potential tool to detect signs of erosion repair, owing to its lower diagnostic capabilities compared with HR-pQCT. The currently available MR imaging units do not allow a systematic evaluation of erosion repair. For this purpose, the development of higher-resolution MR imaging units is needed.

WHAT THE REFERRING PHYSICIAN NEEDS TO KNOW

Clinical use of MR imaging is useful in determining the prognosis on whose basis an aggressive therapy is possibly administered to patients with the most destructive disease.

Early diagnosis and prompt initiation of treatment are important to reduce structural damage and disability, and to improve physical function in patients with RA.[54] At present, the primary goal of treatment for patients with RA is to achieve clinical remission or low levels of disease activity and to stop progression of structural damage.[41]

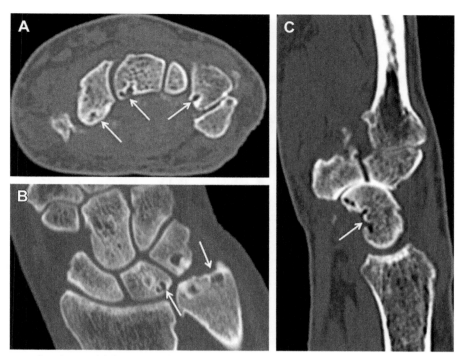

Fig. 4. Bone erosion CT. Axial (*A*) CT scan of the wrist and multiplanar reconstructions in coronal (*B*) and sagittal (*C*) plane. CT clearly depicts cortical bone erosions (*arrows*) with high spatial resolution.

MR imaging is a useful and sensitive imaging technique in early diagnosis of RA. It has been shown that MR imaging may detect the presence of local subclinical inflammation even in undifferentiated arthritis and may predict the RA development.[55,56] A systematic review of the diagnostic and prognostic value of MR imaging in patients with undifferentiated arthritis reported that MR imaging bone edema associated with synovitis and erosion pattern may predict the development of RA from undifferentiated arthritis. On the contrary, the absence on MR imaging of synovitis decreases the probability of developing RA.[57]

Furthermore, MR imaging subclinical inflammation may explain the structural progression on radiography in patients with RA despite clinical remission or low disease activity. Several studies have shown that some patients in clinical remission may develop structural progression on imaging continuing to have synovitis and BME detectable by MR imaging.[58]

The mechanism underlying the association between bone edema and erosion remains to be determined, but bone edema in this context could represent an intraosseous cellular infiltrate capable of eroding cartilage and bone from the subchondral aspect of the joint.[20]

The histologic features associated with bone edema in early RA are yet to be described, owing to difficulty in obtaining material to examine, but Lee and colleagues[52] reported a decrease in bone edema in patients with RA who are in clinical remission, supporting its link to disease activity. Some investigators suggest that synovitis may lead to bone edema and subsequent erosion.[37,43,44,56,58] However, not all patients with baseline synovitis eventually experienced joint erosion.[20]

The clinical relevance of MR imaging findings is emphasized by the fact that many patients in clinical and biochemical remission according to the ACR or EULAR guidelines still have synovitis activity when assessed with both MR imaging and ultrasonography; these findings predict erosive disease progression on radiographs after 1 year.

Recently Døhn and colleagues[47] have shown a good correlation and reproducibility between the volume of bone erosions on MR imaging compared with both to the RAMRIS score as well as the volume on CT as the standard of reference. This study confirms that the RAMRIS score is a valid and reliable scoring method that is well suited and today the best available score to apply to clinical trials. In the Cyclosporine, Methotrexate, Steroid in RA (CIMESTRA) and Golimumab Before Employing Methotrexate as the First-Line Option in the Treatment of Rheumatoid Arthritis of Early Onset (GO-BEFORE) studies, the investigators showed that synovitis and bone edema, at MR imaging, were independent predictors of radiographic progression after 2 years of follow-up.[39,59]

Recently, it has been shown that MR imaging may be used to evaluate the disease activity of patients with RA. In fact, several trials were performed to examine the imaging-detected mechanism of reduction of structural joint damage progression by treatments in patients with RA using MR imaging. In a substudy of a randomized, double-blind, phase 3b study (ACT-RAY) in which 63 patients were randomized to continue methotrexate (MTX) or receive placebo, both in combination with tocilizumab (TCZ), an anti–interleukin (IL)-6 biologic disease-modifying antirheumatic drug (DMARD), the most symptomatic hand was imaged and scored with MR imaging. A rapid suppression of synovitis and osteitis at MR imaging associated with a reduction in structural joint damage progression occurred with TCZ, as monotherapy or in combination with MTX, in 1-year follow-up.[60] Similarly, an MR imaging–verified response to certolizumab pegol (CZP) therapy, an anti–IL-6 biologic DMARD, was performed in a randomized placebo-controlled study enrolling 41 patients with RA. In the CZP group, there were significant reductions from baseline synovitis and osteitis scores at week 16.[61]

SUMMARY

MR and CT imaging in RA allow for a multiplanar visualization and evaluation of the whole joint as well as discrimination and assessment of the intra-articular and periarticular soft tissues. MR imaging is the only modality capable of assessing BME, which is a good predictor of disease progression, and is a safe and well-suited tool to monitor the synovial treatment responses and erosive progression. Many studies demonstrate that clinical evaluation of disease stage and treatment response is not as reliable as imaging, because it is documented that patients who respond clinically and/or are in clinical remission may present imaging signs of inflammation and sometimes even erosive progression.

REFERENCES

1. McInnes IB, Schett G. The pathogenesis of rheumatoid arthritis. N Engl J Med 2011;365(23):2205–19.
2. Smolen JS, Aletaha D, McInnes IB. Rheumatoid arthritis. Lancet 2016;388(10055):2023–38.
3. Østergaard M, Peterfy C, Conaghan P, et al. OMERACT rheumatoid arthritis magnetic resonance imaging studies. Core set of MRI acquisitions, joint pathology definitions, and the OMERACT RA-MRI scoring system. J Rheumatol 2003;30:1385–6.
4. Conaghan P, Bird P, Ejbjerg B, et al. The EULAR–OMERACT rheumatoid arthritis MRI reference image atlas: the metacarpophalangeal joints. Ann Rheum Dis 2005;65(Suppl I):11–21.
5. Splendiani A, Ferrari F, Barile A, et al. Occult neural foraminal stenosis caused by association between disc degeneration and facet joint osteoarthritis: demonstration with dedicated upright MRI system. Radiol Med 2014;119(3):164–74.
6. Salvati F, Rossi F, Limbucci N, et al. Mucoid metaplastic-degeneration of anterior cruciate ligament. J Sports Med Phys Fitness 2008;48(4):483–7.
7. Ripani M, Continenza MA, Cacchio A, et al. The ischiatic region: normal and MRI anatomy. J Sports Med Phys Fitness 2006;46(3):468–75.
8. Masciocchi C, Lanni G, Conti L, et al. Soft-tissue inflammatory myofibroblastic tumors (IMTs) of the limbs: potential and limits of diagnostic imaging. Skeletal Radiol 2012;41(6):643–9.
9. Barile A, Lanni G, Conti L, et al. Lesions of the biceps pulley as cause of anterosuperior impingement of the shoulder in the athlete: potentials and limits of MR arthrography compared with arthroscopy. Radiol Med 2013;118(1):112–22.
10. Barile A, Conti L, Lanni G, et al. Evaluation of medial meniscus tears and meniscal stability: weight-bearing MRI vs arthroscopy. Eur J Radiol 2013; 82(4):633–9.
11. Barile A, Regis G, Masi R, et al. Musculoskeletal tumours: preliminary experience with perfusion MRI. Radiol Med 2007;112(4):550–61.
12. Mariani S, La Marra A, Arrigoni F, et al. Dynamic measurement of patello-femoral joint alignment using weight-bearing magnetic resonance imaging (WB-MRI). Eur J Radiol 2015;84(12):2571–8.
13. Aliprandi A, Di Pietto F, Minafra P, et al. Femoroacetabular impingement: what the general radiologist should know. Radiol Med 2014;119(2):103–12.
14. Cappabianca S, Colella G, Pezzullo MG, et al. Lipomatous lesions of the head and neck region: imaging findings in comparison with histological type. Radiol Med 2008;113(5):758–70.
15. Zappia M, Reginelli A, Russo A, et al. Long head of the biceps tendon and rotator interval. Musculoskelet Surg 2013;97(Suppl 2):S99–108.
16. Aletaha D, Neogi T, Silman AJ, et al. 2010 rheumatoid arthritis classification criteria: an American College of Rheumatology/European League Against Rheumatism collaborative initiative. Arthritis Rheum 2010;62(9):2569–81.
17. Colebatch AN, Edwards CJ, Østergaard M, et al. EULAR recommendations for the use of imaging of the joints in the clinical management of rheumatoid arthritis. Ann Rheum Dis 2013;72(6):804–14.
18. Brunese L, Romeo A, Iorio S, et al. Thyroid B-flow twinkling sign: a new feature of papillary cancer. Eur J Endocrinol 2008;159(4):447–51.

19. Perrotta FM, Astorri D, Zappia M, et al. An ultraso-nographic study of enthesis in early psoriatic arthritis patients naive to traditional and biologic DMARDs treatment. Rheumatol Int 2016;36(11): 1579–83.

20. Mandl P, Naredo E, Wakefield RJ, et al. A systematic literature review analysis of ultrasound joint count and scoring systems to assess synovitis in rheuma-toid arthritis according to the OMERACT filter. J Rheumatol 2011;38(9):2055–62.

21. Boesen M, Østergaard M, Cimmino MA, et al. MRI quantification of rheumatoid arthritis: current knowl-edge and future perspectives. Eur J Radiol 2009; 71:189–96.

22. Freeston JE, Bird P, Conaghan PG, et al. The role of MRI in rheumatoid arthritis: research and clinical is-sues. Curr Opin Rheumatol 2009;21:95–101.

23. Freeston JE, Olech E, Yocum D, et al. A modification of the Omeract RA MRI score for erosions for use with an extremity MRI system with reduced field of view. Ann Rheum Dis 2007;66:1669–71.

24. Aoki T, Yamashita Y, Kazuyoshi SK, et al. Diagnosis of early-stage rheumatoid arthritis: usefulness of un-enhanced and gadolinium-enhanced MR images at 3 T. Clin Imaging 2013;37:348–53.

25. Chand AS, McHaffie A, Clarke AW, et al. Quantifying synovitis in rheumatoid arthritis using computer-assisted manual segmentation with 3 Tesla MRI scanning. J Magn Reson Imaging 2011;33:1106–13.

26. Bird P, Conaghan P, Ejbjerg B, et al. The develop-ment of the EULAR–OMERACT rheumatoid arthritis MRI reference image atlas. Ann Rheum Dis 2005; 64(Suppl I):8–10.

27. Peterfy CG, DiCarlo JC, Olech E, et al. Evaluating joint-space narrowing and cartilage loss in rheuma-toid arthritis by using MRI. Arthritis Res Ther 2012; 14:R131.

28. Østergaard M, Klarlund M. Importance of timing of post-contrast MRI in rheumatoid arthritis: what hap-pens during the first 60 minutes after IV gadolinium-DTPA? Ann Rheum Dis 2001;60:1050–4.

29. Aoki T, Yamashita Y, Oki H, et al. Iterative decompo-sition of water and fat with echo asymmetry and least-squares estimation (IDEAL) of the wrist and finger at 3T: comparison with chemical shift selective fat suppression images. J Magn Reson Imaging 2013;37:733–8.

30. Li X, Yu A, Virayavanich W, et al. Quantitative char-acterization of bone marrow edema pattern in rheu-matoid arthritis using 3 Tesla MRI. J Magn Reson Imaging 2012;35:211–7.

31. Hodgson RJ, Barnes T, Connolly S, et al. Changes underlying the dynamic contrast-enhanced MRI response to treatment in rheumatoid arthritis. Skel-etal Radiol 2008;37:201–7.

32. Hodgson RJ, O'Connor P, Moots R. MRI of rheuma-toid arthritis—image quantitation for the assessment

of disease activity, progression and response to therapy. Rheumatology 2008;47:13–21.

33. Axelsen MB, Stoltenberg M, Poggenborg RP, et al. Dynamic gadolinium-enhanced magnetic reso-nance imaging allows accurate assessment of the synovial inflammatory activity in rheumatoid arthritis knee joints: a comparison with synovial histology. Scand J Rheumatol 2012;41:89–94.

34. Stomp W, Krabben A, van der Heijde D, et al. Aiming for a shorter rheumatoid arthritis MRI protocol: can contrast-enhanced MRI replace T2 for the detection of bone marrow oedema? Eur Radiol 2014;24: 2614–22.

35. McQueen FM. Bone marrow edema and osteitis in rheumatoid arthritis: the imaging perspective. Arthritis Res Ther 2012;14:224.

36. Bøyesen P, Haavardsholm EA, van der Heijde D, et al. Prediction of MRI erosive progression: a com-parison of modern imaging modalities in early rheu-matoid arthritis patients. Ann Rheum Dis 2011;70: 176–9.

37. Gandjbakhch F, Foltz V, Mallet A, et al. Bone marrow oedema predicts structural progression in a 1-year follow- up of 85 patients with RA in remission or with low disease activity with low-field MRI. Ann Rheum Dis 2011;70:2159–62.

38. Haavardsholm EA, Bøyesen P, Østergaard M, et al. Magnetic resonance imaging findings in 84 patients with early rheumatoid arthritis: bone marrow oedema predicts erosive progression. Ann Rheum Dis 2008; 67:794–800.

39. Hetland ML, Ejbjerg B, Hørslev-Petersen K, et al. MRI bone oedema is the strongest predictor of sub-sequent radio- graphic progression in early rheuma-toid arthritis. Results from a 2-year randomised controlled trial (CIMESTRA). Ann Rheum Dis 2009; 68:384–90.

40. McQueen F, Naredo E. The 'disconnect' between sy-novitis and erosion in rheumatoid arthritis: a result of treatment or intrinsic to the disease process itself? Ann Rheum Dis 2011;70:241–4.

41. Smolen JS, Breedveld FC, Burmester GR, et al. Treating rheumatoid arthritis to target: 2014 update of the recommendations of an international task force. Ann Rheum Dis 2016;75(1):3–15.

42. Nieuwenhuis WP, van Steenbergen HW, Stomp W. The course of bone marrow edema in early undiffer-entiated arthritis and rheumatoid arthritis: a longitu-dinal magnetic resonance imaging study at bone level. Arthritis Rheumatol 2016;68(5):1080–8.

43. Lisbona MP, Pàmies A, Almirall M. Association of bone edema with the progression of bone erosions quantified by hand magnetic resonance imaging in patients with rheumatoid arthritis in remission. J Rheumatol 2014;41:1623–9.

44. Chew L, Mohan P, Chan L, et al. Use of magnetic resonance imaging in detecting subclinical synovitis

in rheumatoid arthritis and correlation of imaging findings with interleukin-18 levels. Int J Rheum Dis 2016;19:790–8.

45. Buchbender C, Scherer A, Kröpil P. Cartilage quality in rheumatoid arthritis: comparison of T2* mapping, native T1 mapping, dGEMRIC, ΔR1 and value of pre-contrast imaging. Skeletal Radiol 2012;41: 685–92.

46. Koevoets R, Dirven L, Klarenbeek NB, et al. Insights in the relationship of joint space narrowing versus erosive joint damage and physical functioning of patients with RA. Ann Rheum Dis 2013;72:870–4.

47. Døhn UM, Ejbjerg BJ, Hasselquist M, et al. Rheumatoid arthritis bone erosion volumes on CT and MRI: reliability and correlations with erosion scores on CT, MRI and radiography. Ann Rheum Dis 2007;66: 1388–92.

48. Døhn UM, Terslev L, Szkudlarek M, et al. Detection, scoring and volume assessment of bone erosions by ultrasonography in rheumatoid arthritis: comparison with CT. Ann Rheum Dis 2013;72(4):530–4.

49. Grassi W, Okano T, Di Geso L, et al. Imaging in rheumatoid arthritis: options, uses and optimization. Expert Rev Clin Immunol 2015;11(10):1131–46.

50. Stach CM, Bauerle M, Englbrecht M, et al. Periarticular bone structure in rheumatoid arthritis patients and healthy individuals assessed by high-resolution computed tomography. Arthritis Rheum 2010;62(2):330–9.

51. Fouque-Aubert A, Boutroy S, Marotte H, et al. Assessment of hand bone loss in rheumatoid arthritis by high-resolution peripheral quantitative CT. Ann Rheum Dis 2010;69(9):1671–6.

52. Lee CH, Srikhum W, Andrew J, et al. Correlation of structural abnormalities of the wrist and metacarpophalangeal joints evaluated by high-resolution peripheral quantitative computed tomography, 3 Tesla magnetic resonance imaging and conventional radiographs in rheumatoid arthritis. Int J Rheum Dis 2015;18:628–39.

53. Regensburger A, Rech J, Englbrecht M. A comparative analysis of magnetic resonance imaging and high-resolution peripheral quantitative computed tomography of the hand for the detection of erosion repair in rheumatoid arthritis. Rheumatology (Oxford) 2015;54:1573–81.

54. Ejbjerg B, McQueen F, Lassere M, et al. The EULAR–OMERACT rheumatoid arthritis MRI reference image atlas: the wrist joint. Ann Rheum Dis 2005; 64(Suppl I):i23–47.

55. Krabben A, Stomp W, van der Heijde DM, et al. MRI of hand and foot joints of patients with anticitrullinated peptide antibody positive arthralgia without clinical arthritis. Ann Rheum Dis 2013;72(9):1540–4.

56. Tamai M, Kawakami A, Uetani M, et al. A prediction rule for disease outcome in patients with undifferentiated arthritis using magnetic resonance imaging of the wrists and finger joints and serologic autoantibodies. Arthritis Rheum 2009;61(6):772–8.

57. Machado PM, Koevoets R, Bombardier C, et al. The value of magnetic resonance imaging and ultrasound in undifferentiated arthritis: a systematic review. J Rheumatol Suppl 2011;87:31–7.

58. Dinesh Kumar L, Karthik R, Gayathri N. Advancement in contemporary diagnostic and therapeutic approaches for rheumatoid arthritis. Biomed Pharmacother 2016;79:52–61.

59. Baker JF, Ostergaard M, Emery P, et al. Early MRI measures independently predict 1-year and 2-year radiographic progression in rheumatoid arthritis: secondary analysis from a large clinical trial. Ann Rheum Dis 2014;73(11):1968–74.

60. Conaghan PG, Peterfy C, Olech E, et al. The effects of tocilizumab on osteitis, synovitis and erosion progression in rheumatoid arthritis: results from the ACT-RAY MRI substudy. Ann Rheum Dis 2014; 73(5):810–6.

61. Østergaard M, Jacobsson LT, Schaufelberger C, et al. MRI assessment of early response to certolizumab pegol in rheumatoid arthritis: a randomised, double-blind, placebo-controlled phase IIIb study applying MRI at weeks 0, 1, 2, 4, 8 and 16. Ann Rheum Dis 2015;74(6):1156–63.

Computed Tomography and MR Imaging in Spondyloarthritis

Antonio Leone, MD[a],*, Victor N. Cassar-Pullicino, MD[b],
Paola D'Aprile, MD[c], Michelangelo Nasuto, MD[d],
Giuseppe Guglielmi, MD[d,e]

KEYWORDS

- Spine • Sacroiliac joints • Spondyloarthritis • CT • MR imaging • Ankylosing spondylitis • Psoriasis
- Reiter syndrome

KEY POINTS

- MR imaging may depict bone marrow and soft tissue edema, a feature that helps assess and monitor disease activity.
- With MR imaging, spondyloarthritis can be diagnosed and treated in its early stages long before structural bone damage occurs.
- The application of computed tomography (CT) is limited because of the lack of ability to assess active inflammation, and the high radiation dose.
- CT should be performed when spinal fracture is suspected, and radiography is negative.

INTRODUCTION

Spondyloarthritis (SpA) comprises a group of closely related but phenotypically distinct chronic, inflammatory diseases including ankylosing spondylitis (AS), psoriatic SpA, SpA related to inflammatory bowel disease (eg, Crohn disease or ulcerative colitis), reactive SpA (formerly Reiter syndrome), and undifferentiated SpA.[1–4]

Based on predominant clinical manifestations and in agreement with the Assessment of Spondyloarthritis International Society (ASAS) classification criteria, patients with SpA can also be distinguished as patients with predominantly axial SpA or with predominantly peripheral SpA.[5,6] Although clinical features may allow some differentiation (eg, history of urogenital tract infection in reactive SpA, skin lesions in psoriatic SpA), there remains important clinical overlap so it is difficult to differentiate the various forms in their early phases; furthermore, one form can evolve into another.[7] For these reasons, some investigators[8] suggest a common pathophysiologic mechanism for SpA as a whole and support the concept that SpA is a single multifaceted disorder.

Sacroiliitis is the primary unifying feature. Being made predominantly of fibrous connective tissues and containing very little synovial fluid, the sacroiliac joints may be considered entheses, thus explaining their characteristic involvement in SpA.[9] Unlike rheumatoid arthritis, which affects the synovial membrane, SpA is seronegative for rheumatoid factor and, to varying degrees, is associated with the presence of human leukocyte

Disclosure: The authors have no commercial or financial conflicts of interest.
[a] Institute of Radiology, Fondazione Policlinico Universitario A. Gemelli, Catholic University School of Medicine, Largo A. Gemelli 1, Rome 00168, Italy; [b] Department of Diagnostic Imaging, The Robert Jones and Agnes Hunt Orthopaedic and District Hospital, Gobowen, Oswestry SY10 7AG, UK; [c] Department of Radiology, Ospedale San Paolo, Via Caposcardicchio, Bari 70123, Italy; [d] Department of Radiology, University of Foggia, Viale L. Pinto 1, Foggia 71100, Italy; [e] Casa Sollievo della Sofferenza, Scientific Institute Hospital, Viale Cappucini 1, San Giovanni Rotondo, Foggia 71013, Italy
* Corresponding author.
E-mail address: a.leonemd@tiscali.it

radiologic.theclinics.com

antigen (HLA)–B27.[10] Regardless of subgroup, common clinical and imaging features include inflammatory back pain (Box 1) caused by sacroiliitis or spondylitis, enthesitis, oligoarticular and asymmetric peripheral arthritis predominantly of the lower limbs, and possibly dactylitis or uveitis.[4,11] Laboratory tests are generally nonspecific with increased C-reactive protein level and erythrocyte sedimentation rate.

Imaging is an integral part of the management of patients with SpA because it has become imperative to identify the disease early, before the onset of structural damage, at a phase when disease still may be reversible. Until recently, the definitive diagnosis of SpA relied on radiography, which has been shown to take up to a decade to become diagnostic.[12] Computed tomography (CT) is more sensitive and specific for assessing structural changes; however, only MR imaging allows assessment of acute inflammatory activity in the cartilage, subchondral bone, ligaments, synovium, and capsular region.

This review article focuses on the roles of CT and MR imaging in evaluation of patients with SpA with a specific emphasis on the MR imaging findings of vertebral and sacroiliac involvement, and presents relevant clinical features that assist early diagnosis.

IMAGING MODALITIES AND PROTOCOLS
Computed Tomography

Since 1990, developments in CT technology have led to the current generation of multidetector CT scanners that offer significant increase in imaging acquisition, high spatial resolution, more anatomic coverage, and isotropic data acquisition. With this technique, a high-spatial-resolution thin-section axial data set can be acquired with a wide array of postprocessing reconstruction capabilities, such as high-resolution two-dimensional reformation, and three-dimensional volume rendering techniques, without compromising the spatial resolution of the original axial images. This progress has resulted in the improvement in diagnostic accuracy and the gain is perhaps best exemplified by the surge in the detailed multiplanar reformations in spine imaging.

CT is a widely available and less expensive imaging modality, compared with MR imaging. Bone lesions, such as cortical erosions, subchondral/periarticular sclerosis, joint space widening, and ankylosis are easily detectable by CT, which also represents the reference standard for detection of osteoproductive alterations (Fig. 1). However, early features of SpA, such as bone marrow edema, cannot be distinguished in a CT examination, therefore there is no potential role of this imaging modality in the acute condition. Therapeutic decisions are rarely influenced by structural changes detected on CT.

Compared with MR imaging, CT has the added disadvantage of using ionizing radiation and radiologists are responsible for the radiation exposure. The radiation-free assessment becomes particularly important in the pediatric population, and when repeated follow-up imaging is likely to be necessary. CT may provide additional information on structural damage (eg, incipient erosions or intraarticular ankylosis) if radiography is negative, MR imaging findings are equivocal, or MR imaging cannot be performed.

Computed tomography imaging protocols
CT imaging protocols inevitably vary between institutions, depending on the specific capabilities of the scanner and physician preferences; however, the scan parameters for imaging the spine are generally acquired helically, in high-speed mode, with no gantry tilt, and the studies are usually performed without administration of intravenous contrast material. For image analysis, sagittal and coronal reformations are obtained. Regarding sacroiliac joints, CT examinations should involve coronal oblique images or coronal and axial oblique multiplanar reformation images oriented parallel and perpendicular to the long axis of the sacrum, with a high-resolution algorithm (see Fig. 1).

MR Imaging

MR imaging is currently considered the best noninvasive imaging modality for detecting inflammatory changes of joints, tendons, entheses, and bone marrow. This imaging modality is widely

---

Box 1
Diagnosing inflammatory low back pain

- Onset before the age of 35 to 40 years
- Insidious onset
- Lasting more than 3 months
- Morning stiffness more than 30 minutes
- Improvement with exercise but not with rest
- Awakening with pain in the second half of the night
- Alternating buttock pain (diffuse nonspecific radiation of pain into buttock)
- NSAIDs are very effective in relieving pain and stiffness

Abbreviation: NSAIDs, nonsteroidal antiinflammatory drugs.

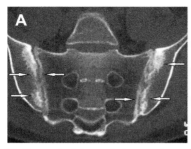
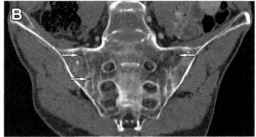

Fig. 1. AS. (*A*) Coronal oblique CT image shows bilateral erosions and sclerosis of both sides of sacroiliac joints with irregular joint spaces (*arrows*). (*B*) Coronal multiplanar reformatted CT image in a different patient showing ankylosis of both sacroiliac joints (*arrows*).

used in clinical practice to assess the early diagnosis of inflammation and disease activity, to show structural lesions early in the disease course, to diagnose disease complications, to provide objective signs based on the therapy that can be initiated, and to monitor and evaluate therapy response.[13]

However, targeted MR imaging cannot be used to assess multifocality. Whole-body MR imaging, including diffusion-weighted imaging, has expanded the potential role of imaging in AS and related SpA, has the benefits of its lack of ionizing radiation, and is being increasingly used for evaluation of multifocal bone lesions and follow-up evaluation. This imaging modality is capable of detecting abnormalities in sacroiliac joints, small spinal joints, peripheral joints, and ligamentous and tendinous attachments by a single MR examination within 30 minutes.[14–16] However, further studies are required before the true management value of whole-body MR imaging as well as of (dynamic) contrast-enhanced MR sequences can be determined.[13]

MR imaging protocols
Mandatory MR imaging sequences for evaluating the spine in adults and children should include sagittal T1-weighted turbo spin-echo (TSE) and fluid-sensitive fat-suppressed sequences (ie, short-tau inversion recovery [STIR] or fat-saturated T2-weighted images), which may depict bone marrow edema, a feature that enables the diagnosis of active lesions in the preradiographic phase. The scanning range for the spine should include the lateral paravertebral segments because the frequently involved costovertebral and costotransverse joints should be investigated.[13] Depending on the findings and their locations, a supplementary transverse fluid-sensitive fat-suppressed sequence may be useful for assessment of the paravertebral soft tissue; posterior spinal elements; or costovertebral, costotransverse, and facet joints.[17,18] Tables 1 and 2 provide the MR

imaging parameters for basic protocols on 1.5-T and 3.0-T scanners, respectively.

An MR imaging protocol for the sacroiliac joints should include coronal oblique TSE T1-weighted and fluid-sensitive fat-suppressed sequences parallel to the long axis of the sacrum. A supplementary 3-mm T1-weighted and fat-suppressed intermediate-weighted spin-echo (SE) transverse oblique sequence, parallel to the upper vertebral end plate of the S1 vertebra, may be useful to avoid pitfalls that might occur on coronal oblique planes because of partial volume effects.[13] **Tables 3 and 4** show the MR imaging parameters for basic protocols on 1.5-T and 3.0-T scanners, respectively. The coronal oblique plane is superior for

Table 1
Mandatory MR imaging sequences for total spine at 1.5-T scanners

Plane of Acquisition/ Sequence	Sagittal/ STIR	Sagittal/ T1 TSE
TR (ms)	5000	846
TE (ms)	108	10
IR	140	—
FOV (mm)	350 × 350	350 × 350
Matrix (Phase × Frequency)	288 × 384	384 × 384
Section Thickness (mm)	3	3
Intersectional Gap (mm)	0.3	0.3

This table reflects the authors' opinions based on the recommendations of the subcommittee on arthritis imaging of the European Society of Skeletal Radiology.

Abbreviations: FOV, field of view; IR, inversion recovery; STIR, short-tau inversion recovery; TE, echo time; TR, repetition time.

Data from Feldtkeller E, Khan MA, van der Heijde D, et al. Age at disease onset and diagnosis delay in HLA-B27 negative vs. positive patients with ankylosing spondylitis. Rheumatol Int 2003;23:61–6.

Table 2
Mandatory MR imaging sequences for total spine at 3.0-T scanners

Plane of Acquisition/ Sequence	Sagittal/ STIR	Sagittal/ T1 TSE
TR (ms)	4266	447
TE (ms)	75	8.2
IR	220	—
FOV (mm)	380 × 380	380 × 380
Matrix (Phase × Frequency)	424 × 300	424 × 304
Section Thickness (mm)	3	3
Intersectional Gap (mm)	0.3	0.4

This table reflects the authors' opinions based on the recommendations of the subcommittee on arthritis imaging of the European Society of Skeletal Radiology.
Data from Feldtkeller E, Khan MA, van der Heijde D, et al. Age at disease onset and diagnosis delay in HLA-B27 negative vs. positive patients with ankylosing spondylitis. Rheumatol Int 2003;23:61–6.

Table 4
Mandatory MR imaging sequences for sacroiliac joints at 3.0-T scanners

Plane of Acquisition/ Sequence	Sagittal/ STIR	Sagittal/ T1 TSE
TR (ms)	4263	625
TE (ms)	75	10
IR	220	—
FOV (mm)	380 × 380	230 × 230
Matrix (Phase × Frequency)	424 × 300	576 × 382
Section Thickness (mm)	3	3
Intersectional Gap (mm)	1	0.4

This table reflects the authors' opinions based on the recommendations of the subcommittee on arthritis imaging of the European Society of Skeletal Radiology.
Data from Feldtkeller E, Khan MA, van der Heijde D, et al. Age at disease onset and diagnosis delay in HLA-B27 negative vs. positive patients with ankylosing spondylitis. Rheumatol Int 2003;23:61–6.

visualization of the subchondral osseous areas. The transverse oblique plane enables a specific distinction between the upper dorsal joint compartment with the interosseous ligaments forming the syndesmosis, and the lower ventral cartilaginous joint compartment, which is a true

Table 3
Mandatory MR imaging sequences for sacroiliac joints at 1.5-T scanners

Plane of Acquisition/ Sequence	Coronal Oblique/ STIR	Coronal Oblique/ T1 TSE
TR (ms)	5030	595
TE (ms)	67	20
IR	150	—
FOV (mm)	320 × 320	320 × 320
Matrix (Phase × Frequency)	320 × 320	384 × 512
Section Thickness (mm)	3	3
Intersectional Gap (mm)	0.6	0.6

This table reflects the authors' opinions based on the recommendations of the subcommittee on arthritis imaging of the European Society of Skeletal Radiology.
Data from Feldtkeller E, Khan MA, van der Heijde D, et al. Age at disease onset and diagnosis delay in HLA-B27 negative vs. positive patients with ankylosing spondylitis. Rheumatol Int 2003;23:61–6.

synovial joint consistent with a symphysis. Therefore, the transverse oblique plane enables assessment of the exact anatomic location of the disorders.[13]

In general, fluid-sensitive fat-suppressed sequences are highly sensitive for detection of musculoskeletal lesions such as spondylitis, sacroiliitis, capsulitis, enthesitis, or synovitis, and the use of contrast medium is not needed.[13] Intravenous contrast material may be administered for initial examination to increase morphologic evaluation of the musculoskeletal system or in doubtful cases; however, it is not required for follow-up evaluation. When a contrast medium is given, images should be acquired with a fat-suppressed, T1-weighted TSE sequence.[13]

CLINICAL AND IMAGING FINDINGS IN SPONDYLOARTHRITIS
Ankylosing Spondylitis

Sacroiliitis
AS is a chronic inflammatory disease of unknown cause that primarily affects the spine and sacroiliac joints. Erosion and ankylosis of the sacroiliac joints are the hallmarks of AS. Sacroiliitis is usually the first manifestation of AS and is characteristically bilateral and symmetric. Erosion of subchondral bone predominates on the iliac side of the cartilaginous joint compartment causing loss of definition of the articular surfaces usually accompanied by variable degrees of

adjacent osteoporosis and surrounding reactive sclerosis (see **Fig. 1**A). Although bone erosion may result in focal joint space widening, as the disease progresses, definition of the joint is completely lost with ankylosis because of new bone formation filling in the erosions and the original cartilaginous joint space (see **Fig. 1**B). Also, the ligamentous joint compartment is frequently affected by bony erosion and entheseal proliferation (**Box 2**).[19]

The earliest signs of sacroiliitis are identified using MR imaging, as recognized by the new classification criteria for axial SpA proposed by the ASAS/Outcome Measures in Rheumatology Clinical Trials (OMERACT) MR imaging group, in patients with greater than or equal to 3 months of back pain who were aged less than 45 years at the onset of back pain.[5] MR imaging of active sacroiliitis is defined as the presence of bone marrow edema on a fluid-sensitive fat-suppressed sequence and located in the subchondral or periarticular bone marrow. It has to be present in at least 2 consecutive images in the case of solitary lesions or just in 1 image if there are multiple lesions. However, this definition should be refined because the bone marrow edema may also be evident in patients with mechanical back pain and even in healthy individuals.[20] Therefore, it is not the presence but the severity of this lesion that is specific to SpA.[20,21] Subchondral bone edema manifests as decrease in signal on T1-weighted images with a corresponding

increase in signal on fluid-sensitive images, and marked enhancement on postcontrast fat-suppressed T1-weighted images (**Fig. 2**). According to these criteria, active sacroiliitis on imaging plus greater than or equal to 1 SpA clinical feature (**Box 3**) is sufficient to make the diagnosis of axial SpA.[5]

In chronic sacroiliitis, subchondral/periarticularly located fat replacement of the bone marrow edema might occur, which is of low signal intensity on fluid-sensitive fat-suppressed sequences and of high signal intensity on T1-weighted sequences.

Spondylitis

The most characteristic spinal feature of early AS is represented by Romanus lesions, which consist of cortical erosions involving one of the vertebral body edges, most commonly one of the anterior edges, at the insertion of the outer fibers of the annulus fibrosus on the ring apophysis of the vertebral endplate (**Fig. 3**). Because such a junction between bone and a ligamentous structure is an enthesis by definition, a Romanus lesion can be considered as an enthesitis of the anterior or

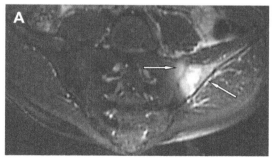
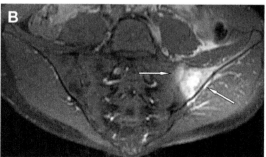

Fig. 2. Active sacroiliitis in a 34-year-old HLA-B27–positive man with 2 years of inflammatory low back pain associated with psoriatic skin and nail changes. (*A*) Coronal fat-suppressed T2-weighted, and (*B*) corresponding contrast-enhanced fat-suppressed MR images show high signal intensity and enhancement respectively, on both sides of the left sacroiliac joint, consistent with bone marrow edema (*arrows*).

Box 2
Progression of imaging findings in ankylosing spondylitis

- Sacroiliitis
  - Subchondral bone marrow edema
  - Small erosions typically beginning on the iliac side of the joint
  - Proliferative changes associated with the enthesitis
  - Subchondral sclerosis
  - Ankylosis of the joint
- Spondylitis
  - Romanus lesion associated with adjacent subchondral bone marrow edema
  - Shiny corners
  - Ossification of the spinal ligaments, intervertebral disks, and zygapophyseal joints
  - Marginal syndesmophytes
  - Bamboo spine

posterior longitudinal ligamentous complexes that progressively causes the squaring of the vertebral bodies.[12,22]

Later in the course of the disease, the vertebral body corner undergoes reactive sclerosis, a finding that appears as a low signal intensity corner on all MR sequences and is referred to as a shiny corner on radiography. The widespread enthesitis promotes ectopic bone formation within the affected structures and progressively leads to ossification of the spinal ligaments, intervertebral disks, and zygapophyseal joints with progressive rigidity and altered biomechanical properties of the spine.

The chronic inflammation at the diskovertebral junction determines the onset of an osteoproliferative process resulting in the formation of marginal syndesmophytes that span the ossified nucleus pulposus at each intervertebral disk level and bridge the adjacent vertebrae until ankyloses (**Fig. 4**).[23] In the late stage of the disease, the ossification of spinal ligaments, the presence of symmetric syndesmophytes along the whole spine, and the squared vertebral bodies lead to the characteristic, rigid hyperkyphosis often referred to as a bamboo spine (see **Box 2**).[24]

Syndesmophytes are classified as to whether they are marginal and symmetric or nonmarginal and asymmetric (**Table 5**). Marginal syndesmophytes are found almost exclusively in AS and SpA related to inflammatory bowel disease. Radiologically, they are characteristically bilateral and symmetric, thin, vertical, and originate at the edge or margin of a vertebral body endplate and extend to the margin of the adjacent vertebral body (see **Fig. 4**). Nonmarginal syndesmophytes are classically found in psoriatic SpA and reactive SpA. They are generally large and bulky, unilateral or asymmetric, parallel to the lateral surface of vertebral bodies, and originate from the midportion

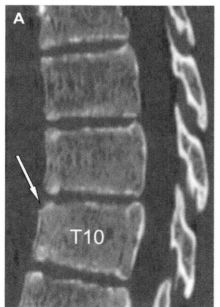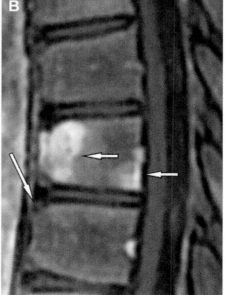

Fig. 3. Romanus lesions in a 37-year-old man. (*A*) Sagittal multiplanar reformatted CT image shows cortical erosion involving the anterosuperior corner of T10 vertebra (*arrow*). (*B*) Corresponding sagittal contrast-enhanced fat-suppressed MR image identifies T10 vertebral body erosion (*arrow*) but also shows postcontrast enhancement in the anterior aspect and posteroinferior corner of the T9 vertebral body (*small arrows*).

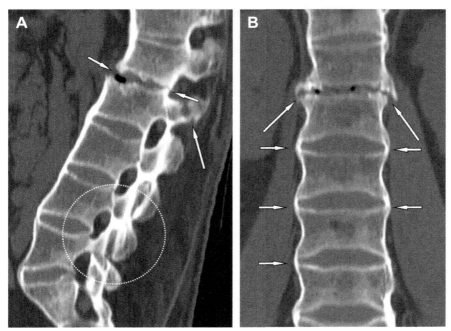

Fig. 4. AS in a 57-year-old man complaining of mechanical back pain during 3 to 4 weeks. (A) Right parasagittal multiplanar reformatted CT image shows transverse intradiskal fracture al L1-L2 level, involving the ossified anterior and posterior longitudinal ligaments (*small arrows*), and extending to posterior elements (*long arrow*). Ankylosis of zygapophyseal joint at L5-S1 level is also evident (*circle*). (B) Corresponding coronal multiplanar reformatted CT image shows symmetric marginal syndesmophytes representing ossification of Sharpey fibers (*small arrows*) and confirms the intradiskal fracture, which also involves marginal syndesmophytes (*long arrows*).

of the vertebral body (Fig. 5). The morphology of syndesmophytes seems to be related to the degree of mobility of the zygapophyseal joints. Reduced joint mobility leads to the development of marginal syndesmophytes (see Fig. 4); in contrast, nonmarginal bulky syndesmophytes develop at levels at which normal joint mobility is maintained because the tensile forces acting on the spine prevent the formation of marginal syndesmophytes.[24]

Table 5
Differential diagnosis between marginal and nonmarginal syndesmophytes

Feature	Marginal	Nonmarginal
Disease	AS SpA related to inflammatory bowel disease	Psoriatic SpA Reactive SpA
Origin	Vertebral body corner	Midvertebral body
Attachment	Attached	Attached or separated
Size	Small	Large
Thickness	Thin	Thick
Symmetry	Symmetric	Asymmetric
Distribution	Continuous	Skips
Definition	Sharp	Fluffy
Bridging	Complete	Incomplete

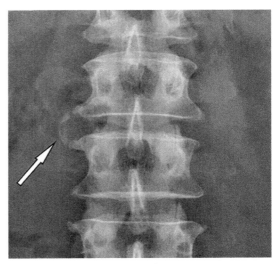

Fig. 5. A 47-year-old man with psoriatic SpA. Anteroposterior radiograph of the lumbar spine showing nonmarginal bulky syndesmophyte at L2-L3 level (*arrow*).

Although CT seems to be more sensitive for depicting erosions, sclerotic changes, and osteoproliferative processes, MR imaging may consistently identify vertebral body corner erosions and may depict edema of the adjacent bone marrow (decreased signal intensity on T1-weighted images, increased signal intensity on fluid-sensitive fat-suppressed images) (see **Fig. 3**).[17] Arthritis of the zygapophyseal and costovertebral/costotransverse joints can be observed in patients with SpA and AS in particular; it is usually associated with periarticular bone marrow edema, erosions, and joint effusion, and affected joints may undergo ankylosis at late phases (**Fig. 6**).

Spinal Fractures

The 2 central features of AS that promote the pathologic remodeling of the spine are inflammation and new bone formation; however, osteoporosis also occurs because of an uncoupling of the bone formation and bone resorption processes.[25–27] Ankylosis and bone resorption promote weakening of the spine as well as increased risk of vertebral fractures, even from trivial trauma.[28]

These fractures are often initially missed because diagnosis can be difficult using radiography alone, and patients attribute acute fracture-type pain to their usual inflammatory pain. Inadequate awareness of these injuries can have severe consequences because vertebral fractures are often unstable.

CT is the most sensitive and specific imaging modality in detecting and defining the extent of spinal fractures (see **Fig. 4**). MR imaging is better than radiography and CT in detecting soft tissues and diskoligamentous injury, furthermore, it may depict bone marrow edema, and it is the modality of choice to detect neurologic complications. Therefore, patients with AS presenting with symptoms of new neck or back pain should be critically evaluated for acute spinal fractures using CT and/or MR imaging, even if radiographs appear normal.[29,30]

Andersson lesion

An infrequent but well-known complication of AS is an extensive inflammatory involvement of the intervertebral disk and adjacent vertebral endplates; the so-called Andersson lesion. This condition is a noninfectious spondylodiskitis that occurs in up to 18% of patients with AS.[31] The etiopathogenesis of Andersson lesions still remains to be elucidated, but probably involves osteoporosis as well as inflammatory and mechanical (stress fractures) factors that prevent healing of lesions and provoke the development of pseudarthrosis.[32]

CT offers considerable contributory advantages compared with radiography in diagnosing Andersson lesions. This imaging modality accurately shows erosions with sclerosing remodeling of the end plates, fractures of the posterior elements, nonfusion of the facet joints, and narrowing of the adjacent disk space if present.

MR imaging, in addition, shows and defines the extent of the surrounding bone marrow edema appearing as high signal on fluid-sensitive sequences. In general, the presence of both high signal on MR fluid-sensitive images and disk space postcontrast enhancement can render the differentiation of the Andersson lesion from infectious spondylodiskitis very difficult. However, absence of an abscess or of epidural involvement, and the presence of productive changes and/or typical vertebral corner erosions in another spinal segment, is suggestive of Andersson lesion.

Psoriatic Spondyloarthritis

Psoriatic SpA has been reported in 30% of patients with psoriasis[33]; its classic peripheral pattern describes an asymmetric oligoarthritis with predominant distal interphalangeal joint involvement. Diagnosis of psoriatic SpA depends on clinical evidence of either characteristic skin lesions or nail changes. Although osteoarticular changes may occur contemporarily or before the onset of skin lesions, the characteristic rash commonly precedes joint disease by months or

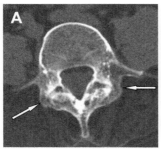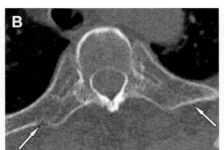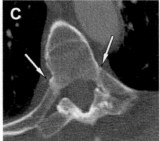

Fig. 6. Same patient as in **Fig. 3**. Axial CT scans clearly show ankylosis of zygapophyseal joints (*arrows* in *A*), costotransverse joints (*arrows* in *B*), and costovertebral joints (*arrows* in *C*).

Table 6
Psoriatic versus infectious sacroiliitis

Feature	Psoriatic Sacroiliitis	Infectious Sacroiliitis
Involvement of the sacroiliac joints	Asymmetric or unilateral	Unilateral
Extension	Bone and joint space	Joint space and adjacent soft tissue
Phlegmon or abscess	Absent	Present

years.[34] Axial psoriatic SpA, characterized by sacroiliitis associated with spondylitis, occurs in approximately 50% of patients with peripheral psoriatic SpA.[35]

The main features related to the axial involvement are (1) unilateral (see **Fig. 2**) or markedly asymmetric sacroiliitis with subchondral bone marrow edema, erosions that are more frequent on the iliac portion of the joint, osteosclerosis, joint space narrowing, and, rarely, ankylosis; (2) sparing or modest involvement of zygapophyseal joints; and (3) nonmarginal bulky syndesmophytes (see **Fig. 5**).

The asymmetric and unilateral involvement of the sacroiliac joints is primarily suggestive of psoriatic sacroiliitis; however, infectious sacroiliitis should be excluded (**Table 6**). In infectious sacroiliitis, the surrounding soft tissue usually is involved.

In contrast, the inflammatory sacroiliitis of SpA is limited to the bone and intraarticular space and does not cross anatomic borders. Therefore, identification of a phlegmon or an abscess in the joint space or in the adjacent soft tissue is helpful for differential diagnosis (**Fig. 7**).[18] Unlike that seen in AS, cervical spine involvement is frequent and includes erosive changes of zygapophyseal joints, and anterior atlantoaxial subluxation (**Fig. 8**).[36]

Spondyloarthritis Related to Inflammatory Bowel Disease

SpA related to the 2 major chronic inflammatory bowel diseases, ulcerative colitis and Crohn disease, can involve both peripheral and axial joints.[37] Peripheral SpA is generally oligoarticular, asymmetric, often transient and migratory, and

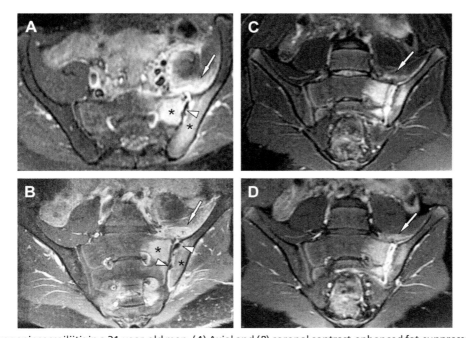

Fig. 7. Pyogenic sacroiliitis in a 31-year-old man. (A) Axial and (B) coronal contrast-enhanced fat-suppressed MR images show enhancement on both sides of the left sacroiliac joint (*asterisks* in A and B) associated with diffuse soft tissue enhancement (*arrow* in A and B). A small abscess in the joint space is also evident (*arrowheads* in A and B). (C) During-treatment coronal fat-suppressed T2-weighted and (D) contrast-enhanced fat-suppressed MR images show improvement in MR findings, with a decrease in soft tissue enhancement in particular (*arrow* in C and D).

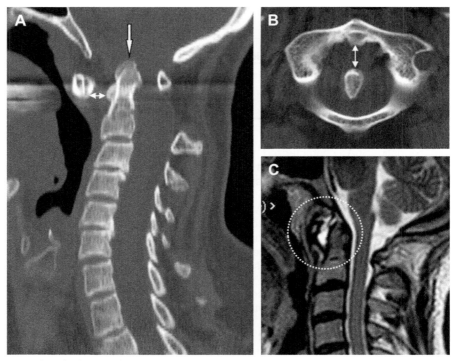

Fig. 8. (*A*) Sagittal multiplanar reformatted CT image in a 56-year-old-woman with psoriatic SpA shows basilar invagination (the odontoid process lies at the level of the foramen magnum) (*arrow*), and anterior atlantoaxial subluxation (>2.5–3 mm between the anterior surface of the odontoid process and the anterior arch of the atlas) (*double-headed arrow*). (*B*) Transverse CT scan through the atlas better shows the anterior atlantoaxial subluxation (*double-headed arrow*). (*C*) Sagittal T2-weighted MR image in a 48-year-old man with psoriatic SpA. Note the anterior atlantoaxial subluxation as well as the fluid collection in the atlantoaxial interval, compatible with slight activity of the disease (*circle*).

predominantly of the lower limbs. Axial SpA may include isolated sacroiliitis or AS. The reported prevalence of SpA in patients with inflammatory bowel disease is widely variable, ranging from 17% to 39%. This wide range may be attributed to differences in research design or diagnostic criteria for spondyloarthritis.[37] Radiological features of both spondylitis and sacroiliitis are similar to those of primitive AS.[38]

Reactive Spondyloarthritis

Reactive SpA (formerly Reiter syndrome) is an aseptic inflammatory arthritis that arises following certain infections of the genitourinary, gastrointestinal, and possibly respiratory tracts.[39] Microbial antigens are thought to represent the trigger for a systemic autoimmune reaction that determines an aseptic inflammatory process involving the axial skeleton or peripheral joints.[40]

A link between human immunodeficiency virus (HIV) infection and reactive SpA, as well as psoriatic SpA and undifferentiated SpA, has been reported; the SpA may occur at any stage of HIV

infection, may be particularly severe, and involves peripheral joints more than axial skeleton.[41]

Reactive SpA is considered a rare disease, predominantly affecting young men aged 25 to 40 years.[42,43] The HLA-B27 gene is present in 45% to 90% of patients and is associated with more severe and prolonged disease.[44]

Clinically, reactive SpA is characterized by the 2 following features: (1) an interval ranging from 1 to 4 weeks between the preceding infection and arthritis, and (2) a typically acute asymmetric, oligoarthritis (involving 1 to 5 joints), commonly affecting the knees, ankles, metatarsophalangeal, and sacroiliac joints. If the hands are involved, the interphalangeal joints are commonly involved with digital tendonitis and enthesitis that give rise to dactylitis. Enthesitis is highly characteristic and both the Achilles tendon and the plantar fascia are commonly affected, often giving rise to heel pain and difficulty walking. Lower back and buttock pain may be caused by sacroiliitis or spondylitis, which are seen more commonly than in psoriatic SpA, with sacroiliitis present in up to 45% of patients and lumbar spondylitis in about

30% of patients.[3,44] Upper thoracic and cervical spine involvement is very rare.

The asymmetric or unilateral involvement of the sacroiliac joints has the same imaging features of psoriatic SpA (Fig. 9). Also, the rare spinal involvement has features similar to those of psoriatic SpA, being represented by nonmarginal bulky syndesmophytes located most frequently in correspondence with the thoracolumbar junction.

Undifferentiated Spondyloarthritis

Patients with typical features of SpA who do not meet the diagnostic criteria for any specific subgroup have been classified as having undifferentiated SpA that shows a mixed axial and peripheral phenotype.[3,4] Although, an important fraction of undifferentiated SpA can progress to AS or other well-defined subgroups of SpA over time, this represents a distinct disease entity based on demographic and clinical differences. Demographically, patients are younger than those with AS and psoriatic SpA, and are more frequently women.

Clinically, the incidence of extra-articular features and HLA-B27 positivity is lower in patients with undifferentiated SpA compared with patients with AS or psoriatic SpA.[45–47] There are no pathognomonic clinical features for undifferentiated SpA; however, inflammatory back pain, peripheral arthritis, and enthesitis are the main clinical features.

Sacroiliitis is below the radiographic cutoff level required by the 1984 modified New York classification criteria (grade 2 sacroiliitis bilaterally or grade 3 or 4 sacroiliitis unilaterally) for the diagnosis of AS[48] and overt radiological spondylitis is usually absent. Peripheral arthritis is typically asymmetric, with ankles and knees as the most frequent joints involved. Enthesitis commonly occurs at the Achilles tendon, and the plantar fascial and tibial tuberosity insertions. Dactylitis can also occur.[45–47]

SUMMARY

The early diagnosis of inflammatory lesions in patients with SpA allows appropriate and effective therapeutic management. Because early inflammation is missed by radiography and CT, the role of MR imaging is particularly important for this purpose. This imaging modality is being increasingly used in practice to assess disease activity, to determine the extent of disease, as well as to monitor and evaluate therapeutic response.

REFERENCES

1. Dougados M, Baeten D. Spondyloarthritis. Lancet 2011;377(9783):2127–37.
2. Mandl P, Navarro-Compán V, Terslev L, et al. EULAR recommendations for the use of imaging in the diagnosis and management of spondyloarthritis in clinical practice. Ann Rheum Dis 2015;74(7):1327–39.
3. Amrami KK. Imaging of the seronegative spondyloarthopathies. Radiol Clin North Am 2012;50(4):841–54.
4. Dougados M, van der Linden S, Juhlin R, et al. The European Spondylarthropathy Study Group preliminary criteria for the classification of spondylarthropathy. Arthritis Rheum 1991;34(10):1218–27.
5. Rudwaleit M, van der Heijde D, Landewé R, et al. The development of Assessment of SpondyloArthritis International Society classification criteria for axial spondyloarthritis (part II): validation and final selection. Ann Rheum Dis 2009;68:777–83.
6. Rudwaleit M, van der Heijde D, Landewé R, et al. The Assessment of SpondyloArthritis International Society classification criteria for peripheral spondyloarthritis and for spondyloarthritis in general. Ann Rheum Dis 2011;70:25–31.
7. Burgos-Vargas R, Casasola-Vargas JC. From retrospective analysis of patients with undifferentiated spondyloarthritis (SpA) to analysis of prospective cohorts and detection of axial and peripheral SpA. J Rheumatol 2010;37(6):1091–5.
8. Baeten D, Breban M, Lories R, et al. Are spondylarthritides related but distinct conditions or a single disease with a heterogeneous phenotype? Arthritis Rheum 2013;65(1):12–20.
9. Puhakka KB, Melsen F, Jurik AG, et al. MR imaging of the normal sacroiliac joint with correlation to histology. Skeletal Radiol 2004;33:15–28.

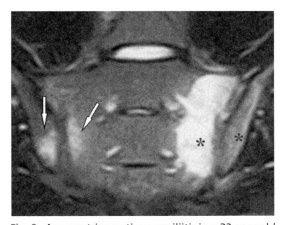

Fig. 9. Asymmetric reactive sacroiliitis in a 33-year-old woman with buttock pain and history of preceding genital infection. Coronal oblique fluid-sensitive fat-suppressed image shows extensive bone marrow edema, particularly on both sides of the left sacroiliac joint (*asterisks*). Moderate bone marrow edema is seen on the sacral and iliac side of the right sacroiliac joint (*arrows*).

10. Khan MA. Update on spondyloarthropathies. Ann Intern Med 2002;136:896–907.

11. Paparo F, Revelli M, Semprini A, et al. Seronegative spondyloarthropathies: what radiologists should know. Radiol Med 2014;119(3):156–63.

12. Feldtkeller E, Khan MA, van der Heijde D, et al. Age at disease onset and diagnosis delay in HLA-B27 negative vs. positive patients with ankylosing spondylitis. Rheumatol Int 2003;23:61–6.

13. Schueller-Weidekamm C, Mascarenhas VV, Sudol-Szopinska I, et al. Imaging and interpretation of axial spondylarthritis: the radiologist's perspective–consensus of the Arthritis Subcommittee of the ESSR. Semin Musculoskelet Radiol 2014;18(3):265–79.

14. Weckbach S, Schewe S, Michaely HJ, et al. Whole-body MR imaging in psoriatic arthritis: additional value for therapeutic decision making. Eur J Radiol 2011;77(1):149–55.

15. Weber U, Hodler J, Jurik AG, et al. Assessment of active spinal inflammatory changes in patients with axial spondyloarthritis: validation of whole body MRI against conventional MRI. Ann Rheum Dis 2010;69(4):648–53.

16. Eshed I, Hermann KG. Novel imaging modalities in spondyloarthritis. Curr Opin Rheumatol 2015;27(4):333–42.

17. Lacout A, Rousselin B, Pelage JP. CT and MRI of spine and sacroiliac involvement in spondyloarthropathy. AJR Am J Roentgenol 2008;191(4):1016–23.

18. Canella C, Schau B, Ribeiro E, et al. MRI in seronegative spondyloarthritis: imaging features and differential diagnosis in the spine and sacroiliac joints. AJR Am J Roentgenol 2013;200(1):149–57.

19. Ostergaard M, Lambert RG. Imaging in ankylosing spondylitis. Ther Adv Musculoskelet Dis 2012;4(4):301–11.

20. Marzo-Ortega H, McGonagle D, O'Connor P, et al. Baseline and 1-year magnetic resonance imaging of the sacroiliac joint and lumbar spine in very early inflammatory back pain. Relationship between symptoms, HLA-B27 and disease extent and persistence. Ann Rheum Dis 2009;68(11):1721–7.

21. Bennett AN, McGonagle D, O'Connor P, et al. Severity of baseline magnetic resonance imaging-evident sacroiliitis and HLA-B27 status in early inflammatory back pain predict radiographically evident ankylosing spondylitis at eight years. Arthritis Rheum 2008;58:3413–8.

22. Leone A, Cassar-Pullicino VN, Casale R, et al. The SAPHO syndrome revisited with an emphasis on spinal manifestations. Skeletal Radiol 2015;44(1):9–24.

23. Jacobs WB, Fehlings MG. Ankylosing spondylitis and spinal cord injury: origin, incidence, management, and avoidance. Neurosurg Focus 2008;24(1):E12.

24. de Vlam K, Mielants H, Verstaete KL, et al. The zygapophyseal joint determines morphology of the enthesophyte. J Rheumatol 2000;27:1732–9.

25. Langlois S, Cedoz JP, Lohse A, et al. Aseptic discitis in patients with ankylosing spondylitis: a retrospective study of 14 cases. Joint Bone Spine 2005;72(3):248–53.

26. Bron JL, de Vries MK, Snieders MN, et al. Discovertebral (Andersson) lesions of the spine in ankylosing spondylitis revisited. Clin Rheumatol 2009;28(8):883–92.

27. Zachariae H. Prevalence of joint disease in patients with psoriasis: implications for therapy. Am J Clin Dermatol 2003;4(7):441–7.

28. Arnett FC. Seronegative spondyloarthropathies. Bull Rheum Dis 1987;37:1–12.

29. Chandran V, Barrett J, Schentag CT, et al. Axial psoriatic arthritis: update on a longterm prospective study. J Rheumatol 2009;36(12):2744–50.

30. Jurik AG. Imaging the spine in arthritis–a pictorial review. Insights Imaging 2011;2(2):177–91.

31. Geusens P, Vosse D, van der Linden S. Osteoporosis and vertebral fractures in ankylosing spondylitis. Curr Opin Rheumatol 2007;19(4):335–9.

32. Smith JA. Update on ankylosing spondylitis: current concepts in pathogenesis. Curr Allergy Asthma Rep 2015;15(1):489.

33. Ghozlani I, Ghazi M, Nouijai A, et al. Prevalence and risk factors of osteoporosis and vertebral fractures in patients with ankylosing spondylitis. Bone 2009;44(5):772–6.

34. Westerveld LA, Verlaan JJ, Oner FC. Spinal fractures in patients with ankylosing spinal disorders: a systematic review of the literature on treatment, neurological status and complications. Eur Spine J 2009;18(2):145–56.

35. Karul M, Bannas P, Schoennagel BP, et al. Fractures of the thoracic spine in patients with minor trauma: comparison of diagnostic accuracy and dose of biplane radiography and MDCT. Eur J Radiol 2013;82(8):1273–7.

36. Wang YF, Teng MM, Chang CY, et al. Imaging manifestations of spinal fractures in ankylosing spondylitis. AJNR Am J Neuroradiol 2005;26(8):2067–76.

37. Arvikar SL, Fisher MC. Inflammatory bowel disease associated arthropathy. Curr Rev Musculoskelet Med 2011;4(3):123–31.

38. Mester AR, Makó EK, Karlinger K, et al. Enteropathic arthritis in the sacroiliac joint. Imaging and differential diagnosis. Eur J Radiol 2000;35:199–208.

39. Wu IB, Schwartz RA. Reiter's syndrome: the classic triad and more. J Am Acad Dermatol 2008;59(1):113–21.

40. Wilson G, Folzenlogen DD. Spondyloarthropathies: new directions in etiopathogenesis, diagnosis and treatment. Mo Med 2012;109(1):69–74.

41. Lawson E, Walker-Bone K. The changing spectrum of rheumatic disease in HIV infection. Br Med Bull 2012;103(1):203–21.

42. Hannu T. Reactive arthritis. Best Pract Res Clin Rheumatol 2011;25(3):347–57.

43. Savolainen E, Kaipiainen-Seppänen O, Kröger L, et al. Total incidence and distribution of inflammatory joint diseases in a defined population: results from the Kuopio 2000 arthritis survey. J Rheumatol 2003;30(11):2460–8.

44. Hamdulay SS, Glynne SJ, Keat A. When is arthritis reactive? Postgrad Med J 2006;82(969):446–53.

45. Zochling J, Brandt J, Braun J. The current concept of spondyloarthritis with special emphasis on undifferentiated spondyloarthritis. Rheumatology (Oxford) 2005;44(12):1483–91.

46. Paramarta JE, De Rycke L, Ambarus CA, et al. Undifferentiated spondyloarthritis vs ankylosing spondylitis and psoriatic arthritis: a real-life prospective cohort study of clinical presentation and response to treatment. Rheumatology (Oxford) 2013;52(10):1873–8.

47. Sampaio-Barros PD, Bortoluzzo AB, Conde RA, et al. Undifferentiated spondyloarthritis: a longterm followup. J Rheumatol 2010;37:1195–9.

48. van der Linden S, Valkenburg HA, Cats A. Evaluation of diagnostic criteria for ankylosing spondylitis. A proposal for modification of the New York criteria. Arthritis Rheum 1984;27:361–8.

Computed Tomography and MR Imaging in Crystalline-Induced Arthropathies

Constantinus Franciscus Buckens, MD, PhD[a],
Maaike P. Terra, MD, PhD[b], Mario Maas, MD, PhD[b,*]

KEYWORDS

- Gout • CPPD • HADD • Crystal arthropathy • Dual-energy computed tomography
- Computed tomography • MR imaging

KEY POINTS

- Computed tomography (CT) is useful for showing crystalline deposits and joint damage in crystalline arthropathies.
- Magnetic resonance is suitable for visualizing joint and soft tissue inflammation in crystalline arthropathies.
- Dual-energy CT has the potential to noninvasively visualize crystalline deposits, particularly monosodium urate deposits in gout.

INTRODUCTION

Conventional radiography remains the first-line imaging modality for crystalline-induced arthropathies, and is frequently used for diagnosis and subsequent monitoring. Existing severity grading schemes reflect this and usually include radiographic parameters. Conventional radiography is limited because of its two-dimensional nature and the inferior soft tissue contrasts achievable.

Computed tomography (CT) and MR imaging provide three-dimensional information on osseous structures, periarticular soft tissue, and tophi with superior spatial resolution. CT provides some soft tissue contrast, which can be enhanced by using intravenous or intra-articular contrast agents. Dual-source CT is a new modality that offers the further advantage of selectively identifying crystalline deposits based on their specific attenuation profiles, by scanning simultaneously with 2 x-ray sources at different voltages, an approach that can be mimicked by scanning with a single source twice (so-called single-source dual-source CT scanning).

MR imaging offers superior soft tissue contrasts and can better characterize the symptom-causing synovitis and soft tissue inflammations that frequently accompany crystalline arthropathies.

The most common crystalline arthropathies are gout (monosodium urate [MSU]deposition) and calcium pyrophosphate dihydrate deposition (CPPD). Other crystal deposition diseases have been described, including hydroxyapatite deposition disease (HADD),[1] calcium oxalate aluminum

Disclosure: The authors have nothing to disclose.
[a] Department of Radiology, Universitair Medisch Centrum Utrecht, Room E01.132, Huispostnummer E01.132, Postbus 85500, Utrecht GA 3508, The Netherlands; [b] Division of Musculoskeletal Radiology, Department of Radiology, Academic Medical Center, Room G1-211, Meibergdreef 9, Amsterdam AZ 1105, The Netherlands
* Corresponding author. Division of Musculoskeletal Radiology, Department of Radiology, Academic Medical Center, University of Amsterdam, Room G1-211, Meibergdreef 9, Amsterdam AZ 1105.
E-mail address: m.maas@amc.uva.nl

Radiol Clin N Am 55 (2017) 1023–1034
http://dx.doi.org/10.1016/j.rcl.2017.04.008
0033-8389/17/© 2017 Elsevier Inc. All rights reserved.

radiologic.theclinics.com

phosphate, cholesterol, xanthine, cysteine, and lysophospholipase deposition, but this article discusses MR and CT imaging of the most common disorders.

TECHNICAL CONSIDERATIONS
Computed Tomography

CT scanning is fast, compared with MR imaging and ultrasonography, and is widely available. Non-enhanced single-source CT provides superior visualization of bony erosions and is excellent for visualizing larger crystal depositions. Typically, the symptomatic joints are included in the scanning volume. In cases of suspected gout, protocols sometimes also routinely screen the hands and the feet, because these are the sites most typically affected and screening them has the highest clinical impact.[2] Both hands and both feet can then be scanned in 2 scanning volumes. A major disadvantage of CT pertains to its use of ionizing radiation. The negative impact of this radiation can be reduced by positioning the (usually peripheral) joints as far as possible from more radiation-sensitive core body structures.[3]

CT scans are typically reconstructed in a bone kernel and stored in reconstructions of 2/2 or 3/3 mm in different planes, depending on the joints scanned and the locally prevailing practice (the authors prefer storing a thinner 1-mm slice thickness reconstruction for higher resolution analysis, and to facilitate on-the-fly multiplanar reconstructions during reading or presentation). Separate reconstructions in soft tissue kernel have an added value for identifying less dense tophi and better visualizing soft tissue inflammation or soft tissue complications. Nonetheless, CT has limited potential for showing soft tissue inflammation.

Intravenous contrast-enhanced CT (CECT) can improve detection of active soft tissue inflammation but is not routinely used in the assessment of crystal arthropathy. It can be considered when MR is contraindicated.

DECT is a recently developed technique that can greatly improve the sensitivity of CT to crystal deposits. It involves scanning the patient with 2 separate energy levels so that crystal deposits can be separated from other mineral deposits (such as calcium in bone) by its distinct spectral profile, in turn determined by the unique atomic number in the crystal deposits. The different spectral attenuation profiles are generated by scanning simultaneously with 2 separate energy sources in DECT, or generated with a single energy source by using rapid voltage switching, or with sequential scanning, or more recently spectral detector solutions with a single x-ray source.[4,5]

MR Imaging

MR generates superior soft tissue contrasts and is suited to showing, without the use of radiation, soft tissue inflammation (synovitis, tenosynovitis, joint effusion, crystal depositions and surrounding soft tissue edema, and bone marrow edema). Structural joint damage (particularly cartilage loss but also bone erosions and deformity) can also be shown. Deeper and less-accessible structures can be visualized, unlike with ultrasonography. Crystal deposits can be measured in 3 dimensions. Because of the cost and the scanning times involved in MR acquisition, imaging is usually confined to the symptomatic joints.

Prevailing standard musculoskeletal MR protocols are usually available specifying patient position, coil choice, and placement. MR sequence selection is usually predetermined as well but should include sequences that can optimally visualize structural joint damage, soft tissue inflammation, and any crystal depositions that may be present, with adequate spatial resolution. T1-weighted and intermediate proton density (PD)–weighted sequences, usually acquired using fast or turbo spin echo techniques, show bone marrow, joint anatomy, and periarticular anatomy. PD or T2-weighted sequences with fat saturation facilitate the detection of bone marrow edema and soft tissue edema, as well as the assessment of cartilage. As ever, sequences should be acquired in multiple planes, or three-dimensional sequences could be included, to permit a multiplanar assessment. The administration of intravenous MR contrast media, with postcontrast T1-weighted sequences with or without fat suppression, can be included to further show active inflammation and differentiate synovial hypertrophy from active synovitis.

GOUT

MSU crystal deposition in joints and periarticular tissues, with concomitant inflammation, characterize gout. Initially it usually presents with intermittent paroxysmal painful episodes but often, left untreated, it eventually progresses to a chronic, debilitating inflammation with bone erosions and tophi. Timely diagnosis is crucial for intervening in the progression of the disease in an early phase but is also challenging. Current diagnostic practice relies heavily on clinical parameters[6,7] and especially the demonstration of MSU crystals in joint aspirations. However, MSU crystals are mostly intracellular during acute attacks of gout and during the intercritical periods, and the sensitivity of the procedure depends not only on a technically successful aspiration but also on adequate crystal concentration in the aspirate, as well as observer skill and experience.[8–10]

Although imaging does not currently play a prominent role in the routine diagnosis of gout, CT and MR imaging can be useful in diagnosing atypical cases. Reflecting this, dual-energy CT (DECT) and ultrasonography have been incorporated into the recent American College of Rheumatology/European League Against Rheumatism gout classification criteria alongside radiographs,[7] but these remain little used in practice.

DECT, CT, and MR imaging also have potential for monitoring disease progression.[11] A working group for the Outcome Measures in Rheumatology (OMERACT) project has identified relevant outcome domains (urate deposition, joint inflammation, and structural joint damage) and evaluated the potential of CT, DECT, and MR imaging (among other modalities) for assessing these domains, broadly concluding that, despite the intrinsic potential, there is as yet insufficient evidence to inform imaging based outcomes monitoring.[12]

Standard Computed Tomography Gout

In the early stages of gout, standard CT has little utility because it is not suitable for imaging the soft tissue inflammation that characterizes early gout. Later in the progression of the disease, bone erosions and tophi can be visualized and quantified (Fig. 1A, B); CT is the gold standard for imaging bone erosions. CT imaging of gout has led to new insights into the pattern and timing of bone erosion in gout, particularly the close relationship between erosions and tophi.[13] Tophi have a characteristic density of around 160 Hounsfield units (HU),[14] and volume and density measurements can be performed using CT.[3] CECT is slightly better than nonenhanced CT at showing major synovitis and soft tissue inflammation.

Dual-energy Computed Tomography Gout

DECT is able to identify MSU deposits based on their characteristic atomic number and mass density. This ability allows even small MSU deposits to be reliably detected on CT, combining MSU detection with the high resolution, fast acquisition times, and superior bone (erosion) visualization already offered by standard CT (Fig. 1C), and holds the potential for earlier diagnosis of gout as well as accurate monitoring of both tophi and bone erosions.[15]

A search of the literature on the diagnostic performance of dual-source DECT for gout involving a PubMed search using terms and synonyms for DECT and gout, which were filtered using inclusion and exclusion criteria limiting the yield to human studies investigating gout or suspected gout from which diagnostic performance could be extracted. Seven studies[2,16–21] were found incorporating 413 patients in whom the sensitivity of DECT for gout ranged from 78% to 100% and the specificity ranged from 50% to 93% (Table 1).

The results from these studies were combined in a bivariate random effects model[22] using the mada package 0.5.7[23] in the R statistical environment (version 3.3.1, R Foundation for Statistical Computing, Vienna, Austria.). This model yielded a pooled estimate of sensitivity of 84% (95% confidence interval, 78%–88%) and a pooled estimate of specificity of 84% (77%–89%) (Fig. 2). There was heterogeneity in the study populations included; patients with chronic tophaceous gout, acute gout, and intercritical gout were variously included, and different reference standards were used across and within studies; crystalproven gout and/or clinical-radiographic criteria. The authors thought that pooling was justified nonetheless -with the use of a random effects model- because this heterogeneity reflects current practice. These diagnostic performance measures are close to those reported in a recent meta-analysis including 3 of these 7 studies,[24] from which a pooled sensitivity of 87% and specificity of 84% was estimated.

Just as in joint aspiration, in which aspiration is negative in 25% of acute-onset gout cases,[8] false-negative results on DECT seem to be particularly frequently observed in recent-onset disease[17] and in cases with small deposits.[20] DECT seems to perform moderately well in cases of intercritical gout (sensitivity of 91% and specificity of 82%; see Table 1).[2]

A recent diagnostic study by Ahmad and colleagues[16] separately reported the diagnostic performance of DECT for gout among patients suspected of gout who were classified using the American College of Rheumatology clinicoradiographic criteria, as well as a subset of these patients in whom a joint aspiration was used as the reference standard. This study exposed a discrepancy in the diagnostic performance of DECT for gout, with DECT having a higher sensitivity (100% vs 82%) but lower specificity (48% vs 97%) when aspiration was used as the reference standard rather than clinicoradiographic criteria. In a separate study, Baer and colleagues[25] showed that MSU deposits are less frequently detected in cases of nontophaceous gout (sensitivity 64% for nontophaceous gout against 100% for tophaceous gout).

Taken together, these intriguing findings suggest that the sensitivity of DECT may be subject

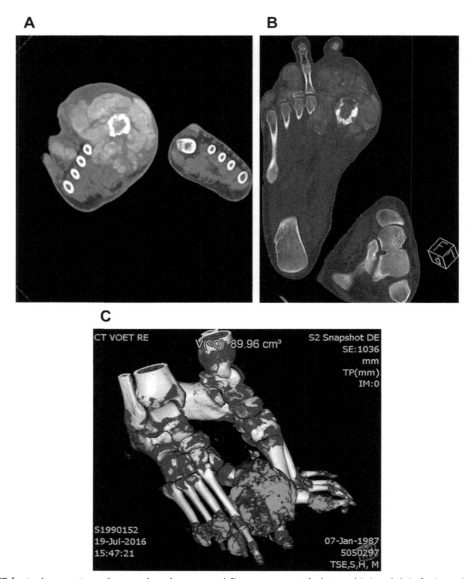

Fig. 1. CT featuring gout erosions and tophus around first metatarsophalangeal joint. (*A*) Soft tissue kernel and window. (*B*) Bone kernel in bone window. (*C*) DECT color-coded volume rendering with MSU deposits in green.

to some of the same limitations as joint aspiration, with both approaches performing less well in cases of recent-onset disease and nontophaceous gout. This finding meets face validity, because both diagnostic approaches rely on the presence of MSU deposits in sufficient number and concentration.

An interesting case report correlating DECT findings with pathology findings seems to support this. Melzer and colleagues[26] found that standard DECT thresholds only reliably show portions of tophi with high concentrations of MSU crystals, a fact that may contribute to the limited sensitivity

of DECT, particularly in early-onset disease when tophi have not yet concentrated. This finding is in keeping with the modest correlation between tophus size measurements on DECT and other measurement means previously reported.[27] DECT technical parameters might also play a role in affecting the sensitivity of DECT for smaller deposits, such as the parameter ratio used to segment the CT data and label MSU deposits,[28] an issue that deserves further investigation.

The lower specificity found in the aspiration arm of the study of Ahmad and colleagues[16] warrants separate consideration, because it suggests

Table 1
Studies investigating the diagnostic performance of dual-energy computed tomography for detecting gout

Lead Author, Year	DECT System	Reference Standard	Number of Subjects	Sensitivity	Specificity	Journal	Study Design
Ahmad et al,[16] 2016	Flash/Siemens	ARA	90	82	89	Int J Rheum Dis	Prospective convenience
Breuer et al,[2] 2016	Flash/Siemens	ARA	50	91	82	Int J Rheum Dis	Retrospective convenience
Bongartz et al,[17] 2015	Flash/Siemens	Aspiration	81	90	83	Ann Rheum Dis	Prospective case control
Gruber et al,[19] 2014	Flash/Siemens	US/aspiration	21	87	50	Rheumatology (Oxford)	Prospective convenience
Huppertz et al,[20] 2014	Flash/Siemens	ARA/Aspiration	60	85	86	Rheumatol Int	Prospective convenience
Choi et al,[21] 2012	Flash/Siemens	Aspiration	80	78	93	Ann Rheum Dis	Prospective case control
Glazebrook et al,[18] 2011	Flash/Siemens	Aspiration	31	100	87	Radiology	Retrospective convenience

Abbreviations: ARA, American Rheumatism Association (now the American College of Rheumatology); US, ultrasonography.

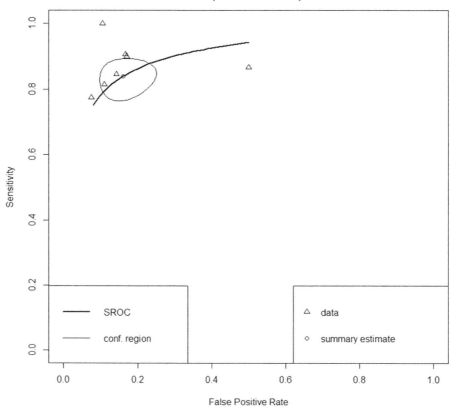

Fig. 2. Summary receiver operating characteristics (SROC) curve for the pooled diagnostic performance of DECT for diagnosing gout.

DECT might detect a high rate of false-positives. False-positive color coding can occur, particularly in osteoarthritic patients, and particularly at the knees,[17] and in nail beds and skin,[29] although in the nail beds and skin this is easy to distinguish from genuine tophi. Troublingly, MSU deposition seems to occur in asymptomatic age-matched and gender-matched individuals, at least in the spine.[30] Together with our pooled specificity of 84%, these findings suggest that perhaps false-positives are to be expected on DECT imaging. Alternatively, the particularly lower specificity found for DECT by Ahmad and colleagues[16] compared with aspiration (49%) might reflect particular limitations of aspiration, rather than a high false-positive rate: false-negative aspirates could conceivably misclassify cases, increasing the apparent false-positive rate of DECT. This issue affects all gout research incorporating aspiration as a gold standard and deserves further investigation.

In addition, DECT has already yielded clues as to the mechanism of bone erosion formation in gout, by showing that tophi form on the surface of bone and within bony erosions but not within intact adjacent bone, suggesting that tophi form outside bone before bone erosion.[31]

There is less information concerning DECT using a single energy source, but these approaches may widen the availability of DECT. A recent publication by Keifer and colleagues[32] using sequential scanning at 2 voltages showed a sensitivity of 71% and a specificity of 96% for gout among a clinically relevant group of patients suspected of gout, a level of performance that deserves further investigation.

MR Imaging Gout

MR offers superior soft tissue contrast, allowing it to better visualize synovitis and soft tissue inflammation as well as tophi and bone erosions. Tophi can reliably and reproducibly be detected on MR imaging[33,34] and have variable signal characteristics, but they are typically low on T1-weighted and intermediate to high on T2-weighted sequences and show heterogeneous enhancement[35] (**Fig. 3**). Besides nodular tophi, amorphous tophi

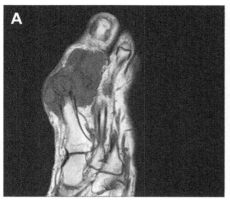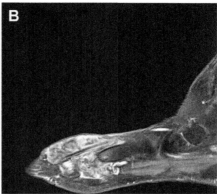

Fig. 3. MR image of gout. (A) Transverse T1-weighted image showing extensive tophus, joint destruction, and bony erosions around first metatarsophalangeal joint. (B) Sagittal T1-weighted image with fat saturation after administration of intravenous contrast agent showing heterogenous enhancement of the tophus.

have also been described using MR imaging.[36] There are few data about the diagnostic performance of MR imaging for gout and MR imaging is not incorporated into recent American College of Rheumatology criteria,[7] although its ability to visualize joint destruction and soft tissue inflammation has obvious potential to monitor disease progression.[12]

Uniquely, MR allows bone marrow edema to be visualized as well, although this does not seem to be a characteristic finding in gout patients, until late-stage disease at least.[33,37,38] This finding in itself has interesting pathophysiologic implications concerning the cause of the characteristic bony erosions observed in gout, along with the aforementioned DECT study showing that tophi appear adjacent to bone and not within intact bone. Notably, MR imaging is sensitive to osteomyelitis, a complication of gout.[37] MR imaging is also more sensitive than ultrasonography to occult destructive arthropathy.[39]

CALCIUM PYROPHOSPHATE DIHYDRATE DEPOSITION

CPPD, also termed pyrophosphate arthropathy or calcium pyrophosphate deposition disease (CPDD) arthropathy,[40] is characterized by the deposition of calcium pyrophosphate crystals in and around joints, causing inflammation, sometimes with paroxysmal goutlike symptoms (a clinical construct termed pseudogout in the past). In contrast, chondrocalcinosis is a nonspecific descriptive term for any observed calcifications within cartilage (whether pyrophosphate or not), and is often asymptomatic. Chondrocalcinosis is often seen in CPPD, along with synovial, ligamentous/tendon, and soft tissue deposits of pyrophosphate.

CPPD tends to be symmetric in distribution. Commonly affected sites include the knee (particularly the patellofemoral compartment), pubic symphysis, wrist (typically associated with scapholunate advanced collapse[41]), and the spine. Characteristically, non–weight-bearing joints such as the shoulder, elbow, and wrist are also affected,[1,42] in contrast with osteoarthritis. CPPD is associated with other metabolic disorders and has a complex relationship with osteoarthritis (sharing many features as well as affecting similar patient groups).[40,43] Differentiating CPPD from osteoarthritis can be difficult, with careful attention to the distribution of affected joints and detection of calcific deposits both distinguishing CPPD[44] (Fig. 4).

Computed Tomography Calcium Pyrophosphate Dihydrate Deposition

Calcium pyrophosphate deposits appear denser on CT than MSU deposits, with attenuation around 450 HU. In contrast with gouty tophi, they characteristically appear fine, punctate, and linear.[44] CT exquisitely shows the calcifications and any pressure erosions in adjacent bone or joint malalignments.[45,46]

Articular structures that are less readily assessed on radiographs benefit particularly from CT, especially the spine.[47,48] CPPD in atypical locations also benefits from CT.[49]

MR Imaging Calcium Pyrophosphate Dihydrate Deposition

MR imaging does not play a role in the diagnosis of CPDD but it may be detected on investigations requested for arthropathy of unknown cause, or be detected incidentally. During bouts of acute

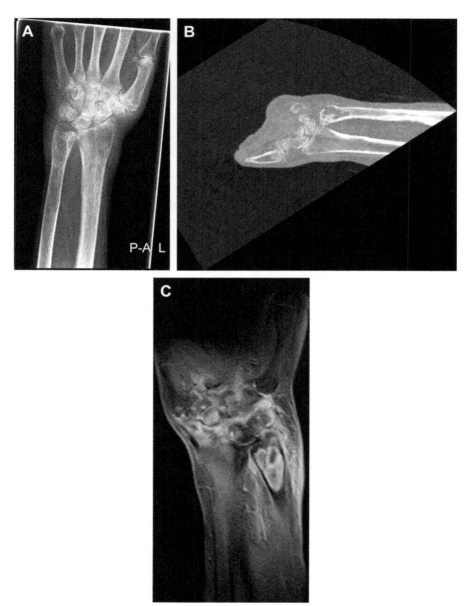

Fig. 4. CPPD. (*A*) Wrist radiograph showing articular calcifications in combination with degenerative joints. (*B*) Coronal oblique CT of same wrist showing subchondral erosion into distal ulna. (*C*) MR CPPD.

inflammation MR shows the joint effusion and soft tissue inflammation (see **Fig. 4**).

Calcium pyrophosphate deposits can be seen as linear or punctate low-signal areas within articular or periarticular structures, with peripheral enhancement.[50]

Chondrocalcinosis (most commonly caused by calcium pyrophosphate) can complicate the interpretation MR imaging performed to evaluate articular structures such as the knee menisci, in which chondrocalcinosis deposits appear as linear areas of (counterintuitively) increased signal intensity.[50–52] It has been posited that the increased signal intensity might be caused by surrounding inflammation/degeneration, or susceptibility artifact.[44,50,51]

CALCIUM HYDROXYAPATITE DEPOSITION DISEASE

Calcium HADD is characterized by periarticular calcium hydroxyapatite depositions, most typically in and about tendons. The depositions are often monoarticular and chondrocalcinosis is

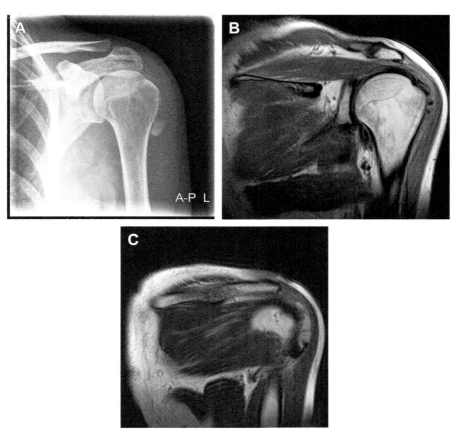

Fig. 5. HADD. (*A*) Shoulder radiograph showing calcifications near insertion of supraspinatus and infraspinatus tendons extending into subdeltoid bursa. (*B* and *C*) Consecutive coronal oblique PD-weighted MR image showing the same.

rare, helping distinguish HADD from CPPD. Furthermore, HADD calcific deposits are often amorphous and homogeneous and not usually linear or punctate as in CPPD, although there is overlap. The pathogenesis is thought to be related to repetitive microtrauma and necrosis followed by dystrophic mineralization.[53]

The shoulder is the most commonly affected site, followed by the hips, elbows, wrists, and knees. Severe arthropathy with bony erosions and calcium hydroxyapatite depositions, termed Milwaukee shoulder, can be considered a rare and severe form of HADD.[54] Acute symptoms of pain and inflammation tend to occur when hydroxyapatite depositions are being resorbed or/and when they migrate out of tendons into bursae or bone[55,56] (**Fig. 5**).

Computed Tomography Hydroxyapatite Deposition Disease

As in CPPD, atypical cases of HADD particularly benefit from the application of tomographic studies, with CT showing globular amorphous deposits, which may be resorbed, during which period they may lose volume and density on longitudinal imaging.[57] CT may show migration of calcific deposits into adjacent tissues, including subcortical erosions and even penetration into adjacent bone.[56,58]

MR Imaging Hydroxyapatite Deposition Disease

MR imaging is not the primary modality for diagnosing HADD but deposits are frequently detected incidentally in tendons and may be seen when MR imaging is requested for arthropathy or periarticular inflammation with unknown cause. Calcium hydroxyapatite depositions appear as low-intensity areas on T1-weighted and T2-weighted sequences[59] (see **Fig. 5**). As in CPPD, adjacent soft tissue and joint inflammation are well visualized during the acute phases of HADD. Bone marrow edema in cases involving osseous involvement can be seen using MR imaging.[56,58] Correlation with radiographs or CT can avoid misdiagnosis in rare cases of osseous involvement.

SUMMARY

Crystalline-induced arthropathies impose substantial morbidity but can be challenging to diagnose, especially in early phases. This article examines how CT and MR imaging can be useful in problematic cases of gout, CPPD, and HADD, but observes that they do not currently play a large role in routine diagnostics or disease monitoring. As a recent technical innovation in CT imaging, DECT deserves special consideration for its potential to highly selectively identify and visualize crystalline deposits based on their unique attenuation profile. DECT seems to perform well, with pooled sensitivity and specificity estimates from recent diagnostic studies for gout of 84%, but it seems to show a lower performance in early gout and during intercritical periods, the very segments that are most challenging to diagnose via traditional means. As ever, further investigation is warranted into the diagnostic potential of DECT for crystalline arthropathies, and the utility of CT, DECT, and MR imaging for disease monitoring.

REFERENCES

1. Resnik CS, Resnick D. Crystal deposition disease. Semin Arthritis Rheum 1983;12(4):390–403.
2. Breuer GS, Bogot N, Nesher G. Dual-energy computed tomography as a diagnostic tool for gout during intercritical periods. Int J Rheum Dis 2016;19(12):1337–41.
3. Dalbeth N, Clark B, Gregory K, et al. Computed tomography measurement of tophus volume: comparison with physical measurement. Arthritis Rheum 2007;57(3):461–5.
4. Johnson TRC. Dual-energy CT: general principles. AJR Am J Roentgenol 2012;199(5 Suppl):S3–8.
5. Omoumi P, Becce F, Racine D, et al. Dual-Energy CT: basic principles, technical approaches, and applications in musculoskeletal imaging (part 1). Semin Musculoskelet Radiol 2015;19(5):431–7.
6. Wallace SL, Robinson H, Masi AT, et al. Preliminary criteria for the classification of the acute arthritis of primary gout. Arthritis Rheum 1977;20(3):895–900.
7. Neogi T, Jansen TLTA, Dalbeth N, et al. 2015 gout classification criteria: an American College of Rheumatology/European League Against Rheumatism collaborative initiative. Arthritis Rheumatol 2015; 67(10):2557–68.
8. Swan A, Amer H, Dieppe P. The value of synovial fluid assays in the diagnosis of joint disease: a literature survey. Ann Rheum Dis 2002;61(6):493–8.
9. Schlesinger N. Diagnosis of gout: clinical, laboratory, and radiologic findings. Am J Manag Care 2005;11(15 Suppl):S443–50 [quiz: S465–8].
10. Von Essen R, Hölttä AM. Quality control of the laboratory diagnosis of gout by synovial fluid microscopy. Scand J Rheumatol 1990;19(3):232–4.
11. Durcan L, Grainger R, Keen HI, et al. Imaging as a potential outcome measure in gout studies: a systematic literature review. Semin Arthritis Rheum 2016;45(5):570–9.
12. Grainger R, Dalbeth N, Keen H, et al. Imaging as an outcome measure in gout studies: report from the OMERACT Gout Working Group. J Rheumatol 2015;42(12):2460–4.
13. Doyle AJ, Dalbeth N, McQueen F, et al. Gout on CT of the feet: a symmetric arthropathy. J Med Imaging Radiat Oncol 2016;60(1):54–8.
14. Gerster JC, Landry M, Dufresne L, et al. Imaging of tophaceous gout: computed tomography provides specific images compared with magnetic resonance imaging and ultrasonography. Ann Rheum Dis 2002; 61(1):52–4.
15. Rajan A, Aati O, Kalluru R, et al. Lack of change in urate deposition by dual-energy computed tomography among clinically stable patients with long-standing tophaceous gout: a prospective longitudinal study. Arthritis Res Ther 2013; 15(5):R160.
16. Ahmad Z, Gupta AK, Sharma R, et al. Dual energy computed tomography: a novel technique for diagnosis of gout. Int J Rheum Dis 2016;19(9):887–96.
17. Bongartz T, Glazebrook KN, Kavros SJ, et al. Dual-energy CT for the diagnosis of gout: an accuracy and diagnostic yield study. Ann Rheum Dis 2015; 74(6):1072–7.
18. Glazebrook KN, Guimarães LS, Murthy NS, et al. Identification of intraarticular and periarticular uric acid crystals with dual-energy CT: initial evaluation. Radiology 2011;261(2):516–24.
19. Gruber M, Bodner G, Rath E, et al. Dual-energy computed tomography compared with ultrasound in the diagnosis of gout. Rheumatology (Oxford) 2014;53(1):173–9.
20. Huppertz A, Hermann KGA, Diekhoff T, et al. Systemic staging for urate crystal deposits with dual-energy CT and ultrasound in patients with suspected gout. Rheumatol Int 2014;34(6):763–71.
21. Choi HK, Burns LC, Shojania K, et al. Dual energy CT in gout: a prospective validation study. Ann Rheum Dis 2012;71(9):1466–71.
22. Reitsma JB, Glas AS, Rutjes AWS, et al. Bivariate analysis of sensitivity and specificity produces informative summary measures in diagnostic reviews. J Clin Epidemiol 2005;58(10):982–90.
23. Doebler P. Mada: meta-analysis of diagnostic accuracy; 2015. Available at: https://CRAN.R-project.org/package=mada. Accessed October 3, 2015.

24. Ogdie A, Taylor WJ, Weatherall M, et al. Imaging modalities for the classification of gout: systematic literature review and meta-analysis. Ann Rheum Dis 2015;74(10):1868–74.
25. Baer AN, Kurano T, Thakur UJ, et al. Dual-energy computed tomography has limited sensitivity for non-tophaceous gout: a comparison study with tophaceous gout. BMC Musculoskelet Disord 2016; 17:91.
26. Melzer R, Pauli C, Treumann T, et al. Gout tophus detection–a comparison of dual-energy CT (DECT) and histology. Semin Arthritis Rheum 2014;43(5): 662–5.
27. Dalbeth N, Aati O, Gao A, et al. Assessment of tophus size: a comparison between physical measurement methods and dual-energy computed tomography scanning. J Clin Rheumatol 2012; 18(1):23–7.
28. McQueen FMF, Doyle AJ, Reeves Q, et al. DECT urate deposits: now you see them, now you don't. Ann Rheum Dis 2013;72(3):458–9.
29. Mallinson PI, Coupal T, Reisinger C, et al. Artifacts in dual-energy CT gout protocol: a review of 50 suspected cases with an artifact identification guide. AJR Am J Roentgenol 2014;203(1):W103–9.
30. Carr A, Doyle AJ, Dalbeth N, et al. Dual-energy CT of urate deposits in costal cartilage and intervertebral disks of patients with tophaceous gout and age-matched controls. AJR Am J Roentgenol 2016; 206(5):1063–7.
31. Towiwat P, Doyle AJ, Gamble GD, et al. Urate crystal deposition and bone erosion in gout: "inside-out" or "outside-in"? A dual-energy computed tomography study. Arthritis Res Ther 2016;18(1):208.
32. Kiefer T, Diekhoff T, Hermann S, et al. Single source dual-energy computed tomography in the diagnosis of gout: diagnostic reliability in comparison to digital radiography and conventional computed tomography of the feet. Eur J Radiol 2016;85(10):1829–34.
33. McQueen FM, Doyle A, Reeves Q, et al. Bone erosions in patients with chronic gouty arthropathy are associated with tophi but not bone oedema or synovitis: new insights from a 3 T MRI study. Rheumatol Oxf Engl 2014;53(1):95–103.
34. Schumacher HR, Becker MA, Edwards NL, et al. Magnetic resonance imaging in the quantitative assessment of gouty tophi. Int J Clin Pract 2006; 60(4):408–14.
35. Chen CK, Yeh LR, Pan HB, et al. Intra-articular gouty tophi of the knee: CT and MR imaging in 12 patients. Skeletal Radiol 1999;28(2):75–80.
36. Popp JD, Bidgood WD, Edwards NL. Magnetic resonance imaging of tophaceous gout in the hands and wrists. Semin Arthritis Rheum 1996;25(4):282–9.
37. Poh YJ, Dalbeth N, Doyle A, et al. Magnetic resonance imaging bone edema is not a major feature of gout unless there is concomitant osteomyelitis:

38. 10-year findings from a high-prevalence population. J Rheumatol 2011;38(11):2475–81.
38. Cimmino MA, Zampogna G, Parodi M, et al. MRI synovitis and bone lesions are common in acute gouty arthritis of the wrist even during the first attack. Ann Rheum Dis 2011;70(12):2238–9.
39. Carter JD, Kedar RP, Anderson SR, et al. An analysis of MRI and ultrasound imaging in patients with gout who have normal plain radiographs. Rheumatol Oxf Engl 2009;48(11):1442–6.
40. Zhang W, Doherty M, Bardin T, et al. European League Against Rheumatism recommendations for calcium pyrophosphate deposition. Part I: terminology and diagnosis. Ann Rheum Dis 2011;70(4): 563–70.
41. Chen C, Chandnani VP, Kang HS, et al. Scapholunate advanced collapse: a common wrist abnormality in calcium pyrophosphate dihydrate crystal deposition disease. Radiology 1990;177(2):459–61.
42. Resnick D, Niwayama G, Goergen TG, et al. Clinical, radiographic and pathologic abnormalities in calcium pyrophosphate dihydrate deposition disease (CPPD): pseudogout. Radiology 1977;122(1):1–15.
43. Ea HK, Nguyen C, Bazin D, et al. Articular cartilage calcification in osteoarthritis: insights into crystal-induced stress. Arthritis Rheum 2011;63(1):10–8.
44. Steinbach LS, Resnick D. Calcium pyrophosphate dihydrate crystal deposition disease: imaging perspectives. Curr Probl Diagn Radiol 2000;29(6): 209–29.
45. Mizutani H, Ohba S, Mizutani M, et al. Tumoral calcium pyrophosphate dihydrate deposition disease with bone destruction in the shoulder. CT and MR findings in two cases. Acta Radiol 1998;39(3): 269–72.
46. Misra D, Guermazi A, Sieren JP, et al. CT imaging for evaluation of calcium crystal deposition in the knee: initial experience from the Multicenter Osteoarthritis (MOST) study. Osteoarthritis Cartilage 2015;23(2): 244–8.
47. Baysal T, Baysal O, Kutlu R, et al. The crowned dens syndrome: a rare form of calcium pyrophosphate deposition disease. Eur Radiol 2000;10(6):1003–5.
48. Scutellari PN, Galeotti R, Leprotti S, et al. The crowned dens syndrome. Evaluation with CT imaging. Radiol Med (Torino) 2007;112(2):195–207.
49. Brunot S, Fabre T, Lepreux S, et al. Pseudotumoral presentation of calcium pyrophosphate dihydrate crystal deposition disease. J Rheumatol 2008; 35(4):727–9.
50. Beltran J, Marty-Delfaut E, Bencardino J, et al. Chondrocalcinosis of the hyaline cartilage of the knee: MRI manifestations. Skeletal Radiol 1998; 27(7):369–74.
51. Kaushik S, Erickson JK, Palmer WE, et al. Effect of chondrocalcinosis on the MR imaging of knee menisci. AJR Am J Roentgenol 2001;177(4):905–9.

52. Burke BJ, Escobedo EM, Wilson AJ, et al. Chondro-calcinosis mimicking a meniscal tear on MR imaging. AJR Am J Roentgenol 1998;170(1):69–70.

53. Steinbach LS. Calcium pyrophosphate dihydrate and calcium hydroxyapatite crystal deposition diseases: imaging perspectives. Radiol Clin North Am 2004;42(1):185–205, vii.

54. Halverson PB, McCarty DJ, Cheung HS, et al. Milwaukee shoulder syndrome: eleven additional cases with involvement of the knee in seven (basic calcium phosphate crystal deposition disease). Semin Arthritis Rheum 1984;14(1):36–44.

55. Omoumi P, Zufferey P, Malghem J, et al. Imaging in gout and other crystal-related arthropathies. Rheum Dis Clin North Am 2016;42(4):621–44.

56. Moseley HF, Jean JP. Shoulder lesions. 3rd edition. Baltimore (MD): Williams and Wilkins; 1969.

57. Malghem J, Omoumi P, Lecouvet F, et al. Intraosseous migration of tendinous calcifications: cortical erosions, subcortical migration and extensive intramedullary diffusion, a SIMS series. Skeletal Radiol 2015;44(10):1403–12.

58. Flemming DJ, Murphey MD, Shekitka KM, et al. Osseous involvement in calcific tendinitis: a retrospective review of 50 cases. AJR Am J Roentgenol 2003;181(4):965–72.

59. Zubler C, Mengiardi B, Schmid MR, et al. MR arthrography in calcific tendinitis of the shoulder: diagnostic performance and pitfalls. Eur Radiol 2007;17(6):1603–10.

SAPHO and Recurrent Multifocal Osteomyelitis

Simon Greenwood, MBChB, MSc, MRCP, FRCR[a], Antonio Leone, MD[b],
Victor N. Cassar-Pullicino, MD, FRCR[a],*

KEYWORDS

- SAPHO • CRMO • Hyperostosis • Osteitis • Pediatric • Whole-body MR imaging

KEY POINTS

- SAPHO and CRMO are complex inflammatory disorders in which multifocal osteitis is the dominant feature, with varying degrees of associated synovitis, hyperostosis, and cutaneous lesions.
- SAPHO tends to affect 30 to 50 year olds, whereas CRMO is invariably seen in the pediatric population, both with a marked female predominance.
- The conditions are typically multifocal with predilections for certain anatomic sites; SAPHO the anterior chest wall and CRMO the metaphyses of the tibia and distal femur, but affected sites are not always symptomatic, with several only being evident on imaging.
- Conventional radiographs are often normal at initial presentation and early MR imaging is invaluable in making a prompt diagnosis, including whole-body MR imaging to assess for subclinical sites and demonstrate the typical multifocal pattern of involvement.
- Treatment options include simple analgesics, nonsteroidal anti-inflammatory drugs, corticosteroids, bisphosphonates, and biologic agents, including TNF-α antagonists.

INTRODUCTION

SAPHO and recurrent multifocal osteomyelitis are complex inflammatory conditions whose features center on a variety of osteoarticular and cutaneous manifestations (Fig. 1). The understanding of these conditions has evolved over several decades, with progressive advances being made in terms of their clinical course, pathogenesis, radiologic features, and therapeutic options. Nonetheless, an understanding of several aspects of these diverse conditions is still developing, and with such a wide range of clinical and radiologic appearances, it can require great skill to make the diagnoses. There is a reliance on imaging in both conditions, so the onus is often on the clinical radiologist to recognize the complex and often subtle diagnostic features. A good understanding of the evolution of disease, pathogenesis, and advanced imaging features helps to facilitate timely diagnoses in what is a diagnostically challenging patient group.

EVOLUTION OF TERMS

For more than 50 years, an association has been well documented between certain musculoskeletal and skin conditions. In 1961, Windom and colleagues first described a case report linking acne conglobata and peripheral arthritis.[1] This then sparked a flurry of literature over the subsequent decades describing similar cases. There have been wide variations reported in the presentation and clinical course of these cases, such as patient demographics, musculoskeletal sites affected, and types of skin condition. This, in turn, has led

Disclosure Statement: No commercial or financial conflicts of interest and no funding sources.
[a] Department of Diagnostic Imaging, The Robert Jones and Agnes Hunt Orthopaedic Hospital NHS Foundation Trust, Twmpath Lane, Gobowen, Oswestry SY10 7AG, UK; [b] Emergency/Musculoskeletal Section, Institute of Radiology, Catholic University, School of Medicine, Policlinico A. Gemelli, Largo A. Gemelli, 1, Rome 00135, Italy
* Corresponding author.
E-mail address: victor.pullicino@rjah.nhs.uk

Radiol Clin N Am 55 (2017) 1035–1053
http://dx.doi.org/10.1016/j.rcl.2017.04.009
0033-8389/17/© 2017 Elsevier Inc. All rights reserved.

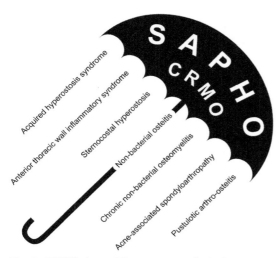

Fig. 1. SAPHO (synovitis, acne, pustulosis, hyperostosis, and oseitis) and chronic recurrent multifocal osteomyelitis (CRMO) are umbrella terms covering a range of previously described conditions, all under the same unifying concept.

to a wide variety of terms used in their description. Acquired hyperostosis syndrome, subacute and chronic symmetric osteomyelitis, pustulotic arthro-osteitis, bilateral clavicular osteomyelitis with palmoplantar pustulosis (PPP), sterno-costo-clavicular hyperostosis, intersterno-costo-clavicular ossification, and nonbacterial osteitis are just some of the more than 50 terms that have been used to date, with the common denominator each time being the presence of an inflammatory osteitis.[2–8]

It was in 1987 and 1988 that a group of French authors coined the acronym, SAPHO.[9,10] In their original article titled, "le syndrome acné-pustulose-hyperostose-ostéite," they described their findings in 85 patients in whom they saw associations between musculoskeletal lesions, pustulosis palmaris et planataris, and acne. Their subsequent article then changed the "S" in the acronym from "syndrome" to "synovitis," creating "synovitis, acne, pustulosis, hyperostosis and osteitis" (SAPHO). The term has since been commonly used as an encompassing umbrella term, covering all the associated entities. It therefore covers a wide range of related conditions, and suggestions have been made to formalize this with specific diagnostic criteria.[10,11] Whether or not these sorts of criteria are implemented, the fundamental importance is that radiologists and other clinicians have a good understanding of the range of clinical and imaging features of SAPHO, so that it is diagnosed correctly, and in a timely manner.

In this article, we adopt SAPHO as the term to encompass all the associated entities, with the one exception being that of chronic recurrent multifocal osteomyelitis (CRMO). Although this has sometimes been included under the SAPHO umbrella, there are a few common variations between the two, which we highlight separately (**Table 1**).

The term CRMO evolved from initial reports of a chronic symmetric osteomyelitis,[3] which was renamed to CRMO when further reports showed that the lesions were not always symmetric.[12,13] In fact, CRMO does not even have to be chronic, recurrent, or multifocal, a point that highlights the diverse range of disease manifestations. Consequently, cases under this umbrella have also been described using such terms as chronic nonbacterial osteomyelitis, and nonbacterial osteitis.[14–16]

THE DIAGNOSTIC CONUNDRUM

SAPHO and CRMO cover a complex group of conditions with a wide array of clinical presentations. It has therefore not been uncommon for their diagnoses to be delayed by several years, with their symptoms often being wrongly attributed to other conditions before the final diagnosis is made.[16–20] It is also suspected that the true prevalence of these conditions is much higher than the 1 in 10,000 that has been previously estimated.[17,20–22] However, as an understanding and awareness of this group of conditions develops, it is hoped that the diagnoses will be considered progressively earlier in the clinical course of these patients.

The most common disease mimics are those of infection and neoplasia, two differential diagnoses important to rule out when considering the diagnoses of SAPHO and CRMO. However, most often there are clinical and radiologic findings typical of SAPHO and CRMO that help point to the correct diagnosis. Although diagnostic criteria have been proposed, they have not yet been validated.

In practice, the diagnosis is made by a wide range of clinical teams, rheumatologists being the most frequent, followed by radiologists, pediatricians, general practitioners, orthopedic surgeons, and other specialities.[17] This is because the diagnoses cannot be made based solely on either clinical or radiologic findings. Instead, it is the combination of often subtle clinical and radiologic findings that clinch the diagnoses.

Many of the radiologic subtleties center on the main diagnostic features of hyperostosis and osteitis, both of which can have varying radiologic appearances. Hyperostosis affects the cortical bone,

Table 1
Characteristic features of SAPHO and CRMO

		SAPHO	CRMO
Shared characteristic features	Relapsing and remitting	+++	+++
	Multifocal involvement	+++	+++
	Several subclinical sites	++	++
	Early bone marrow edema	+++	+++
	Osteitis	+++	+++
	Skin manifestations	+++	+
Distinguishing characteristic features	Sternocostal involvement	+++	−
	Sole clavicular involvement	−	++
	Long bone metaphyses	−	+++
	Synovitis	+++	−
	Ankylosis	++	−
	Paravertebral enthesopathy	++	−
	Vertebra nigra	+	−
	Vertebra plana	−	+

+++, most commonly seen; ++, seen with moderate frequency; +, less commonly seen; −, not a recognized feature.

with bone hypertrophy extending from the endosteum and the periosteum. This results in narrowing of the medullary canal, cortical thickening, and bone expansion. Osteitis affects the cancellous bone in the medullary cavity. Here, inflammation leads to a range of osteolytic and osteosclerotic appearances, with the most common outcome being that of sclerosis with intervening areas of lucency. Both of these processes are seen in varying combinations at any involved site, and because the radiologic appearance of these processes evolves through time, there is a wide range of possible findings on imaging.

PATIENT DEMOGRAPHICS

There is a marked female predominance in SAPHO and CRMO, and although they can present at any age, as a general rule they tend to affect more specific age groups.[17–19,23,24] SAPHO tends to affect young adults, typically 30 to 50 year olds, whereas CRMO is invariably seen in pediatric patients.[25–27] Indeed, many refer to CRMO as the pediatric manifestation of SAPHO.[28,29]

To date, a disproportionate number of cases in the literature have originated from specific regions, including Japan and Northern Europe. However, this is not thought to relate to increased disease incidence in these regions, rather, it is caused by increased awareness and an earlier documentation of cases in the literature. There is currently no known geographic or ethnic factor in disease prevalence.

PRESENTING SYMPTOMS

In both conditions, it is possible for patients to have only one affected osteoarticular site.[23,30,31]

However, in most cases there are multiple sites affected at presentation, even if several of these are subclinical and only evident radiologically.[21,23,27,28,32] There can be symmetric involvement, especially in the anterior chest wall in SAPHO, and in the femora and tibiae in CRMO, but overall, the disease distributions tend to be asymmetrical.[18–20,23] Presenting symptoms of affected sites include pain, swelling, tenderness, and limited range of movement.[17,19,23] Patients tend to be afebrile with normal white cell count and C-reactive protein levels, but the erythrocyte sedimentation rate is usually raised.[14,16,23,33]

AFFECTED SITES
SAPHO

In SAPHO, the most common site to be affected is the upper, anterior chest wall, which is involved in approximately 75% of cases.[9,18,19,27] This site includes the medial ends of the clavicles, sternoclavicular joints, sternocostal junctions, and sternomanubrial joint.

Spinal involvement is also common, seen in approximately 50% of cases.[19,34] It is usually multifocal, but centered on the thoracic spine, and often with a segment of contiguous vertebral involvement.[35,36] Within each affected vertebra, there is a propensity to affect the anterior vertebral body corners, although several of these sites may remain subclinical despite abnormalities on imaging.[21,37]

With decreasing frequency, other sites affected include the sacroiliac joints (~25%), long bones (~25%), and mandible (~10%).[19,27,38] In addition, as rare sites of involvement, there have been individual case reports of extraosseous soft tissue and intracranial involvement.[39,40]

Chronic Recurrent Multifocal Osteomyelitis

By contrast, CRMO most commonly affects the long bone metaphyses, seen in approximately 75% of cases and almost always involving the tibia or femur.[23,41,42] Other less frequently involved sites include the spine (~25%), clavicle (~20%), pelvis (~20%), and mandible (~10%).[16,23,43,44]

CLINICAL COURSE

In SAPHO and CRMO, the usual clinical course is one of relapsing and remitting rheumatologic flares.[19,33,45] A small proportion of patients only have a single, self-limiting episode lasting less than 6 months. However, most follow a course of recurrent exacerbations, with variability as to whether or not complete remission is gained between episodes.[16,18,43] In the chronic course, it is common to see progressive involvement of additional sites as the recurrent exacerbations progress through time.[18,19,34,44]

Typically, there is a fairly slow progression of the osteoarticular manifestations at any particular site, and in both conditions a high proportion of patients do not experience long-term debilitating sequelae.[17,19,43,46,47] However, there is still a significant proportion of patients who suffer longstanding effects on their quality of life. In SAPHO, this is most commonly in the form of arthralgia, whereas in CRMO it is often pain and deformity.[43,48] In CRMO especially, there is a growing appreciation that the disease is not as indolent as previously thought, with a higher proportion of patients now being shown to have long-term sequelae and disease activity into adulthood.[43,49,50]

ASSOCIATION WITH SKIN LESIONS
SAPHO

In SAPHO, the correlation between cutaneous and musculoskeletal lesions is highly variable, adding to the diagnostic difficulty.[4,19] The most common skin manifestations are those of PPP and severe acne,[9,26,27,51,52] with females presenting more commonly with PPP and males more commonly with severe acne.[17,19]

PPP presents as a relapsing and remitting skin condition, characterized by small, sterile, yellowish pustules on the palms and soles.[32] An association with PPP has been reported in greater than 50% of patients diagnosed with SAPHO, whereas osseous changes have been reported in approximately 20% of patients diagnosed with PPP.[17,19,27,51,53] Manifestations of severe acne include acne

conglobata, acne fulminans, and hydradenitis suppurativa. These have been reported in approximately 20% of patients with SAPHO.[9,27] Pustular psoriasis is another skin condition with a recognized association with SAPHO, but the reported frequency of this association varies widely.

Skin lesions may present before, at the same time as, or after osteoarticular lesions.[4,27] Studies have reported this with slightly varying frequency, but on the whole they show that approximately 60% to 70% of patients who present with osteoarticular manifestations either have a history of skin lesions or have active skin lesions at the time of presentation.[18,27] This still leaves a significant percentage of patients whose initial presentation is with osteoarticular lesions, but without any skin manifestations. Several of these patients subsequently go on to develop skin manifestations, a high proportion of which are within the following 2 years.[4] However, latency periods of several decades have also been reported.[4,19] To that end, the absence of skin manifestations does not exclude the diagnosis.[9,32]

Chronic Recurrent Multifocal Osteomyelitis

The association with skin lesions is much stronger in SAPHO than in CRMO, where it is only seen in approximately 20% of cases.[16,43] When there is skin involvement in CRMO cases, PPP is again the most common manifestation, followed by acne.[16,20,54]

INCLUSION CRITERIA

The link between osteoarticular lesions and typical skin manifestations features heavily when diagnostic inclusion criteria have been proposed for SAPHO. Examples include, 'osteoarticular manifestations associated with PPP or severe acne', and, 'isolated sterile hyperostosis/osteitis'.[10,11] Suggested exclusion criteria are simply based on the confirmation of one of the differential diagnoses, particularly isolating an infective cause of the osteitis, or confirming a neoplastic cause.[11] Diagnostic criteria have also been proposed for CRMO, such as multifocal bone lesions over a prolonged course that are not responsive to antibiotics.[55] In line with these proposed criteria, the diagnoses of SAPHO and CRMO are straightforward when the presenting features adhere to typical clinical and radiologic patterns. Unfortunately, the imaging spectrum of both diseases is so wide that it often creates diagnostic difficulty, especially in atypical cases, which can fall foul of the lack of specificity of any diagnostic criteria. This is particularly the case in monostotic involvement.

IMAGING FEATURES

The diagnoses of SAPHO and CRMO are straightforward when typical imaging findings are coupled with typical skin lesions. However, these cases still require good communication between the clinical team and radiologist. In the more diagnostically challenging cases, this cohesive clinical teamwork is even more essential.

From an imaging perspective, we outline the typical imaging findings, as well as the less typical imaging findings, for both SAPHO and CRMO. When considering these diagnoses, it is worth noting that often only a specific symptomatic site is imaged at presentation. This therefore does not take into account old, previously affected sites, or concurrently active subclinical sites, which have different imaging features. Consequently, in diagnostically difficult cases, it is of huge benefit to image other commonly affected sites, even in the absence of symptoms. The logic for this is based on the fact that a high proportion of patients with SAPHO and CRMO have several concurrent subclinical sites of inflammation, the demonstration of which is invaluable in making the diagnosis.[21,23] It is also important to note that in SAPHO and CRMO, several of the early radiologic findings are not demonstrated on all imaging modalities.[42,56] For example, in patients with SAPHO, only 10% to 20% of conventional radiographs have been shown to be abnormal at initial presentation, despite 100% then being abnormal later in the course of the disease.[34,42]

Several studies have shown the benefits of using fluid-sensitive MR imaging sequences to look for early signs of disease in clinical and subclinical sites.[23,42,57–59] This has the obvious advantage over whole-body bone scintigraphy of avoiding the use of ionizing radiation.[21,60,61] Another advantage of whole-body MR imaging over whole-body bone scintigraphy is that some lesions are masked on scintigraphy by other areas of increased uptake. This is particularly true in pediatric cases where the typical juxtaphyseal lesions of CRMO can easily be seen on MR imaging, but obscured on scintigraphy by normal physiologic increased uptake of the adjacent physis.[23]

GENERAL IMAGING FEATURES
SAPHO

The imaging features of SAPHO relate to the processes of synovitis, hyperostosis, and osteitis. Synovitis is invariably caused by extension of osteitis to involve the adjacent intra-articular structures, so the pattern of affected sites mirrors that of the osteitis; the upper anterior chest wall and sternoclavicular joints being most commonly affected.[10,27,32] It can present as a monoarthritis, but is usually multifocal.[9,18,19] At the affected sites, the imaging findings are difficult to distinguish from seronegative spondyloarthropathies, with joint space narrowing, subchondral erosions, periarticular osteopenia, and ankylosis all seen.[32,34] In hyperostosis, the features are of bone hypertrophy and cortical thickening with associated narrowing of the medullary canal.[2,32,62] This is as a result of corticoperiosteal osteogenesis caused by chronic endosteal and periosteal inflammatory reactions. Osteitis refers directly to the inflammation of bone, and it can involve the cortical and cancellous portions. Radiologic findings include bone marrow edema, osteolysis and osteosclerosis, but its appearances can vary hugely, depending on the extent of bone involvement and the stage of disease.[35,63]

In established cases of SAPHO, the combination of synovitis, hyperostosis, and osteitis can therefore result in varying amounts of expanded and osteosclerotic bone with intervening areas of osteolysis and erosion.[32,62] These findings are readily evident on imaging, with computed tomography (CT) of the anterior chest wall being particularly useful in their demonstration.[35,64] However, in the early stages of disease, the only salient imaging feature may be the bone marrow edema of early osteitis, strengthening the case for fluid-sensitive MR imaging sequences to aid early diagnosis.[42,65]

Chronic Recurrent Multifocal Osteomyelitis

The imaging features in CRMO also center around the process of osteitis, but there are some distinctions between the findings seen in CRMO and those seen in SAPHO. This is at least in part caused by the overwhelming tendency for CRMO lesions to center on the metaphysis of long bones, without epiphyseal or joint involvement. The disease is most commonly bilateral and multifocal. Lesions can be symmetric, but most patients demonstrate multiple asymmetrical lesions.[20,23] The progression of radiologic findings at affected sites is through bone edema, osteolysis, and reactive sclerosis, with the most common appearance at the time of diagnosis being a mixed lucent and sclerotic juxtaphyseal lesion.[15,44,50]

In the early stages of disease, there can be subtle widening of the growth plate on conventional radiographs.[23,50] However, the most sensitive early imaging finding is the demonstration of bone marrow edema on MR imaging, which is seen when the radiographs still have normal appearances.[16,23] The edema can extend into the epiphysis, but there is rarely extension to involve the adjacent joint, hence much lower rates of associated synovitis.[23,42] Hyperostosis is an associated feature with periosteal reaction and inflammation of the adjacent soft tissues, but abscess formation and soft tissue fistulae are not seen.[23,25,39,44,58,66] The most common clinical course is relapsing and remitting, with relapses often recurring at the same sites, as well as new sites becoming involved.[33,44,45,67] However, it is also possible to see resolution of radiologic findings and remodeling to normal bone with prolonged remission.[44,66]

ANTERIOR CHEST WALL
SAPHO

The anterior chest wall is by far the most common site of involvement in SAPHO.[27,68] Any component of the anterior chest wall can be involved, but the findings here are almost always bilateral, although usually more florid on one side than the other.[9,18,19] SAPHO tends to initially develop in the region of the costoclavicular ligaments. Indeed, costoclavicular enthesopathy and small hyperostotic foci at the first costosternal junction are considered key early diagnostic features.[2] Typically, there are then a further two well-described stages of disease progression at this site.[7,69] In stage 2, the costoclavicular ligament involvement spreads to the sternoclavicular joints and adjacent structures: the medial ends of the clavicles, adjacent sternum, costal cartilages, and first ribs. The findings are typically of an erosive arthropathy in the sternoclavicular joints with erosions, sclerosis, and hyperostosis of the adjacent bones (Fig. 2). In stage 3, there is further progression, with the sclerosis and hyperostosis extending laterally in the clavicles, including affecting the superior borders. The sternum, manubrium, and upper ribs also undergo similar progressive changes, and in advanced cases it is possible to see ankylosis across the sternoclavicular and first sternocostal joints.[7,35]

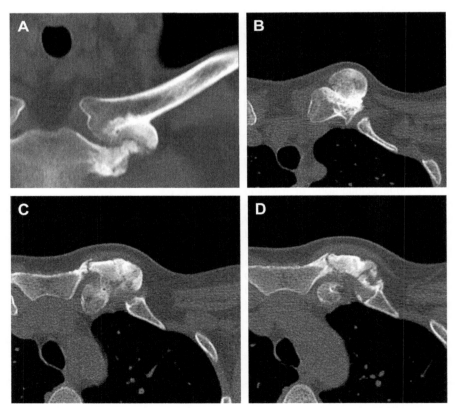

Fig. 2. SAPHO of the anterior chest wall showing marked hyperostosis and enthesopathy across the sterno-costoclavicular junction. (*A*) Coronal CT reconstruction showing exuberant hyperostosis extending from the inferior aspect of the medial left clavicle and the adjacent sternum. (*B*) Axial CT showing the hyperostosis to extend from the dorsal and ventral surfaces of the clavicle. (*C*, *D*) Slices extending more caudally showing associated involvement of the left first sternocostal junction where there is erosion and sclerosis.

This typical progression of disease is what results in the bull's-head appearance on technetium bone scans.[51] This sign has proved to be a highly specific finding in the diagnosis of SAPHO, despite an occasional exception to the rule.[51,70] However, its sensitivity levels are much lower than its specificity, and with increasing use of MR imaging in the early diagnosis of SAPHO, it may well become of less diagnostic significance in the future (Fig. 3).[68] In association with the bone and joint changes in the anterior chest wall, CT and MR imaging can also show exuberant soft tissue inflammation, which has been known to cause thoracic inlet venous compression and mimic neoplasia.[19,34,71]

Chronic Recurrent Multifocal Osteomyelitis

In CRMO, the only anterior chest wall site typically involved is the clavicle.[15,23,67] There is a notable predilection for the medial third, where the most common findings are of sclerosis and marked hyperostosis.[44,66] Associated periosteal reaction is seen in approximately 40% of patients.[23,44] On MR imaging, bone marrow edema and involvement of the adjacent soft tissues are also common

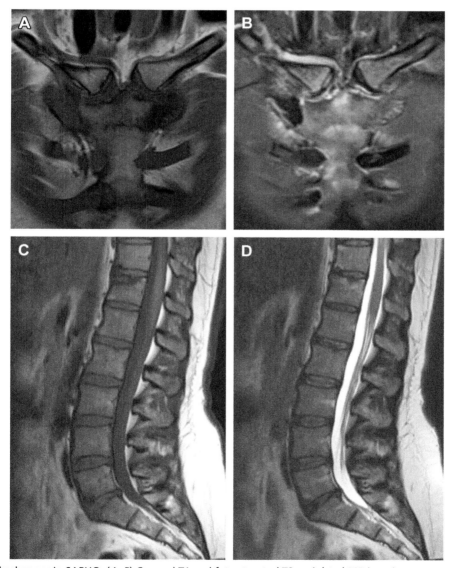

Fig. 3. Early changes in SAPHO. (A, B) Coronal T1 and fat-saturated T2-weighted MR imaging sequences through the anterior chest wall showing subtle multifocal, bilateral marrow edema. (C, D) Sagittal T1 and T2-weighted MR imaging sequences showing involvement of anterior vertebral body corners at T11, T12, L5, and S1.

features.[58,72] Invariably, the sternum and ribs are not involved, neither is there costoclavicular enthesopathy nor bony ankylosis across the sternoclavicular joint (**Fig. 4**).[28,72,73]

AXIAL SKELETON
SAPHO

The spine is the second most common site involved in SAPHO. Early changes here are often subclinical.[36] However, in other cases, it is the initial presenting site.[74–76] When there is involvement of the spine, it is most commonly centered on the thoracic spine.[37] There may only be one level involved. However, the usual findings are of multifocal, multilevel disease, with a high proportion of patients showing a pattern of contiguous vertebral body involvement (**Fig. 5**).[21,36,37,77]

There may be several different imaging findings at affected levels, and these can occur in varying combinations. Vertebral body corner lesions are common and are almost always seen anteriorly.[36] The pathologic process is one of enthesitis, similar to that seen with Romanus lesions in spondylarthropathies.[36,78] The earliest finding is of marrow edema on fluid-sensitive MR imaging sequences and this precedes any plain film or CT findings.[42,65] The active edema and hyperemia also result in enhancement of the affected area on postcontrast

T1 sequences.[36,79] In the subacute phase, the affected vertebral corners can undergo progressive fatty degeneration.[77] At more chronically affected sites, sclerosis and erosions are also commonly seen.[64]

When trying to differentiate the vertebral corner lesions in SAPHO from other potential diagnoses, there are a few key features to help make the distinction. The presence of prevertebral soft tissue thickening and involvement of two or more contiguous vertebrae are features that favor a diagnosis of SAPHO over spondylarthropathy.[35,37] Furthermore, the vertebral corner lesions in SAPHO extend to involve the adjacent vertebral end plate or anterior cortex.[35,37]

When there is multilevel spinal involvement in SAPHO, the main differential diagnosis is metastatic disease.[80] In these patients, multiple lesions all centered on the anterior vertebral corners favors the diagnosis of SAPHO over metastases, in which a more random distribution of involvement is seen.[36,81]

Another spinal manifestation of SAPHO is that of nonspecific spondylodiscitis, with the main differential diagnosis for these radiologic findings being infective spondylodiscitis.[36] Focal erosions, sclerotic remodeling of the end plates and associated bone marrow edema are all shared features.[35] Features that favor a diagnosis of SAPHO over

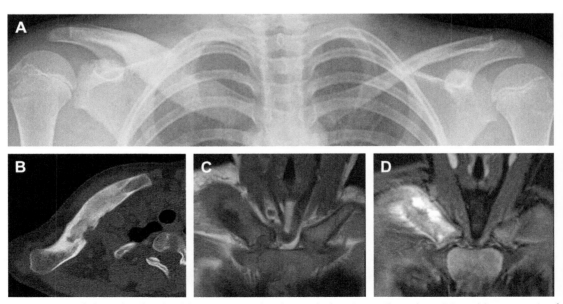

Fig. 4. CRMO of the right clavicle. (*A*) Conventional radiograph showing unilateral osteitis and hyperostosis of the right clavicle. Note the involvement extending laterally from the medial end with sparing of the lateral clavicle. (*B*) Axial-oblique reformatted CT through the right clavicle showing the hyperostosis with typical areas of intervening lucency. (*C*, *D*) Coronal T1 and fat-saturated T2-weighted sequences showing the right clavicular hypertrophy with associated edema. Also note the extension up to the right sternoclavicular joint, but not beyond, sparing the remaining anterior chest wall.

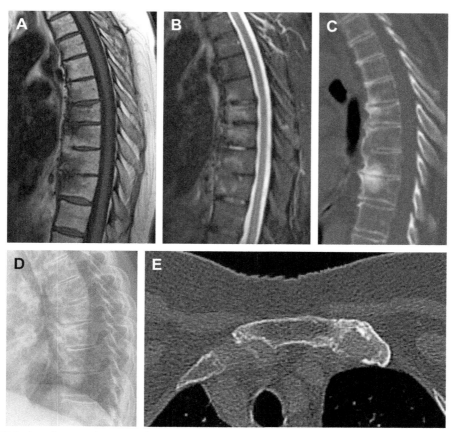

Fig. 5. SAPHO. (*A*, *B*) Sagittal T1 and fat saturated T2-weighted MR imaging sequences showing contiguous involvement of consecutive thoracic vertebral bodies, with sclerosis and edema at multiple levels, and anterior fusion between the T8 and T9 vertebral bodies. Note the lesions centered anteriorly across the discovertebral junction with involvement of the anterior cortex, and the absence of abscess formation. (*C*) The osteitis, fusion, and sclerosis are optimally appreciated on the corresponding sagittal CT reconstruction, compared with the lateral radiograph (*D*). (*E*) Elsewhere, there is concurrent involvement of the anterior chest wall, including anky-losis across the left first sternocostal junction.

infective spondylodiscitis include multilevel verte-bral involvement and lesions centered anteriorly in the discovertebral junction. Also, an absence of such features as abscess and sequestra forma-tion, disk edema, and disk and epidural enhance-ment favor a diagnosis of SAPHO.[36,37,65,82] There invariably are clinically and biochemically distin-guishing features between these diagnoses. How-ever, if biopsy is required to exclude an infective cause, then involved disk material in patients with SAPHO is classically sterile, with chronic in-flammatory and mild fibrotic changes only.[31,65]

In more chronic cases, the reactive sclerosis around the end plate can progress to involve the whole vertebral body, resembling an ivory vertebra (**Fig. 6**).[36,83] There may also be associ-ated hyperostosis.[36] Differential diagnoses for these appearances include Paget disease and osteoblastic metastases. If typical imaging signs

are concurrently present elsewhere, then the diag-nosis of SAPHO is more straightforward, but differ-entiation on imaging alone is more difficult when only one level is osteosclerotic.[31]

Paravertebral ossifications are seen in more chronic cases of SAPHO.[18] The patterns of para-vertebral ossification include enthesophytes, mar-ginal syndesmophytes, and nonmarginal, asymmetrical syndesmophytes, which can resemble the syndesmophytosis seen in seroneg-ative spondyloarthropathies, particularly psoria-sis.[18,53,84] The ossification can progress to anterior bony bridging at multiple levels, with asso-ciated kyphosis.[21,28] Another factor that can contribute to anterior kyphosis in chronic SAPHO cases is ankylosis of the vertebral bodies. As adja-cent vertebral bodies become hyperostotic, they can fuse across the discovertebral junction anteri-orly, fixing the anterior kyphosis.[21,28] It has been

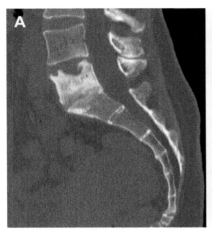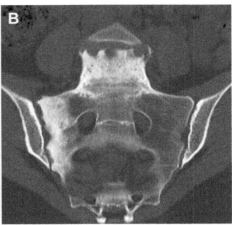

Fig. 6. Chronic changes in SAPHO. (*A*) Reformatted sagittal CT showing dense sclerosis of the L5 vertebral body with erosions of the superior end plate, ankylosis across the L5/S1 disk, and sclerosis of the superior aspect of S1. There are also early changes at the C1-C2 coccygeal junction. (*B*) Reformatted coronal CT showing additional involvement of the right sacroiliac joint, where there is dense sclerosis and erosion on the sacral side.

observed that once this ankylosis has occurred, the associated hyperostosis can resolve.[85] Paravertebral soft tissue masses are less common, but can occasionally be seen in chronic cases of SAPHO involving the spine, usually with a high fat content in chronic cases.[37,86]

Other sites of involvement related to the axial skeleton are the mandible and the sacroiliac joint.[18,19] Findings in the mandible tend to affect the posterior body and ramus.[18] They follow a progressive course from initial osteolysis, periosteal reaction, and overlying soft tissue inflammation through to more chronic sclerosis and hyperostosis of the affected bone.[18,19,47] There can be extension to the adjacent temporomandibular joint where appearances can resemble an inflammatory arthropathy (**Fig. 7**).[87,88] The sacroiliac joint is commonly affected and is usually unilateral.[18,19,34] Radiologic findings are of erosive inflammation surrounded by osteosclerosis and hyperostosis (see **Fig. 6**).[18,19] A useful distinguishing feature between sacroiliitis secondary to spondylarthropathy and sacroiliac involvement in SAPHO is the degree of involvement of the ilium, with extensive sclerosis of the adjacent ilium favoring a diagnosis of SAPHO.[28,46]

Chronic Recurrent Multifocal Osteomyelitis

The two main spinal findings in CRMO are vertebral corner lesions and osteolytic lesions, with the thoracic spine most commonly affected.[67,89,90] Spinal involvement is usually multifocal, but compared with SAPHO, a smaller proportion of patients have involvement of two or more contiguous vertebral bodies.[23,67] The vertebral corner

lesions typically show early edematous change on MR imaging, but there is not the progression to focal erosions and sclerosis seen in patients with SAPHO.[35,44] Similarly, osteosclerosis, paravertebral ossifications and focal end plate erosions are all far less commonly seen in patients with CRMO.[14,66,90] Instead, osteolytic lesions are more commonly seen radiographically, occasionally with a rim of reactive sclerosis and with a high incidence of associated vertebral body collapse.[14,89] An insufficiency fracture line has been described in the involved vertebral body on MR imaging, and complete vertebra plana is not an uncommon finding.[58,91,92] Occasionally, this can lead to complications, such as spinal canal stenosis and cord injury.[93] In patients with partial vertebral body collapse, the causative osteolytic lesion can undergo healing, usually with a degree of residual kyphosis (**Fig. 8**).[90,94] Where there has been progression to vertebra plana, there is no subsequent reconstitution of vertebral height.[23,89]

The mandible and pelvis can occasionally be involved in CRMO.[23,58] Mandibular involvement is similar to spinal involvement, in that they both result in a high proportion of deforming changes on long-term follow-up.[23,95] Involvement of the pelvis most commonly takes the form of lesions at the synchondroses, the disease predominating at these metaphyseal-equivalent sites. However, unilateral sacroiliitis can also be seen.[58,96]

APPENDICULAR SKELETON
SAPHO

It is unusual for SAPHO to affect the appendicular skeleton, featuring in only 5% of cases.[27] When it

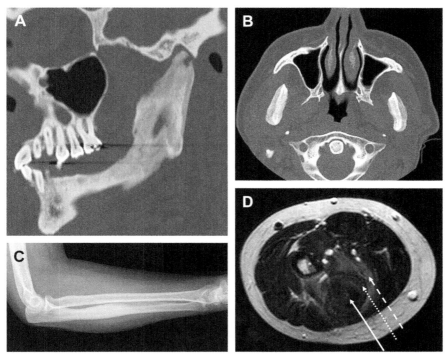

Fig. 7. SAPHO. (A) Sagittal CT reformat showing marked hyperostosis of the mandible with extension up to the temporomandibular joint and associated erosion on the mandibular side. (B) Axial CT scan showing the degree of hyperostosis on both sides of the mandible. There is also associated swelling of the overlying masseter muscles, particularly on the right side. (C, D) Lateral radiograph of the forearm in the same patient and corresponding axial T2-weighted MR imaging sequence showing focal bone expansion of the mid ulnar diaphysis. The MR image demonstrates the osteitic bone as dense low signal in the medullary cavity (solid arrow), the hyperostotic bone causing expansion of the cortex (dotted arrow) and the associated edema in the adjacent soft tissues (dashed arrow).

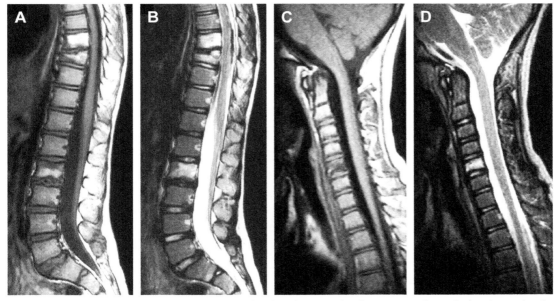

Fig. 8. CRMO of the spine. (A–D) Sagittal T1-weighted and T2-weighted sequences through the thoracolumbar and cervical spine showing multilevel vertebral involvement, including varying degrees of edema and fat conversion in the T8, T9, L2, and C5 vertebral bodies. In addition, a characteristic feature in CRMO is the associated vertebral body collapse, seen here in T9 and, to a lesser extent, in C5.

is involved, the classical features of synovitis, hyperostosis, and osteitis can all be seen, either in combination or in isolation, and invariably at the diametaphysis (see **Fig. 7**).

Chronic Recurrent Multifocal Osteomyelitis

By contrast, the appendicular skeleton is by far the most common site involved in CRMO, particularly the metaphyses of the tibia and distal femur.[23,41,43] Here, the earliest finding is of bone marrow edema on MR imaging.[44,58,66] Subtle widening of the physis on plain radiographs can also be seen, but is a less sensitive sign.[23,50] The findings then progress into juxta-articular osteolysis, with or without associated periosteal reaction, hyperostosis, and soft tissue inflammation (**Fig. 9**).[15,23,44]

The size of the osteolytic lesion is variable, and the imaging appearances at any one particular site can be indistinguishable from infective osteomyelitis, especially when there is associated soft tissue involvement and periosteal reaction.[92] The presence of hyperostosis and multifocal involvement in typical sites are useful findings to help distinguish an osteolytic CRMO lesion from infective osteomyelitis. To that end, there is a trend toward the use of whole-body MR imaging scanning instead of biopsy in diagnostically difficult cases.[57,89]

The associated soft tissue involvement can rarely appear masslike, making distinction from malignancy difficult.[39] Again, demonstration of multifocal involvement in typical locations is a useful distinguishing feature. Despite this, biopsy often is required to rule out the most common differential diagnoses of infection and malignancy. When this is undertaken, the histology typically shows inflammatory changes consistent with the stage of disease, including fibrous replacement of marrow with associated plasma cells, lymphocytes, and polymorphs.[97–100] In the subacute

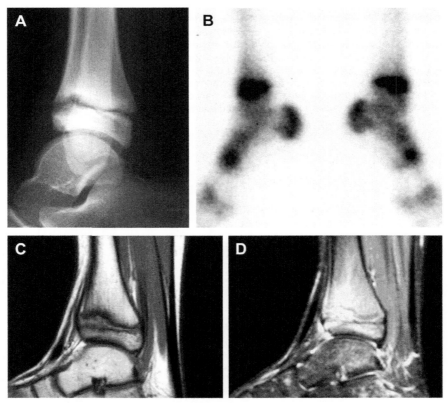

Fig. 9. CRMO at the metaphysis. (*A–D*) Sagittal radiograph, technetium bone scan, and T1 and fat saturated T2-weighted MR imaging sequences. The conventional radiograph shows subtle widening of the distal right tibial physis, particularly anteriorly. The appearances are more marked on the MR imaging sequences, where the physeal widening is demonstrated with florid surrounding edema. Note how the edema can extend into the epiphysis, but the adjacent joint is not affected. Also of important note is the relative masking of the appearances on the technetium bone scan by the normal physiologic increased uptake in the physis.

phase, a rim of reactive sclerosis forms around the osteolytic lesion, which then progresses to a thicker sclerotic rim, as well as heterogeneous sclerosis of the lesion itself.[15,44,50] The healing of long bone lesions is variable. Several patients see good resolution, including normalization of radiographic appearances.[58,94,101] The long-term prognosis of long bone lesions certainly tends to be better than those in the spine and mandible, where chronic bony remodeling is more common.[23,89,90,95] However, a significant proportion of patients with long bone involvement also experience chronic deforming sequelae, including significant limb length discrepancies.[43,49,102]

HOST FACTORS

There is almost certainly a genetic susceptibility for the exaggerated inflammatory response seen in patients with SAPHO and CRMO. This determines the onset and expressivity of the disease. Studies have confirmed hereditary links in both conditions and in CRMO, a specific genetic association has been shown with chromosome 18q.[103–106] There are also variants of both conditions in which specific genetic mutations are already known. For example, pyogenic sterile arthritis, pyoderma gangrenosum, and acne syndrome is an autosomal-dominant condition related to a mutation on the PSTPIP1 gene located on chromosome 15, and Majeed syndrome, which consists of CRMO, neutrophilic dermatosis, and congenital dyserythropoetic anemia, is an autosomal-recessive disorder related to mutations in the LPIN2 gene.[107–109] There is also a higher incidence of inflammatory bowel disease in patients with SAPHO and CRMO, suggesting possible shared genetic mutations, such as NOD2.[103,110–112] Rheumatoid factor and human leukocyte antigen-B27 are invariably negative in both conditions.[14,17,18] There is a suggestion that both SAPHO and CRMO sit at the undifferentiated end of the spondyloarthropathy spectrum, particularly given the frequently reported association of SAPHO with pustular psoriasis.[17,19] It has also been demonstrated that a large proportion of patients with CRMO eventually develop features that would meet certain diagnostic criteria for spondylarthropathy.[96,113]

The fact that there is such a multifactorial cause for SAPHO and CRMO, much of which is still unknown, supports a multitherapy approach to treatment. It also emphasizes the need for the clinical teams, including rheumatologists, dermatologists, general practitioners, orthopedic surgeons, histopathologists, and radiologists to collaborate well together when considering the diagnoses.

TREATMENT OPTIONS AND THEIR THEORETIC PRINCIPLES

Several different treatment options have been trialed over the years, with varying amounts of success. These include antibiotics, analgesics, nonsteroidal anti-inflammatory drugs (NSAIDs), oral corticosteroids, bisphosphonates, and various biologic agents, including tumor necrosis factor (TNF)-α antagonists.

The relative rarity of SAPHO and CRMO, and the difficulty in making their diagnosis in atypical cases, mean that randomized controlled trials comparing these different treatment options have not been possible thus far. It is certainly an area that would benefit from further research. Nonetheless, there have been numerous studies reporting outcomes from each different therapeutic option and these provide as robust an opinion as possible at this stage, given the small patient groups.

Antibiotics

In SAPHO and CRMO, the microbiology result from biopsies of osteoarticular lesions is usually sterile.[22,23,37,114,115] The main purpose of the biopsy is to exclude infective osteomyelitis or neoplasia. The only organism that has occasionally been isolated from osteoarticular biopsies in patients with classical features of SAPHO is *Propionibacterium acnes*.[116,117] This is a slow-growing anaerobe that is a normal part of the skin flora, and is also found more focally in acne lesions.[118]

Isolating this bacterium from osteoarticular lesions in patients with SAPHO led to trials of antibiotic use in these patients. There have been some reported improvements with this therapy.[18,119,120] However, there is also evidence refuting this, with several trials failing to show any improvement with antibiotic therapy and others showing that any observed benefits receded after treatment was stopped.[18,19,116,121]

Likewise, in CRMO, antibiotics have proved to be an ineffective treatment option.[43,50,54] This disappointing response to antibiotic therapy has led to more recent theories proposing that the *P acnes* bacterium may simply be the trigger for an autoimmune inflammatory cascade in these patients, with the osteoarticular changes being a result of the inflammatory reaction, rather than the bacteria itself.[53,117,118,122–125] The main cytokines implicated in this response are TNF-α and various interleukins (IL), including IL-1, IL-6, IL-8, and IL-18.[117,122,124,126–128] This proposal is further supported by the fact that more promising responses to treatment have been achieved with the use of therapies specifically targeting the inflammatory nature of these diseases.

Analgesics, Nonsteroidal Anti-inflammatory Drugs, and Corticosteroids

NSAIDs and simple analgesics have long been considered first-line treatment options for SAPHO and CRMO, with other therapies only being added in refractory cases.[24,129] In more than half of all patients, this first-line treatment achieves adequate symptomatic control.[14,17,20,130]

For cases refractory to the use of simple analgesics and NSAIDs, a course of oral corticosteroids has been shown to have good effect in some patients with SAPHO, as has selective intra-articular injection of corticosteroids.[19,131] However, the main research focus in recent years has been on the use of bisphosphonates and biologic agents.

Bisphosphonates

The theoretic effects of bisphosphonates in patients with SAPHO and CRMO are two-fold. First, they act by suppressing the osteoclastic bone resorption seen in osteitis, and second, they lessen the systemic inflammatory response by suppressing the production of IL-1ß, IL-6, and TNF-α.[21,132,133]

In practice, this has resulted in numerous studies reporting the efficacious use of a variety of bisphosphonates in patients with CRMO and SAPHO, most notably with pamidronate, but also including zolendronic acid and risedronate.[85,133–139] There is a rapidly growing body of evidence supporting their earlier use in the clinical course of both conditions.

Biologic Agents

TNF-α is one of several inflammatory cytokines released in systemic acute phase reactions and its overexpression has been shown on bone biopsy of affected sites in patients with SAPHO.[126,140] TNF-α antagonists not only block the activity of TNF, but they also induce apoptosis of TNF-α-producing T cells. The use of TNF-α antagonists has shown some promising results, particularly with the use of infliximab in refractory cases of SAPHO and CRMO.[141–144] Improvements have been shown in the burden of skin lesions, as well as in the symptoms of musculoskeletal manifestations.[141,145] However, these therapies are not without their side effects, and have therefore tended to be reserved only as second-line therapies.[146]

Another second-line biologic agent trialed in the treatment of SAPHO is the IL-1 receptor antagonist, anakinra. Its use was supported by the demonstration of P2X7 receptor–inflammasone axis in these patients, with separate groups of authors showing promising early results.[147,148]

When assessing response to treatment, the measurement has invariably been a symptomatic response to the musculoskeletal manifestations of disease. Unfortunately, there is little known about the specific imaging response to correlate with these symptomatic improvements.

SUMMARY

SAPHO and CRMO cover a range of disease manifestations, based on the presence of inflammatory osteoarticular lesions, and often associated with cutaneous manifestations. They are great disease mimickers and require skillful collaboration between several clinical teams to make the diagnosis. Although both conditions have shared characteristic features, there are also several features that allow distinction between the two (see **Table 1**).

Clinical radiologists play a huge part in this process, because several of the key diagnostic features are only evident on imaging. In particular, whole-body MR imaging has an increasing part to play in their early diagnosis.

The value of the clinical radiologist in SAPHO and CRMO is not only in making the diagnoses when typical cutaneous and imaging findings are present, but also in considering the diagnoses early in the clinical course of the more diagnostically challenging cases, thus facilitating prompt treatment and helping to reduce the overall morbidity of these diseases.

REFERENCES

1. Windom R, Sandford J, Ziff M. Acne conglobata and arthritis. Arthritis Rheum 1961;4:632–5.
2. Dihlmann W, Dihlmann SW. Acquired hyperostosis syndrome: spectrum of manifestations at the sternocostoclavicular region. Radiologic evaluation of 34 cases. Clin Rheumatol 1991;10:250–63.
3. Giedion A, Holthusen W, Masel L, et al. Subacute and chronic "symmetrical" osteomyelitis. Ann Radiol (Paris) 1972;15:329–42.
4. Sonozaki H, Mitsui H, Miyanaga Y, et al. Clinical features of 53 cases with pustulotic arthro-osteitis. Ann Rheum Dis 1981;40:547–53.
5. Kato T, Kambara H, Hoshi E. Case of bilateral clavicular osteomyelitis with palmar and plantar pustulosis. Seikei Geka 1968;19:590–3 [in Japanese].
6. Köhler H, Uehlinger E, Kutzner J, et al. Sterno-costoclavicular hyper-ostosis: a hitherto undescribed entity (author's transl). Dtsch Med Wochenschr 1975; 100:1519–23 [in German].

7. Sonozaki H, Azuma A, Okai K, et al. Clinical features of 22 cases with "inter-sterno-costo-clavicular ossification". A new rheumatic syndrome. Arch Orthop Trauma Surg 1979;95:13–22.

8. Edlund E, Johnsson U, Lidgren L, et al. Palmoplantar pustulosis and sternocostoclavicular arthroosteitis. Ann Rheum Dis 1988;47:809–15.

9. Chamot A, Benhamou C, Kahn M, et al. Acne-pustulosis-hyperostosis-osteitis syndrome. Results of a national survey. 85 cases. Rev Rhum Mal Osteoartic 1987;54:187–96 [in French].

10. Benhamou C, Chamot A, Kahn M. Synovitis-acnepustulosis-hyperostosis-osteomyelitis syndrome (SAPHO). A new syndrome among the spondyloarthropathies? Clin Exp Rheumatol 1988;6:109–12.

11. Kahn M, Khan M. The SAPHO syndrome. Baillieres Clin Rheumatol 1994;8(2):333–62.

12. Gustavson KH, Wilbrand HF. Chronic symmetrical osteomyelitis. Report of a case. Acta Radiol Diagn (Stockh) 1974;15:551–7.

13. Probst F, Bjorkstein B, Gustavson K. Radiological aspect of chronic recurrent multifocal osteomyelitis. Ann Radiol 1978;21:115–25.

14. Jansson A, Renner E, Ramser J, et al. Classification of non-bacterial osteitis: retrospective study of clinical, immunological and genetic aspects in 89 children. Rheumatology 2007;46:154–60.

15. Gikas P, Islam L, Aston W, et al. Nonbacterial osteitis: a clinical, histopathological, and imaging study with a proposal for protocol-based management of patients with this diagnosis. J Orthop Sci 2009; 14(5):505–16.

16. Kaiser D, Bolt I, Hofer M, et al. Chronic nonbacterial osteomyelitis in children: a retrospective multicenter study. Paediatric Rheumatol Online J 2015; 13(1):25.

17. Witt M, Meier J, Hammitzsch A, et al. Disease burden, disease manifestations and current treatment regimen of the SAPHO syndrome in Germany: results from a nationwide patient survey. Semin Arthritis Rheum 2014;43(6):745–50.

18. Colina M, Govoni M, Orzincolo C, et al. Clinical and radiologic evolution of synovitis, acne, pustulosis, hyperostosis, and osteitis syndrome: a single center study of a cohort of 71 subjects. Arthritis Rheum 2009;61:813–21.

19. Hayem G, Bouchaud-Chabot A, Benali K, et al. SAPHO syndrome: a long term follow-up study of 120 cases. Semin Arthritis Rheum 1999;29(3):159–71.

20. Walsh P, Manners P, Vercoe J, et al. Chronic recurrent multifocal osteomyelitis in children: nine years' experience at a stateside tertiary paediatric rheumatology referral centre. Rheumatology 2015; 54(9):1688–91.

21. Magrey M, Khan MA. New insights into synovitis, acne, pustulosis, hyperostosis, and osteitis (SAPHO) syndrome. Curr Rheumatol Rep 2009;11:329–33.

22. Hayem G. Valuable lessons from SAPHO syndrome. Joint Bone Spine 2007;74:123–6.

23. Falip C, Alison M, Boutry N, et al. Chronic recurrent multifocal osteomyelitis (CRMO): a longitudinal case series review. Pediatr Radiol 2013;43(3): 355–75.

24. Schultz C, Holterhus PM, Seidel A, et al. Chronic recurrent multifocal osteomyelitis in children. Pediatr Infect Dis J 1999;18:1008–13.

25. Iyer RS, Thapa MM, Chew FS. Chronic recurrent multifocal osteomyelitis: review. AJR Am J Roentgenol 2011;196:S87–91.

26. Van Doornum S, Barraclough D, McColl G, et al. SAPHO: rare or just not recognized? Semin Arthritis Rheum 2000;30:70–7.

27. Li C, Zuo Y, Wu N, et al. Synovitis, acne, pustulosis, hyperostosis and osteitis syndrome: a single centre study of a cohort of 164 patients. Rheumatology (Oxford) 2016;55:1023–30.

28. Earwaker J, Cotten A. SAPHO: syndrome or concept? Imaging findings. Skeletal Radiol 2003; 32:311–27.

29. Beretta-Piccoli BC, Sauvain MJ, Gal I, et al. Synovitis, acne, pustulosis, hyperostosis, osteitis (SAPHO) syndrome in childhood: a report of ten cases and review of the literature. Eur J Pediatr 2000;159:594–601.

30. Karadag-Saygi E, Gunduz O, Gumrukcu G, et al. SAPHO syndrome: misdiagnosed and operated. Acta Reumatol Port 2008;33:460–3.

31. Court C, Charlez C, Molina V, et al. Isolated thoracic spine lesion: is this the presentation of a SAPHO syndrome? A case report. Eur Spine J 2005;14:711–5.

32. Boutin RD, Resnick D. The SAPHO syndrome: an evolving concept for unifying several idiopathic disorders of bone and skin. AJR Am J Roentgenol 1998;170:585–91.

33. Handrick W, Hörmann D, Voppmann A, et al. Chronic recurrent multifocal osteomyelitis. Report of eight children. Pediatr Surg Int 1998;14:195–8.

34. Maugars Y, Berthelot J, Ducloux J, et al. SAPHO syndrome: a follow-up study of 19 cases with special emphasis on enthesis involvement. J Rheumatol 1995;22:2135–41.

35. Leone A, Cassar-Pullicino VN, Casale R, et al. The SAPHO syndrome revisited with an emphasis on spinal manifestations. Skeletal Radiol 2015;44:9–24.

36. Laredo J, Vuillemin-Bodaghi V, Boutry N, et al. SAPHO syndrome: MR appearance of vertebral involvement. Radiology 2007;242(3):825–31.

37. McGauvran AM, Kotsenas AL, Diehn FE, et al. SAPHO syndrome: imaging findings of vertebral involvement. AJNR Am J Neuroradiol 2016;37: 1567–72.

38. Zemann W, Pau M, Feichtinger M, et al. SAPHO syndrome with affection of the mandible: diagnosis,

treatment, and review of literature. Oral Surg Oral Med Oral Pathol Oral Radiol Endod 2011;111: 190–5.

39. Sundaram M, McDonald D, Engel E, et al. Chronic recurrent multifocal osteomyelitis: an evolving clinical and radiological spectrum. Skeletal Radiol 1996;25:333–6.

40. Abul-Kasim K, Nilsson T, Turesson C. Intracranial manifestations in SAPHO syndrome: the first case report in literature. Rheumatol Int 2012;32(6): 1797–9.

41. Mandell GA, Contreras SJ, Conard K, et al. Bone scintigraphy in the detection of chronic recurrent multifocal osteomyelitis. J Nucl Med 1998;39: 1778–83.

42. Fritz J, Tzaribatschev N, Claussen CD, et al. Chronic recurrent multifocal osteomyelitis: comparison of whole-body MR imaging with radiography and correlation with clinical and laboratory data. Radiology 2009;252:842–51.

43. Huber A, Lam P, Duffy C, et al. Chronic recurrent multifocal osteomyelitis: clinical outcomes after more than 5 years of follow-up. J Pediatr 2002; 141:198–203.

44. Khanna G, Sato T, Ferguson P. Imaging of chronic recurrent multifocal osteomyelitis. Radiographics 2009;29(4):1159–77.

45. Girschick HJ, Raab P, Surbaum S, et al. Chronic nonbacterial osteomyelitis in children. Ann Rheum Dis 2005;64:279–85.

46. Sallés M, Olivé A, Perez-Andres R, et al. The SAPHO syndrome: a clinical and imaging study. Clin Rheumatol 2011;30:245–9.

47. Nguyen MT, Borchers A, Selmi C, et al. The SAPHO syndrome. Semin Arthritis Rheum 2012; 42:254–65.

48. Catalano-Pons C, Comte A, Wipff J, et al. Clinical outcome in children with chronic recurrent multifocal osteomylitis. Rheumatology (Oxford) 2008; 47:1397–9.

49. Voit AM, Arnoldi AP, Douis H, et al. Whole-body magnetic resonance imaging in chronic recurrent multifocal osteomyelitis: clinical longterm assessment may underestimate activity. J Rheumatol 2015;42(8):1455–62.

50. Freyschmidt J, Sternberg A. The bullhead sign: scintigraphic pattern of sternocostoclavicular hyperostosis and pustulotic arthroosteitis. Eur Radiol 1998;8:807–12.

51. Cotten A, Flipo RM, Mentre A, et al. SAPHO syndrome. Radiographics 1995;15:1147–54.

52. Sugimoto H, Tamura K, Fujii T. The SAPHO syndrome: defining the radiologic spectrum of diseases comprising the syndrome. Eur Radiol 1998; 8:800–6.

53. Paller AS, Pachman L, Rich K, et al. Pustulosis palmaris et plantaris: its association with chronic recurrent multifocal osteomyelitis. J Am Acad Dermatol 1985;12:927–30.

54. King SM, Laxer R, Manson D, et al. Chronic recurrent multifocal osteomyelitis: a noninfectious inflammatory process. Pediatr Infect Dis J 1987;6: 907–11.

55. Surendra G, Shetty U. Chronic recurrent multifocal osteomyelitis: a rare entity. J Med Imaging Radiat Oncol 2015;59(4):436–44.

56. Guha A, Brown M, Jacobs B. G357 Chronic recurrent multifocal osteomyelitis (CRMO): the value of whole body MRI demonstrated by a series of 13 adult and 34 paediatric patients. Arch Dis Child 2015;100:A146.

57. Jurik AG, Egund N. MRI in chronic recurrent multifocal osteomyelitis. Skeletal Radiol 1997;26:230–8.

58. Arnoldi A, Schlett C, Douis L, et al. Whole-body MRI in patients with non-bacterial osteitis: radiological findings and correlation with clinical data. Eur Radiol 2017;27(6):2391–9.

59. Guérin-Pfyffer S, Guillaume-Czitrom S, Tammam S, et al. Evaluation of chronic recurrent multifocal osteitis in children by whole-body magnetic resonance imaging. Joint Bone Spine 2012;79(6):616–20.

60. Weckbach S. Whole-body MRI for inflammatory arthritis and other multifocal rheumatoid diseases. Semin Musculoskelet Radiol 2012;16(5):377–88.

61. Matzaroglou CH, Velissaris D, Karageorgos A, et al. SAPHO syndrome diagnosis and treatment: report of five cases and review of the literature. Open Orthop J 2009;3:100–6.

62. Depasquale R, Kumer N, Lalam R, et al. SAPHO: what radiologists should know. Clin Radiol 2012; 67:195–206.

63. Lacout A, Rousselin B, Pelage J. CT and MRI of spine and sacroiliac involvement in spondyloarthropathy. Am J Roentgenol 2008;191:1016–23.

64. Toussirot E, Dupond J, Wendling D. Spondylodiscitis in SAPHO syndrome. A series of eight cases. Ann Rheum Dis 1997;56:52–8.

65. Manson D, Wilmot D, King S, et al. Physeal involvement in chronic recurrent multifocal osteomyelitis. Pediatr Radiol 1989;20(1):76–9.

66. Jurriaans E, Singh NP, Finlay K, et al. Imaging of chronic recurrent multifocal osteomyelitis. Radiol Clin North Am 2001;39:305–27.

67. Mortensson W, Edeburn G, Fries M, et al. Chronic recurrent multifocal osteomyelitis in children. A roentgenologic and scintigraphic investigation. Acta Radiol 1988;29:565–70.

68. Fu Z, Liu M, Li Z, et al. Is the bullhead sign on bone scintigraphy really common in the patient with SAPHO syndrome? A single-centre study of a 16-year experience. Nucl Med Commun 2016;37(4):387–92.

69. Watts R, Crisp A, Hazelman B, et al. Arthro-osteitis: a clinical spectrum. Br J Rheumatol 1993;32: 403–7.

70. Ni J, Ping T. An unusual bone metastasis mimicking SAPHO (synovitis, acne, pustulosis, hyperostosis and osteitis) syndrome on bone scintigraphy. Clin Nucl Med 2016;41(2):173–5.

71. Van Holsbeeck M, Martel W, Dequeker J, et al. Soft tissue involvement, mediastinal pseudotumor, and venous thrombosis in pustulotic arthroosteitis. A study of eight new cases. Skelet Radiol 1989;18:1–8.

72. Girschick H, Krauspe R, Tschammler A, et al. Chronic recurrent osteomyelitis with clavicular involvement in children: diagnostic value of different imaging techniques and therapy with non-steroidal anti-inflammatory drugs. Eur J Pediatr 1998;157:28–33.

73. Reith J, Bauer T, Schils J. Osseous manifestations of SAPHO (synovitis, acne, pustulosis, hyperostosis, osteitis) syndrome. Am J Surg Pathol 1996;20:1368–77.

74. Kotilainen P, Gullichsen R, Saario R, et al. Aseptic spondylitis as the initial manifestation of the SAPHO syndrome. Eur Spine J 1997;6(5):327–9.

75. Ellis B, Shier C, Leisen J, et al. Acne-associated spondylarthropathy: radiographic features. Radiology 1987;162:541–5.

76. Sweeney S, Kumar V, Tayar J, et al. Case 181: synovitis acne pustulosis hyperostosis osteitis (SAPHO) syndrome. Radiology 2012;263(2):613–7.

77. Nachtigal A, Cardinal E, Bureau N, et al. Vertebral involvement in SAPHO syndrome: MRI findings. Skeletal Radiol 1999;28:163–8.

78. Romanus R, Yden S. Destructive and ossifying spondylitic changes in rheumatoid ankylosing spondylitis (pelvospondylitis ossificans). Acta Orthop Scand 1952;22:88–99.

79. Hermann K, Althoff C, Schneider U, et al. Spinal changes in patients with spondyloarthritis: comparison of MR imaging and radiographic appearances. Radiographics 2005;253:559–69.

80. Mann B, Shaerf D, Sheeraz A, et al. SAPHO syndrome presenting as widespread bony metastatic disease of unknown origin. Rheumatol Int 2012;32(2):505–7.

81. Yuh W, Quets J, Lee H, et al. Anatomic distribution of metastases in the vertebral body and modes of hematogenous spread. Spine 1996;21(19):2243–50.

82. Takigawa T, Tanaka M, Nakahara S, et al. SAPHO syndrome with rapidly progressing destructive spondylitis: two cases treated surgically. Eur Spine J 2008;17(Suppl 2):S331–7.

83. Takeuchi K, Matsusita M, Takagishi K. A case of SAPHO (synovitis-acne-pustulosis-hyperostosis-osteomyelitis) syndrome in which [18F]fluorodeoxyglucose positron emission tomography was useful for differentiating from multiple metastatic bone tumors. Mod Rheumatol 2007;17(1):67–71.

84. Kahn M. Psoriatic arthritis and synovitis, acne, pustulosis, hyperostosis, and osteitis syndrome. Curr Opin Rheumatol 1993;5(4):428–35.

85. Colina M, La Corte R, Trotta F. Sustained remission of SAPHO syndrome with pamidronate: a follow-up of fourteen cases and review of the literature. Clin Exp Rheumatol 2009;27:112–5.

86. Inoue K, Yamaguchi T, Ozawa H, et al. Diagnosing active inflammation in the SAPHO syndrome using 18FDG-PET/CT in suspected metastatic vertebral bone tumors. Ann Nucl Med 2007;21(8):477–80.

87. Kodama Y, Tanaka R, Kurokawa A. Severe destruction of the temporomandibular joint with complete resorption of the condyle associated with synovitis, acne, pustulosis, hyperostosis, and osteitis syndrome. Oral Surg Oral Med Oral Pathol Oral Radiol 2013;116(2):128–33.

88. Müller-Richter U, Roldán J, Mörtl M, et al. SAPHO syndrome with ankylosis of the temporomandibular joint. Int J Oral Maxillofac Surg 2009;38(12):1335–41.

89. Anderson S, Heini P, Sauvain M, et al. Imaging of chronic recurrent multifocal osteomyelitis of childhood first presenting with isolated primary spinal involvement. Skeletal Radiol 2003;32:328–36.

90. Hospach T, Langendoerfer M, von Kalle T, et al. Spinal involvement in chronic recurrent multifocal osteomyelitis (CRMO) in childhood and effect of pamidronate. Eur J Pediatr 2010;169:1105–11.

91. Yu L, Kasser J, O'Rourke E, et al. Chronic recurrent multifocal osteomyelitis: association with vertebra plana. J Bone Joint Surg Am 1989;71:105–12.

92. Demharter J, Bohndorf K, Michl W, et al. Chronic recurrent multifocal osteomyelitis: a radiological and clinical investigation of five cases. Skeletal Radiol 1997;26:579–88.

93. Baulot E, Bouillien D, Giroux E, et al. Chronic recurrent multifocal osteomyelitis causing spinal cord compression. Eur Spine J 1998;7:340–3.

94. Carr A, Cole W, Robertson D, et al. Chronic multifocal osteomyelitis. J Bone Joint Surg Br 1993;75B:583–91.

95. Suei Y, Taguchi A, Tanimoto K. Diffuse sclerosing osteomyelitis of the mandible: its characteristics and possible relationship to synovitis, acne, pustulosis, hyperostosis, osteitis (SAPHO) syndrome. J Oral Maxillofac Surg 1996;54:1194–9.

96. Vittecoq O, Said L, Michot C, et al. Evolution of chronic recurrent multifocal osteitis towards spondylarthropathy over the long term. Arthritis Rheum 2000;43(1):109–19.

97. Chow L, Griffith J, Kumta SM, et al. Chronic recurrent multifocal osteomyelitis: a great clinical and radiological mimic in need of recognition by the pathologist. APMIS 1999;107(4):369–79.

98. Tyrrell P, Cassar-Pullicino V, Eisenstein S, et al. Back pain in childhood. Ann Rheum Dis 1996;55:789–93.

99. Björkstén B, Boquist L. Histopathological aspects of chronic recurrent multifocal osteomyelitis. J Bone Joint Surg Br 1980;62(3):376–80.

100. Girschick H, Han-Iko H, Dag H, et al. Chronic recurrent multifocal osteomyelitis in children: diagnostic value of histopathology and microbial testing. Hum Pathol 1999;30(1):59–65.

101. Jurik A, Helmig O, Ternowitz T, et al. Chronic recurrent multifocal osteomyelitis: a follow-up study. J Pediatr Orthop 1988;8:49–58.

102. Duffy C, Lam P, Ditchfield M, et al. Chronic recurrent multifocal osteomyelitis: review of orthopaedic complications at maturity. J Pediatr Orthop 2002; 22(4):501–5.

103. Hurtado-Nedelec M, Chollet-Martin S, Chapeton D, et al. Genetic susceptibility factors in a cohort of 38 patients with SAPHO syndrome: a study of PSTPIP2, NOD2, and LPIN2 genes. J Rheumatol 2010;37:401–9.

104. El-Shanti H, Ferguson P. Chronic recurrent multifocal osteomyelitis: a concise review and genetic update. Clin Orthop Relat Res 2007;462:11–9.

105. Ferguson P, Sandu M. Current understanding of the pathogenesis and management of chronic recurrent multifocal osteomyelitis. Curr Rheumatol Rep 2012;14:130–41.

106. Golla A, Jansson A, Ramser J, et al. Chronic recurrent multifocal osteomyelitis (CRMO): evidence for a susceptibility gene located on chromosome 18q21.3-18q22. Eur J Hum Genet 2002;10(3):217–21.

107. Yeon H, Lindor N, Seidman J, et al. Pyogenic arthritis, pyoderma gangrenosum, and acne syndrome maps to chromosome 15q. Am J Hum Genet 2000;66:1443–8.

108. Ferguson P, Chen S, Tayeh M, et al. Homozygous mutations in LPIN2 are responsible for the syndrome of chronic recurrent multifocal osteomyelitis and congenital dyserythropoietic anaemia (Majeed syndrome). J Med Genet 2005;42:551–7.

109. Al-Mosawi Z, Al-Saad K, Ijadi-Maghsoodi R, et al. A splice site mutation confirms the role of LPIN2 in Majeed syndrome. Arthritis Rheum 2007;56:960.

110. Siau K, Laversuch C. SAPHO syndrome in an adult with ulcerative colitis responsive to intravenous pamidronate: a case report and review of the literature. Rheumatol Int 2010;30:1085–8.

111. Bousvaros A, Marcon M, Treem W, et al. Chronic recurrent multifocal osteomyelitis associated with chronic inflammatory bowel disease in children. Dig Dis Sci 1999;44(12):2500–7.

112. Bognar M, Blake W, Agudelo C. Chronic recurrent multifocal osteomyelitis associated with Crohn's disease. Am J Med Sci 1998;315(2):133–5.

113. Dougado M, van der Linden S, Juhlin R, et al. The European Spondyarthropathy Study Group preliminary criteria for the classification of spondyloarthropathy. Arthritis Rheum 1991;34:1218–27.

114. Colina M, Lo Monaco A, Khodeir M, et al. *Propionibacterium acnes* and SAPHO syndrome: a case report and literature review. Clin Exp Rheumatol 2007;25:457–60.

115. Pelkonen P, Ryöppy S, Jääskeläinen J, et al. Chronic osteomyelitislike disease with negative bacterial cultures. Am J Dis Child 1988;142(11): 1167–73.

116. Assmann G, Kueck O, Kirchhoff T, et al. Efficacy of antibiotic therapy for SAPHO syndrome is lost after its discontinuation: an interventional study. Arthritis Res Ther 2009;11(5):R140.

117. Govoni M, Colina M, Massara A, et al. SAPHO syndrome and infections. Autoimmun Rev 2009;8:256–9.

118. Brüggemann H, Henne A, Hoster F, et al. The complete genome sequence of *Propionibacterium acnes*, a commensal of human skin. Science 2004;305(5684):671–3.

119. Ballara S, Siraj Q, Maini R, et al. Sustained response to doxycycline therapy in two patients with SAPHO syndrome. Arthritis Rheum 1999;42: 819–21.

120. Schilling F, Wagner A. Azithromycin: an anti-inflammatory effect in chronic recurrent multifocal osteomyelitis? A preliminary report. Z Rheumatol 2000;59:352–3.

121. Aljuhani F, Tournadre A, Tatar Z, et al. The SAPHO syndrome: a single-center study of 41 adult patients. J Rheumatol 2015;42(2):329–34.

122. Assmann G, Simon P. The SAPHO syndrome: are microbes involved? Best Pract Res Clin Rheumatol 2011;25(3):423–37.

123. Amital H, Govoni M, Maya R, et al. Role of infectious agents in systemic rheumatic diseases. Clin Exp Rheumatol 2008;26(1 Suppl 48):S27–32.

124. Barton GM, Medzhitov R. Toll-like receptor signaling pathways. Science 2003;300(5625):1524–5.

125. Rozin A. SAPHO syndrome: is a range of pathogen-associated rheumatic diseases extended? Arthritis Res Ther 2009;11(6):131.

126. Wagner A, Andresen J, Jendro M, et al. Sustained response to tumor necrosis factor alpha-blocking agents in two patients with SAPHO syndrome. Arthritis Rheum 2002;46:1965–8.

127. Rozin A. From molecular mimicry to cross-reactivity or pathogen expansion? A hypothesis. Clin Rheumatol 2007;26:285–8.

128. Kalis C, Gumenscheimer M, Freudenberg N, et al. Requirement of TLR9 in the immunomodulatory activity of *Propionibacterium acnes*. J Immunol 2005; 174:4295–300.

129. Firinu D, Garcia-Larsen V, Manconi P, et al. SAPHO syndrome: current developments and approaches to clinical treatment. Curr Rheumatol Rep 2016; 18:35.

130. Beck C, Morbach H, Beer M, et al. Chronic nonbacterial osteomyelitis in childhood: prospective

follow-up during the first year of anti-inflammatory treatment. Arthritis Res Ther 2010;12(2):R74.

131. Jung J, Molinger M, Kohn D, et al. Intra-articular glucocorticosteroid injection into sternocostoclavicular joints in patients with SAPHO syndrome. Semin Arthritis Rheum 2012;42(3):266–70.

132. Rogers M, Gordon S, Benford H, et al. Cellular and molecular mechanisms of action of bisphosphonates. Cancer 2000;88(12):S2961–78.

133. Amital H, Applbaum Y, Aamar S, et al. SAPHO syndrome treated with pamidronate: an open-label study of 10 patients. Rheumatology 2004;43(5):658–61.

134. Solau-Gervais E, Soubrier M, Gerot I, et al. The usefulness of bone remodelling markers in predicting the efficacy of pamidronate treatment in SAPHO syndrome. Rheumatology 2006;45:339–42.

135. Morbach H, Stenzel M, Girschick H. Bisphosphonate treatment for patients with chronic nonbacterial osteomyelitis. Nat Clin Pract Rheumatol 2008;4:570–1.

136. Kerrison C, Davidson J, Cleary A, et al. Pamidronate in the treatment of childhood SAPHO syndrome. Rheumatology 2004;43:1246–51.

137. Simm P, Allen R, Zacharin M. Bisphosphonate treatment in chronic recurrent multifocal osteomyelitis. J Pediatr 2008;152:571.

138. Gorecki P, Stockmann P, Distler J, et al. Implication of bisphosphonate use in the treatment of SAPHO syndrome: case report and discussion of current literature. J Med Hypotheses Ideas 2015;9(2):72–8.

139. Zwaenepoel T, de Vlam K. SAPHO: treatment options including bisophphonates. Semin Arthritis Rheum 2016;46(2):168–73.

140. Laveti D, Kumar M, Hemalatha R, et al. Anti-inflammatory treatments for chronic diseases: a review. Inflamm Allergy Drug Targets 2013;12(5):349–61.

141. Ben Abdelghani K, Dran D, Gottenberg J, et al. Tumor necrosis factor alpha blockers in SAPHO syndrome. J Rheumatol 2010;37:1699–704.

142. Moll C, Hernández M, Cañete J, et al. Ilium osteitis as the main manifestation of the SAPHO syndrome: response to infliximab therapy and review of the literature. Semin Arthritis Rheum 2008;37(5):299–306.

143. Burgemeister L, Baeten D, Tas S. Biologics for rare inflammatory diseases: TNF blockade in the SAPHO syndrome. Neth J Med 2012;70(10):444–9.

144. Deutschmann A, Mache C, Bodo K, et al. Successful treatment of chronic recurrent multifocal osteomyelitis with tumor necrosis factor-alpha blockage. Pediatrics 2005;116:1231–3.

145. Adisen E, Gurer M. Therapeutic options for palmoplantar pustulosis. Clin Exp Dermatol 2010;35(3):219–22.

146. Massara A, Cavazzini P, Trotta F. In SAPHO syndrome anti-TNF-alpha therapy may induce persistent amelioration of osteoarticular complaints, but may exacerbate cutaneous manifestations. Rheumatology 2006;45(6):730–3.

147. Colina M, Pizzirani C, Khodeir M, et al. Dysregulation of P2X7 receptor-inflammasome axis in SAPHO syndrome: successful treatment with anakinra. Rheumatology 2010;49:1416–8.

148. Wendling D, Prati C, Aubin F. Anakinra treatment of SAPHO syndrome: short-term results of an open study. Ann Rheum Dis 2012;71(6):1098–100.

Imaging of Myopathies

Lukas Filli, MD[a],*, Sebastian Winklhofer, MD[b],
Gustav Andreisek, MD, MBA[c,d], Filippo Del Grande, MD, MBA, MHEM[d,e]

KEYWORDS

• MR imaging • Skeletal muscle • Myopathy • Myositis • Muscle dystrophy

KEY POINTS

• MR imaging features in common myopathies are generally nonspecific, but their distribution pattern can be suggestive of specific types and subtypes of disease.
• MR imaging plays a central role in guiding muscle biopsy, which still remains the gold standard for the diagnosis of myopathy.
• Advanced MR imaging methods may be able to better differentiate and characterize myopathies in the near future.

THE ROLE OF MR IMAGING IN IMAGING OF MYOPATHIES

Introduction

The purpose of this review article is to clarify the current role of MR imaging in the assessment of myopathies. Typical MR imaging findings are discussed for different forms of myopathies, including idiopathic inflammatory myopathies, muscular dystrophies, and congenital myopathies. The last section deals with advanced MR imaging techniques and their role in further characterization of muscular disease.

General MR imaging Findings

Given its excellent soft tissue contrast, MR imaging is the most specific and sensitive imaging method for detecting skeletal muscle abnormalities related to myopathies. In order to detect both acute and chronic disease, MR protocols should include both T1- and T2-weighted fat-suppressed sequences. Short-tau inversion recovery (STIR) can be used in place of T2-weighted sequences.[1–3]

In general, high-signal intensity on T2-weighted or STIR images most commonly indicates muscle edema in the acute stage of disease, whereas high-signal intensity on T1-weighted images usually represents fatty degeneration in chronic stage of the disease.[4] The value of additional contrast-enhanced sequences remains controversial.[3]

Whole-Body MR Imaging

Muscle edema and fatty degeneration are rather nonspecific manifestations of myopathy,[5,6] which can be seen in inflammatory myopathies, neuromuscular disorders, or muscular dystrophy.[7] However, their distribution in the body may be suggestive of certain subtypes of disease. Therefore, it is important to identify distinct distribution patterns of skeletal muscle involvement. In order to assess the entire musculoskeletal system, whole-body MR imaging has become increasingly important during the last years.[1–3,8–10]

Whole-body MR imaging, besides revealing specific distribution patterns of certain forms of myopathies, can also detect clinically silent involvement of muscle groups, and potential

Disclosures: The authors have nothing to disclose.
[a] Institute of Diagnostic and Interventional Radiology, University Hospital Zurich, University of Zurich, Raemistrasse 100, 8091 Zurich, Switzerland; [b] Department of Neuroradiology, University Hospital Zurich, University of Zurich, Frauenklinikstrasse 10, 8091 Zurich, Switzerland; [c] Department of Radiology, Kantonsspital Münsterlingen, Spitalcampus 1, 8596 Münsterlingen, Switzerland; [d] University of Zurich, Raemistrasse 71, 8006 Zurich, Switzerland; [e] Department of Radiology, Ospedale Regionale di Lugano, Via Tesserete 46, Lugano 6900, Switzerland
* Corresponding author.
E-mail address: Lukas.Filli@usz.ch

Radiol Clin N Am 55 (2017) 1055–1070
http://dx.doi.org/10.1016/j.rcl.2017.04.010
0033-8389/17/

isolated involvement of those muscles that cannot be individually assessed by clinical testing.[11,12] Furthermore, MR imaging helps localize the most suitable site for muscle biopsy.[13] In patients with established diagnosis, serial whole-body MR imaging allows the assessment of not only treatment response (**Fig. 1**) but also early detection of adverse side effects (eg, avascular necrosis

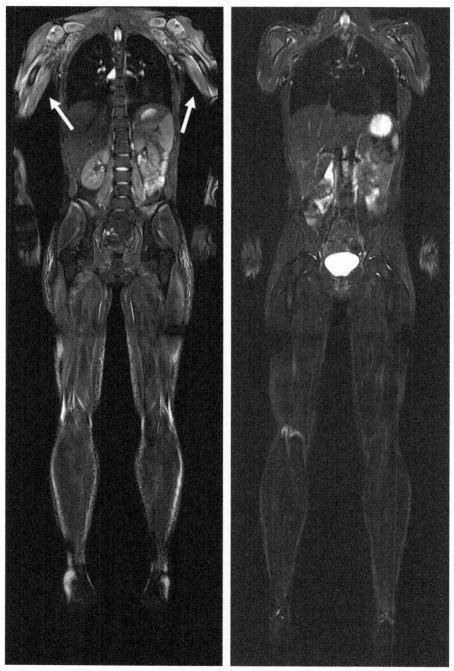

Fig. 1. (*Left*) Whole-body MR imaging (coronal STIR) of a 20-year-old female patient with polymyositis. Symmetric hyperintensity of the upper and lower limb muscles with punctum maximum in the upper arms (*arrows*). (*Right*) Subtotal regression of the hyperintensities in the corresponding follow-up examination 6 months after high-dose steroid and methotrexate therapy.

related to steroid therapy).[14] One limitation of whole-body MR imaging is the patient size, because if the patient is too big with respect to the bore width, fat-suppression artifacts may hamper the evaluation of the shoulder girdle and/ or upper arms. Another limitation is the duration of the examination, which should be kept as short as possible.[3]

IDIOPATHIC INFLAMMATORY MYOPATHIES

Idiopathic inflammatory myopathies are a heterogeneous group of rare immune-mediated myopathies of unknown cause.[15] The 3 most common subtypes in the adult population are dermatomyositis, polymyositis, and inclusion body myositis. Early diagnosis is important because idiopathic inflammatory myopathies can be treated successfully and, unlike in many other myopathies, fatty degeneration may be prevented.

A common feature of idiopathic inflammatory myopathies is their clinical presentation with muscle weakness. In more than 85% of cases, MR imaging reveals edema in symptomatic muscles.[16] However, because muscle edema is a rather unspecific finding, the diagnosis of inflammatory myopathy cannot be based solely on MR imaging. Still, MR imaging is a useful tool in diagnostic decision making. First, it is important to guide biopsy (which remains the diagnostic gold standard) and substantially reduce the rate of false-negative biopsies.[7,17,18] Second, it helps to narrow the differential diagnosis by revealing specific distribution patterns.

Muscle edema is a common finding in the early stage of disease. In chronic disease, muscle atrophy and fatty degeneration can occur. Isolated edema (ie, without atrophy or fatty infiltration) is more commonly seen in dermatomyositis and polymyositis rather than inclusion body myositis.[19]

Dermatomyositis and Polymyositis

Dermatomyositis and polymyositis commonly lead to symmetric involvement of the proximal muscles of the upper and lower extremities and relatively spare the muscles of the body trunk.[3,17,20] Both are more common in women and may be associated with malignancy. A common MR finding in patients with dermatomyositis is edema along the muscle fascia and in the subcutaneous fat, which is less commonly seen in patients with polymyositis.[5] Histologically, inflammatory cells in polymyositis are predominantly endomysial as opposed to perimysial location in patients with dermatomyositis.[8] Dermatomyositis is additionally associated with skin manifestations such as heliotrope rash or Gottron papules.

In the early stage of disease, patients with dermatomyositis may present with muscle weakness, but serum creatine kinase levels and muscle strength might still be normal.[21] In these situations, MR imaging is important to facilitate early diagnosis by already showing inflammatory muscle changes in most of these patients.[21] In addition, MR imaging helps to determine a suitable site for muscle biopsy, thereby reducing the false-negative biopsy rate,[13,17] and has proven to be cost-effective in patients with polymyositis.[18] Furthermore, once the diagnosis has been established and treatment has been initiated, MR imaging represents a useful tool for the assessment of treatment response[22] (see **Fig. 1**; **Figs. 2–4**).

Inclusion Body Myositis

Inclusion body myositis is a slowly progressive degenerative muscle disease usually seen in patients older than 50 years. Muscle atrophy and fatty degeneration are the predominant finding in these patients.[21] Inflammatory changes are usually less pronounced than in patients with polymyositis[19] and may be secondary to muscle degeneration rather than a primary autoimmune process.[23] Unlike dermatomyositis and polymyositis, inclusion body myositis is not associated with malignancy.[24]

Sporadic inclusion body myositis demonstrates a specific distribution pattern of muscle involvement: It mainly involves anteriorly located muscle

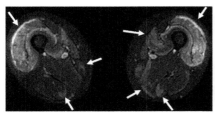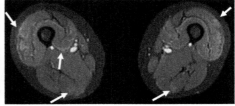

Fig. 2. Axial fat-suppressed T2-weighted (*left*) and corresponding T1-weighted postcontrast MR imaging (*right*) of the thighs of a 56-year-old female with histologically proven dermatomyositis. Bilateral symmetric T2 hyperintensities and mild contrast enhancement (*arrows*) are visible in the quadriceps femoris, sartorius, semi-membranosus and semitendinosus muscles.

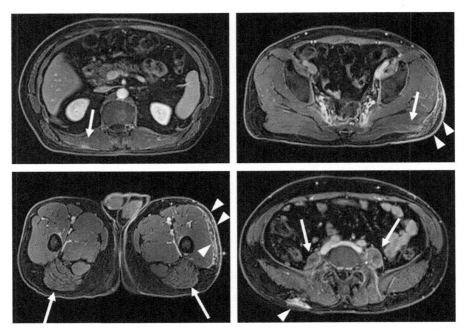

Fig. 3. Axial fat-suppressed T1-weighted postcontrast MR imaging of a 51-year-old male patient with a long history of dermatomyositis. Mild contrast enhancement (*arrows*) of the lumbar paraspinal muscles (*upper left*) and the left gluteus maximus muscle (*upper right*). Subcutaneous fluid collections and diffuse contrast enhancement in the left gluteal region and along the left vastus lateralis muscle representing a typical finding in dermatomyositis (*arrowheads in all images*). Moderate bilateral atrophy of the gluteus maximus and psoas muscles (*bottom images; arrows*).

groups of the legs, particularly the quadriceps muscle (with relative sparing of the rectus femoris muscle), the distal sartorius muscle, and the ankle dorsiflexors[19,25,26] (**Fig. 5**). The anterior predominance is also seen in the upper extremity, with common involvement of the wrist and deep finger flexors.[26] An exception to this rule is the observed severe atrophy of the medial head of the gastrocnemius muscle.[25] The adductor and abductor muscles of the shoulder and pelvic girdles are relatively spared.[25,27] Some studies reported that asymmetrical involvement is more common in inclusion body myositis than in dermatomyositis and polymyositis,[19,28] whereas others could not confirm this observation.[26]

Although most patients show the distribution pattern described above, other patients show incomplete clinical or radiologic manifestation of disease. Therefore, inclusion body myositis may be initially misdiagnosed, particularly as polymyositis.[26] Furthermore, other forms of myopathies that lead to fatty degeneration of the quadriceps muscle, such as limb girdle muscular dystrophy (LGMD) or Becker dystrophy, need to be considered. However, as opposed to inclusion body myositis, these also commonly involve the biceps femoris, semimembranosus, and thigh adductor muscles.[29]

Whole-body MR imaging can help to recognize the typical involvement pattern in the lower

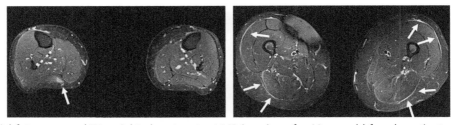

Fig. 4. Axial fat-suppressed T1-weighted postcontrast MR imaging of a 44-year-old female patient with known polymyositis. (*Left*) Subtle contrast enhancement in the lateral head of the right gastrocnemius muscle. (*Right*) Bilateral hyperintense epifascial signal alterations (*arrows*) along the vastus lateralis, rectus femoris, and ischiocrural muscles of the thighs.

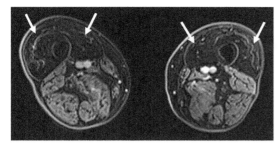

Fig. 5. Axial fat-suppressed T1-weighted postcontrast MR imaging of a 75-year-old male patient with sporadic inclusion body myositis. There is severe bilateral and symmetric muscle atrophy with fatty degeneration of the quadriceps femoris muscle (*arrows*). The involvement of anteriorly located muscle groups represents a typical pattern for inclusion body myositis.

extremities and find the optimal site for biopsy. In addition, the treatment response of muscle changes as assessed by MR imaging correlates with clinical improvement of muscle function.[30] With regard to the involvement of wrist and deep finger flexor muscles, according to the authors' experience, current whole-body MR imaging protocols are not useful, because these muscles cannot be reliably assessed; although not routinely performed in the diagnostic workup,[26] additional dedicated MR imaging of the hand and wrist may be considered in these cases.

Muscle Involvement in Other Forms of Rheumatologic Disease

Along with idiopathic inflammatory myopathies, muscle involvement is also present in other types of rheumatologic disease, such as connective tissue disease. The most common subtype with inflammatory muscle changes is systemic sclerosis.[21]

Systemic sclerosis is characterized by inflammation of the connective tissue leading to tenosynovitis, synovitis, joint effusion, and bone erosions.[31] In most cases, skeletal muscles are affected by inflammatory changes as well, in particular, the proximal muscles of the upper and lower extremities[32] (**Fig. 6**). It is important to detect involvement of skeletal muscle in order to improve staging and to assess response to treatment. However, MR imaging probably cannot distinguish between inflammatory and noninflammatory myopathy.[31]

MUSCULAR DYSTROPHIES

Muscular dystrophies are a heterogeneous group of slowly progressive myopathies. This article describes MR imaging findings and distribution patterns for the most common forms.

Duchenne Muscular Dystrophy

Duchenne muscular dystrophy is an X-chromosomal recessive disorder and the most common

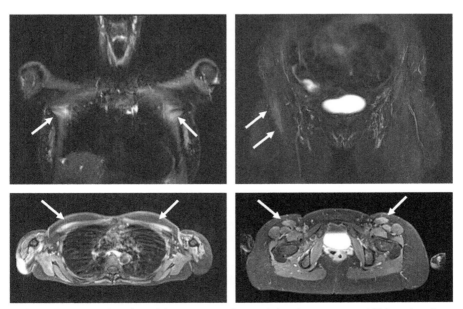

Fig. 6. Coronal STIR (*upper row*) and axial fat-suppressed T1-weighted postcontrast MR imaging (*lower row*) of a 38-year-old female patient with systemic sclerosis. Edema and contrast enhancement of the pectoralis major and the sartorius muscles (*arrows*). Inflammatory changes of the proximal muscles of the upper and lower extremities are a typical finding in cases of muscle involvement in systemic sclerosis.

form of muscular dystrophy in childhood, characterized by absent production of dystrophin,[33] a protein that is important for muscle fiber strength by linking actin filaments to structural proteins.

As their muscle tissue is replaced by fat and connective tissue, patients with Duchenne muscular dystrophy suffer from progressive muscle weakness, beginning in the proximal lower extremities. Boys usually become symptomatic at less than 5 years of age and show a rapid decline during the second decade of life.[34] The diagnosis is established based on physical examination, serum creatine phosphokinase levels, and genetic analysis.

MR imaging plays a role in assessing the extent of muscle atrophy and fatty degeneration both qualitatively and quantitatively and is able to detect subclinical muscle involvement.[11] Individual muscle groups may show different progression during the disease course, which can be monitored with MR imaging.

Qualitative assessment by MR imaging can be performed muscle-wise using the 4-point Mercuri score (Table 1), which was originally introduced for patients with rigid spine muscular dystrophy.[35]

Quantitative MR imaging–based evaluation of muscle involvement in Duchenne muscular dystrophy has been increasingly used in the last years.[36–44] Several MR imaging methods have been proposed in patients with Duchenne muscular dystrophy in order to detect and monitor pathologic changes in muscle tissue:

- T1-weighted imaging: As the T1 values are much shorter for fat than for water, fatty muscle atrophy during disease progression leads

to decreased T1 values.[33] This allows monitoring of disease progression.
- Dixon technique: Fat and water signal can be separated voxel-wise by using the Dixon technique.[45] This technique allows for the quantification of the fat signal fraction (FSF) in individual muscle groups[46] and is more precise and reliable than qualitative MR imaging–based assessment in patients with Duchenne muscular dystrophy.[47] FSF values correlate better with disease severity than clinical muscle strength measures.[38]
- T2-weighted imaging (along with T2 mapping) is used to estimate muscle damage and fatty infiltration. T2 values increase with disease progression in Duchenne muscular dystrophy[48] and show a significant correlation with the qualitative Mercuri score and clinical measures of disease severity.[49]
- Fat-suppressed sequences such as STIR are very sensitive to fluid and allow early detection of muscle edema in patients with Duchenne muscular dystrophy. This is particularly helpful in younger boys, in whom fatty atrophy is not yet a prominent feature.[50]
- Muscle cross-sectional area (CSA): Compared with age-matched control subjects, patients with Duchenne muscular dystrophy have an approximately 60% higher CSA of the calf muscles. The quadriceps CSA is higher during the first decade of life but lower afterward.[51] The limitation of CSA measurements is their lack of discrimination between normal muscle tissue and fatty atrophy.

Table 1
Qualitative scoring of muscle degeneration as published by Mercuri and colleagues

Stage	Findings
0	Normal appearance
1	Early moth-eaten appearance, with scattered small areas of decreased density on CT or increased density on the T1 MR sequence
2a	Late moth-eaten appearance, with numerous discrete areas of decreased density (CT) or increased density (MR imaging) with beginning confluence, comprising <30% of the volume of the individual muscle
2b	Late moth-eaten appearance, with numerous discrete areas of decreased density (CT) or increased density (MR imaging) with beginning confluence, comprising 30%–60% of the volume of the individual muscle
3	Washed-out appearance, fuzzy appearance due to confluent areas of decreased density (CT) or increased density (MR imaging) with muscle still present at the periphery
4	End-stage appearance, muscle replaced by lower density (CT) or increased density (MR imaging) connective tissue and fat, with only a rim of fascia and neurovascular structures distinguishable

Data from Mercuri E, Talim B, Moghadaszadeh B, et al. Clinical and imaging findings in six cases of congenital muscular dystrophy with rigid spine syndrome linked to chromosome 1p (RSMD1). Neuromuscul Disord 2002;12(7–8):631–8.

The gold standard for assessing potential treatment response in preclinical trials in Duchenne muscular dystrophy is muscle biopsy. However, this procedure is invasive, prone to errors with specimen processing, may not reliably represent the overall disease progression, and could even lead to false negative results.[33] Thus, MR imaging may be used as an alternative surrogate outcome measure.[41,52–54]

A recent study revealed a distinctive pattern of lower extremity muscle involvement in Duchenne muscular dystrophy as observed on MR imaging.[55] The gluteus medius, minimus, and adductor magnus muscles were most severely involved at all stages. Moderate to severe changes in the gluteus maximus and quadriceps muscles were observed, whereas the gracilis, Sartorius, and semimembranosus muscles were entirely spared (Fig. 7).

Becker Muscular Dystrophy

Patients with Becker muscular dystrophy suffer from insufficient production of dystrophin (as opposed to complete absence of dystrophin in Duchenne muscular dystrophy). The clinical presentation can be very variable, ranging from minimal symptoms (weakness, cramps) to severe disease with loss of ambulation.[56]

Similar to Duchenne muscular dystrophy, there is a highly symmetric distribution pattern of muscle involvement. The gluteus, quadriceps, and semimembranosus muscles are commonly involved, and this pattern is consistently seen in most symptomatic patients (Fig. 8); however, muscle involvement is generally milder than in patients with Duchenne muscular dystrophy.[28,29,56] The upper extremities are less commonly affected, with early involvement of the teres major, triceps, and biceps muscles.[57] Furthermore, MR imaging can detect muscle involvement in clinically asymptomatic patients. MR findings correlate with clinical function.[58] In preclinical trials, MR imaging has been used as surrogate marker for treatment response.[59]

Other myopathy forms should be considered in the differential diagnosis of Becker muscular dystrophy, mainly LGMD and idiopathic inflammatory myopathies. There are some differences in the distribution patterns on MR imaging. In Becker muscular dystrophy, the gastrocnemius muscle is relatively spared as opposed to some forms of

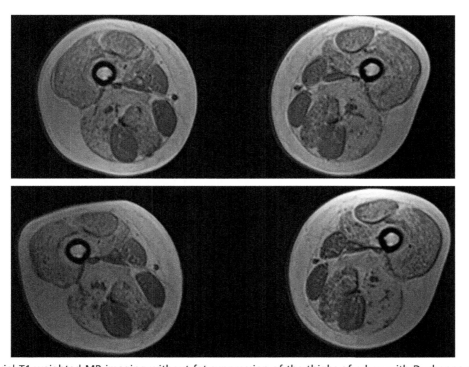

Fig. 7. Axial T1-weighted MR imaging without fat suppression of the thighs of a boy with Duchenne muscular dystrophy. (*Upper image*) Typical distribution pattern with severe symmetric fatty degeneration of the quadriceps, adductor, and biceps femoris muscles as well as sparing of the gracilis, sartorius, and semimembranosus muscles. (*Lower image*) Two-year follow-up MR imaging shows no significant morphologic changes over time. (*Courtesy of* Arne Fischmann, MD, Klinik St. Anna, Lucerne, Switzerland.)

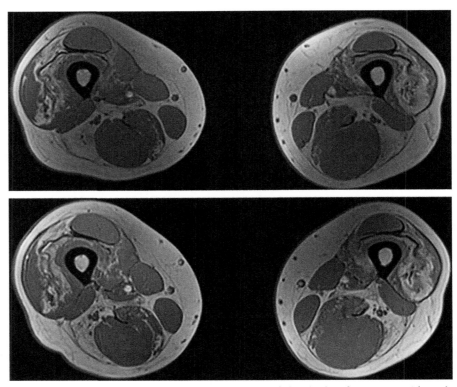

Fig. 8. Axial T1-weighted MR imaging without fat suppression of the thighs of a patient with Becker muscular dystrophy. (*Upper image*) Typical distribution pattern with symmetric fatty degeneration of the quadriceps, adductor, and biceps femoris muscles. Muscle involvement is generally milder than in patients with Duchenne muscular dystrophy. (*Lower image*) Two-year follow-up MR imaging shows no significant morphologic changes over time. (*Courtesy of* Arne Fischmann, MD, Klinik St. Anna, Lucerne, Switzerland.)

LGMD[60]; by contrast, there is relative sparing of the quadriceps muscle in patients with LGMD.[56,61] In Becker muscular dystrophy, fatty atrophy is more pronounced in the hamstring and thigh adductor muscles than in polymyositis or inclusion body myositis.[62]

Limb Girdle Muscular Dystrophy

The term limb girdle muscular dystrophy comprises a heterogeneous group of hereditary myopathies, which most commonly affect the pelvic girdle and leg muscles. Distribution patterns of muscle involvement recognized on MR imaging may help establish a diagnosis and differentiate LGMD from other types of myopathy. Muscle biopsy may be nonspecific in some cases.[63]

Recent whole-body MR imaging study on patients with LGMD2B[64] and LGMD2L[65] revealed a characteristic distribution pattern of skeletal muscle involvement. MR imaging showed mild to moderate involvement of pelvic muscles as well as severe involvement of the thigh muscles. The sartorius and gracilis muscles are less affected

or even spared, similar to the pattern observed in Duchenne muscular dystrophy. Regarding the lower leg, the posterior compartment is most predominantly affected on MR imaging[66] (**Figs. 9** and **10**).

Asymmetry is more commonly seen in LGMD2L than in LGMD2B.[65] In LGMD2A, characteristic findings are early involvement of the gluteus maximus muscle, sparing of the vastus lateralis muscle, and predominant involvement of the medial head of the gastrocnemius muscle.[60–62] The reason for this selective involvement is unknown yet. Despite these characteristic findings in different subtypes of LGMD, MR imaging currently seems unable to reliably distinguish between them given the huge overlap of distribution patterns.

Myotonic Dystrophy

Myotonic dystrophy type 1 and type 2 are autosomal-dominant myopathies. They show different distribution patterns of clinically recognizable skeletal muscle involvement but both lead to generalized muscle weakness over time.[67,68]

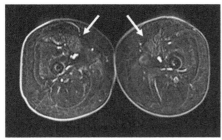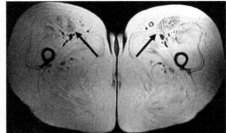

Fig. 9. A 52-year-old female patient with a long history of LGMD. Axial fat-suppressed T1-weighted postcontrast MR imaging (*left*) and axial T1-weighted image without fat suppression (*right*) demonstrate severe fatty degeneration of the muscles of the pelvis and the thighs with relative sparing of the sartorius muscles (*arrows*).

In patients with myotonic dystrophy type 1, there is predominant involvement of the anterior thigh muscles with relative sparing of the rectus femoris muscle,[67,69] similar to other forms of muscle dystrophies and idiopathic inflammatory myopathies. In addition, early degeneration of the medial head of the gastrocnemius muscle is frequently seen in myotonic dystrophy type 1,[67] which is also a common finding in patients with inclusion body myositis and LGMD2A. The tibialis posterior muscle is entirely spared.

In myotonic dystrophy type 2, the extent and severity of fatty degeneration are generally less severe than in type 1, and MR imaging may often appear normal despite clinical symptoms.[67]

CONGENITAL MYOPATHIES

Congenital myopathies are a heterogeneous group of rare autosomal-dominant or autosomal-recessive myopathies with muscle weakness at birth or onset of symptoms during childhood. Diagnosis is based on genetic analysis, and the required biopsy can be targeted based on MR imaging.[62] Furthermore, typical distribution patterns of muscle involvement have been found for several forms of disease. For example, in patients with ryanodine receptor (RYR1) mutations, the quadriceps muscle is commonly affected with relative sparing of the rectus femoris muscle[70,71] (Fig. 11). By contrast, other types of congenital myopathies predominantly involve posterior thigh muscles.[62]

Table 2 provides a selection of different congenital myopathies with respective distribution patterns seen on MR imaging, based on the comprehensive review article recently published by Quijano-Roy and colleagues.[72] It shows the heterogeneous patterns of muscle involvement, which may help narrow the differential diagnosis before biopsy and thereby tailor the required genetic analyses to individual cases.

OUTLOOK: ADVANCED IMAGING METHODS

In previous sections, emphasis was on the high sensitivity but low specificity of MR imaging to inflammatory changes, atrophy, and fatty degeneration of skeletal muscle. Furthermore, the importance of pattern recognizing for narrowing the differential diagnosis was discussed; nevertheless, there are still substantial overlaps on MR imaging among different forms of myopathy.

In search of more specific tools for characterization of skeletal muscle physiology and abnormality, advanced MR imaging techniques have been increasingly investigated in recent years. These advanced techniques give insight into functional processes, such as metabolism, diffusion, or microvascular perfusion. Thus, they provide information beyond what can be depicted on conventional MR imaging and could help to assess the disease course and treatment response in more detail.

In this last section, the most commonly used techniques are discussed, some of which might enter clinical routine in the near future.

Arterial Spin Labeling

Arterial spin labeling is an advanced technique for measuring local perfusion of skeletal muscle without the need for intravenous contrast injection. First, water molecules in arterial blood are magnetically labeled proximal to a slice of interest. Second, the labeled blood flows into the slice of interest and alters tissue magnetization. Local perfusion can then be estimated based on the tissue magnetization in the slice of interest.

Arterial spin labeling of skeletal muscle has been validated many years ago,[73] but reports of clinical application in myopathies are sparse.[74] Important limitations include its sensitivity to motion artifacts, low contrast-to-noise ratio, and relatively long acquisition times.

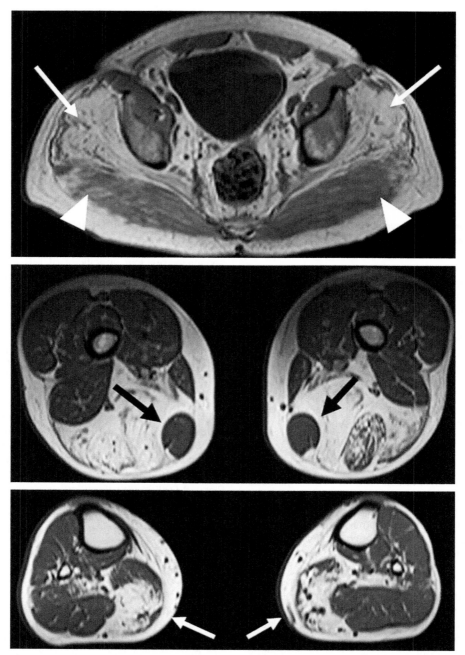

Fig. 10. Axial T1-weighted MR imaging without fat suppression of a 55-year-old male patient with LGMD. (*Top*) Severe bilateral symmetric fatty atrophy of the medial and minimal gluteus muscles (*arrows*) as well as moderate fatty degeneration of the gluteus maximus muscles (*arrowheads*). (*Middle*) Bilateral severe fatty atrophy of the hamstring with compensatory hypertrophy of the gracilis muscles (*arrows*). (*Bottom*) Bilateral fatty atrophy of the medial head of the gastrocnemius muscle (*arrows*). In contrast to inclusion body myositis, where the anterior involvement of anterior muscles groups is commonly affected, in LGMD, typically the posterior compartments of the lower extremities are involved.

Blood Oxygenation Level–Dependent Imaging

Blood oxygenation level–dependent (BOLD) MR imaging depends on alterations of hemoglobin oxygen saturation in the microvasculature. Although oxyhemoglobin is diamagnetic, deoxyhemoglobin is paramagnetic and thus decreases the magnetic susceptibility of surrounding water protons. Thus, BOLD MR imaging has been recognized as a

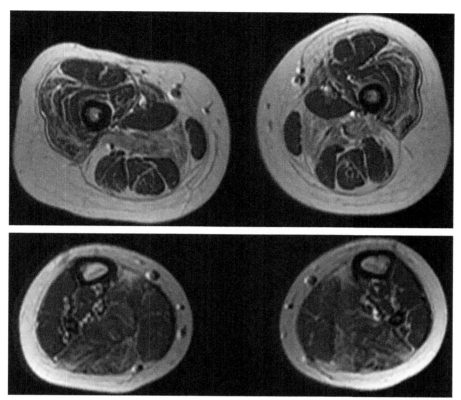

Fig. 11. Axial T1-weighted MR imaging (without fat suppression) showing the typical pattern of muscle involvement in an 8-year-old male patient with RYR1-related myopathy. In the upper legs (*upper image*), involvement of the vasti, sartorius, and adductor magnus muscles is noted, whereas the rectus femoris, adductor longus, gracilis, and hamstring muscles are relatively spared. In the lower legs (*lower image*), there is symmetric fatty infiltration of the soleus muscle, whereas the medial gastrocnemius muscles as well as the anterior and lateral compartments are relatively spared. (*Data from* Refs.[70–72]; and *Courtesy of* Andrea Klein, MD, University Children's Hospital Basel (UKBB), Basel, Switzerland.)

new potential tool to evaluate muscle abnormalities.[75] The BOLD signal is influenced (and potentially biased) by numerous factors, such as microvascular density, muscle blood volume, and metabolic factors.[76,77] However, perfusion-related changes of muscle tissue oxygenation still are the predominant factor.[78]

Recently, the usefulness of BOLD MR imaging has been evaluated in patients with systemic sclerosis.[79] The results indicated impaired microcirculation in skeletal muscle even in asymptomatic patients. Further studies on patients with myopathies are needed to fully elucidate the clinical potential of BOLD MR imaging.

Diffusion-Weighted Imaging and Related Methods

Diffusion-weighted imaging (DWI) is a powerful tool to visualize the diffusion of water molecules in skeletal muscle. It allows calculating the

apparent diffusion coefficient (ADC), which is a quantitative marker of diffusion. Diffusion is increased in active inflammation and decreased in the case of fatty degeneration. As a consequence, DWI can be used in the assessment of idiopathic inflammatory myopathies and may serve as a biomarker for disease course and response to treatment.[80,81]

Diffusion tensor imaging (DTI) is a further development of DWI. By measuring the diffusion of water molecules along different gradient directions, the fractional anisotropy and main direction of diffusion can be determined (**Fig. 12**). New developments allow DTI of skeletal muscle within shorter acquisition times and increase its clinical applicability.[82] Potential clinical applications of DTI in patients with myopathies are still under investigation. In patients with polymyositis or dermatomyositis, DTI revealed no significant differences in fractional anisotropy between edematous and normal-appearing muscle

Table 2
Selection of different congenital myopathies with respective distribution patterns of skeletal muscle involvement seen on MR imaging

Congenital Myopathy	Commonly Involved Muscles (Selection)	Relatively Spared Muscles (Selection)
RYR 1-related myopathies	Gluteus maximus, adductor magnus, vasti, semitendinosus, sartorius, soleus, peroneus	Rectus femoris, adductor longus, gracilis, biceps femoris, gastrocnemius, tibialis anterior, tibialis posterior
Selenoprotein 1-related myopathies	Gluteal muscles, sartorius, hamstring, gastrocnemius, sternocleidomastoideus	Rectus femoris, adductor longus, gracilis, soleus, tibialis anterior
Dynamin 2-related myopathies	Gluteus minimus, adductor longus, vastus intermedius, hamstring, soleus, medial gastrocnemius, temporal, lateral pterygoid	Vastus medialis and lateralis, sartorius, gracilis, tibialis posterior, masseter, medial pterygoid
MTM1-related myopathy	Hamstring, adductor magnus, vastus intermedius, vastus medialis	Adductor longus, sartorius, gracilis, rectus femoris, vastus lateralis
Nebulin-related nemaline myopathy	Tibialis anterior, soleus, medial gastrocnemius, lateral pterygoid	Lateral gastrocnemius, peroneus, thigh muscles
ACTA1-related myopathies	Sartorius, adductor magnus, tibialis anterior, tibialis posterior, peroneus	Quadriceps, gastrocnemius

Data from Quijano-Roy S, Carlier RY, Fischer D. Muscle imaging in congenital myopathies. Semin Pediatr Neurol 2011;18(4):221–9.

tissue.[81] In a recent study on patients with Duchenne muscular dystrophy, DTI measures correlated with muscle strength and adiposity and may be able to detect early changes.[83]

Intravoxel incoherent motion imaging (IVIM) is based on the assumption that part of the signal measured on DWIs actually comes from microvascular perfusion ("pseudodiffusion").[84] IVIM allows simultaneous quantification of diffusion and microperfusion. In patients with polymyositis or dermatomyositis, IVIM showed decreased fractional volume of capillary perfusion in inflamed skeletal muscle.[80] IVIM can also detect dynamic changes in perfusion of skeletal muscle[85] and may be a powerful alternative to other methods such as arterial spin labeling or BOLD imaging in the future.

Magnetic Resonance Spectroscopy

Different metabolites in skeletal muscle can be quantified with phosphorous (^{31}P) MR spectroscopy. In addition, this method allows indirect calculation of the intracellular pH.[86–88]

In patients with inflammatory myopathies, ^{31}P MR spectroscopy revealed impaired phosphorous metabolism during exercise, which normalizes after treatment with steroids.[89,90] In patients with Duchenne muscular dystrophy, MR spectroscopy can be applied both to evaluate

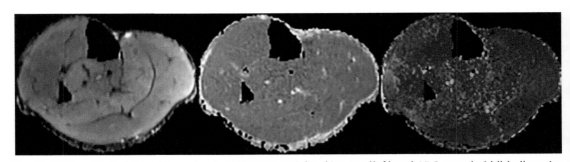

Fig. 12. DWI and DTI of the calf muscles. In DWI, trace-weighted images (*left*) and ADC maps (*middle*) allow visualization and quantification of the diffusion of water molecules in tissue. DTI additionally provides color-coded maps of the main direction of diffusion (*right*).

intramuscular lipid composition[86] and to assess muscle metabolism.[91]

To date, no pathognomonic MR spectroscopy pattern could be found for specific myopathies because all of them eventually lead to fatty degeneration.[88] Nevertheless, MR spectroscopy may be a promising tool in the assessment of potential treatment response.

Magnetic Resonance Elastography

MR elastography induces shear waves, which are propagated through skeletal muscle, which allows quantification of regional tissue elasticity. In patients with active inflammatory myopathies, reduced stiffness was found in the vastus medialis muscle.[92] The usefulness of MR elastography in clinical routine has to be proven yet.

Body Composition Analysis and Profiling

Body composition profiling has been developed as a cloud-based computer-aided solution to determine fat and muscle volume based on whole-body MR imaging scans. Software distinguishes human tissue, mainly fat from muscle and organs, and automatically calculates various quantitative parameters such as visceral adipose tissue, abdominal subcutaneous adipose tissue, and thigh muscle volume. Additional parameters that can be derived are liver fat fraction, lean muscle tissue volume, and total adipose tissue, as well as volumetric data of additional muscle groups, if needed.

These new software solutions could be the basis for characterization and staging of myopathies based on normative values from larger cohorts of healthy subjects.[93–95] Currently, several companies are going on the market with respective solutions.

SUMMARY

MR features in common myopathies are generally nonspecific, but their distribution pattern can be suggestive of specific types and subtypes of disease. Furthermore, MR imaging plays a central role in guiding muscle biopsy, which still remains the gold standard for the diagnosis of myopathy. Advanced MR imaging methods may be able to better differentiate and characterize myopathies in the near future; however, further studies are required in order to better understand their role in clinical practice.

ACKNOWLEDGMENTS

The authors thank Andrea Klein, MD (University Children's Hospital Basel UKBB, Switzerland) and Arne Fischmann, MD (Klinik St. Anna, Lucerne, Switzerland) for their highly valuable support by providing figures of patients with RYR1-related myopathy and muscular dystrophies.

REFERENCES

1. Lenk S, Fischer S, Kotter I, et al. Possibilities of whole-body MRI for investigating musculoskeletal diseases. Radiologe 2004;44(9):844–53 [in German].
2. Schmidt GP, Reiser MF, Baur-Melnyk A. Whole-body imaging of the musculoskeletal system: the value of MR imaging. Skeletal Radiol 2007; 36(12):1109–19.
3. Filli L, Maurer B, Manoliu A, et al. Whole-body MRI in adult inflammatory myopathies: do we need imaging of the trunk? Eur Radiol 2015;25(12):3499–507.
4. Schulze M, Kotter I, Ernemann U, et al. MRI findings in inflammatory muscle diseases and their noninflammatory mimics. AJR Am J Roentgenol 2009; 192(6):1708–16.
5. Garcia J. MRI in inflammatory myopathies. Skeletal Radiol 2000;29(8):425–38.
6. May DA, Disler DG, Jones EA, et al. Abnormal signal intensity in skeletal muscle at MR imaging: patterns, pearls, and pitfalls. Radiographics 2000;20: S295–315.
7. Van De Vlekkert J, Maas M, Hoogendijk JE, et al. Combining MRI and muscle biopsy improves diagnostic accuracy in subacute-onset idiopathic inflammatory myopathy. Muscle Nerve 2015;51(2): 253–8.
8. Del Grande F, Carrino JA, Del Grande M, et al. Magnetic resonance imaging of inflammatory myopathies. Top Magn Reson Imaging 2011;22(2):39–43.
9. Boutry N, Hachulla E, Zanetti-Musielak C, et al. Imaging features of musculoskeletal involvement in systemic sclerosis. Eur Radiol 2007;17(5):1172–80.
10. Schick F. Whole-body MRI at high field: technical limits and clinical potential. Eur Radiol 2005;15(5): 946–59.
11. Sookhoo S, Mackinnon I, Bushby K, et al. MRI for the demonstration of subclinical muscle involvement in muscular dystrophy. Clin Radiol 2007;62(2):160–5.
12. Shelly MJ, Bolster F, Foran P, et al. Whole-body magnetic resonance imaging in skeletal muscle disease. Semin Musculoskelet Radiol 2010;14(1):47–56.
13. Connor A, Stebbings S, Anne Hung N, et al. STIR MRI to direct muscle biopsy in suspected idiopathic inflammatory myopathy. J Clin Rheumatol 2007; 13(6):341–5.
14. Bashir WA, O'Donnell P. The myositides: the role of imaging in diagnosis and treatment. Semin Musculoskelet Radiol 2010;14(2):217–26.
15. Dalakas MC. Inflammatory muscle diseases. N Engl J Med 2015;373(4):393–4.

16. Dobloug C, Garen T, Bitter H, et al. Prevalence and clinical characteristics of adult polymyositis and dermatomyositis; data from a large and unselected Norwegian cohort. Ann Rheum Dis 2015;74(8): 1551–6.

17. O'Connell MJ, Powell T, Brennan D, et al. Whole-body MR imaging in the diagnosis of polymyositis. AJR Am J Roentgenol 2002;179(4):967–71.

18. Schweitzer ME, Fort J. Cost-effectiveness of MR imaging in evaluating polymyositis. AJR Am J Roentgenol 1995;165(6):1469–71.

19. Dion E, Cherin P, Payan C, et al. Magnetic resonance imaging criteria for distinguishing between inclusion body myositis and polymyositis. J Rheumatol 2002;29(9):1897–906.

20. Harris-Love MO, Shrader JA, Koziol D, et al. Distribution and severity of weakness among patients with polymyositis, dermatomyositis and juvenile dermatomyositis. Rheumatology 2009;48(2):134–9.

21. Maurer B, Walker UA. Role of MRI in diagnosis and management of idiopathic inflammatory myopathies. Curr Rheumatol Rep 2015;17(11):67.

22. Tomasova Studynkova J, Charvat F, Jarosova K, et al. The role of MRI in the assessment of polymyositis and dermatomyositis. Rheumatology 2007; 46(7):1174–9.

23. Greenberg SA. Inclusion body myositis. Curr Opin Rheumatol 2011;23(6):574–8.

24. Kissel JT. Misunderstandings, misperceptions, and mistakes in the management of the inflammatory myopathies. Semin Neurol 2002;22(1):41–51.

25. Cox FM, Reijnierse M, van Rijswijk CS, et al. Magnetic resonance imaging of skeletal muscles in sporadic inclusion body myositis. Rheumatology 2011; 50(6):1153–61.

26. Tasca G, Monforte M, De Fino C, et al. Magnetic resonance imaging pattern recognition in sporadic inclusion-body myositis. Muscle Nerve 2015;52(6): 956–62.

27. Badrising UA, Maat-Schieman ML, van Houwelingen JC, et al. Inclusion body myositis. Clinical features and clinical course of the disease in 64 patients. J Neurol 2005;252(12):1448–54.

28. Degardin A, Morillon D, Lacour A, et al. Morphologic imaging in muscular dystrophies and inflammatory myopathies. Skeletal Radiol 2010;39(12):1219–27.

29. Lamminen AE. Magnetic resonance imaging of primary skeletal muscle diseases: patterns of distribution and severity of involvement. Br J Radiol 1990; 63(756):946–50.

30. Amato AA, Sivakumar K, Goyal N, et al. Treatment of sporadic inclusion body myositis with bimagrumab. Neurology 2014;83(24):2239–46.

31. Schanz S, Henes J, Ulmer A, et al. Magnetic resonance imaging findings in patients with systemic scleroderma and musculoskeletal symptoms. Eur Radiol 2013;23(1):212–21.

32. Low AH, Lax M, Johnson SR, et al. Magnetic resonance imaging of the hand in systemic sclerosis. J Rheumatol 2009;36(5):961–4.

33. Finanger EL, Russman B, Forbes SC, et al. Use of skeletal muscle MRI in diagnosis and monitoring disease progression in Duchenne muscular dystrophy. Phys Med Rehabil Clin N Am 2012;23(1): 1–10, ix.

34. Mazzone E, Vasco G, Sormani MP, et al. Functional changes in Duchenne muscular dystrophy: a 12-month longitudinal cohort study. Neurology 2011; 77(3):250–6.

35. Mercuri E, Talim B, Moghadaszadeh B, et al. Clinical and imaging findings in six cases of congenital muscular dystrophy with rigid spine syndrome linked to chromosome 1p (RSMD1). Neuromuscul Disord 2002;12(7–8):631–8.

36. Forbes SC, Willcocks RJ, Triplett WT, et al. Magnetic resonance imaging and spectroscopy assessment of lower extremity skeletal muscles in boys with Duchenne muscular dystrophy: a multicenter cross sectional study. PLoS One 2014;9(9):e106435.

37. Forbes SC, Lott DJ, Finkel RS, et al. MRI/MRS evaluation of a female carrier of Duchenne muscular dystrophy. Neuromuscul Disord 2012;22(Suppl 2): S111–21.

38. Wren TA, Bluml S, Tseng-Ong L, et al. Three-point technique of fat quantification of muscle tissue as a marker of disease progression in Duchenne muscular dystrophy: preliminary study. AJR Am J Roentgenol 2008;190(1):W8–12.

39. Garrood P, Hollingsworth KG, Eagle M, et al. MR imaging in Duchenne muscular dystrophy: quantification of T1-weighted signal, contrast uptake, and the effects of exercise. J Magn Reson Imaging 2009;30(5):1130–8.

40. Fischmann A, Hafner P, Gloor M, et al. Quantitative MRI and loss of free ambulation in Duchenne muscular dystrophy. J Neurol 2013;260(4):969–74.

41. Willcocks RJ, Arpan IA, Forbes SC, et al. Longitudinal measurements of MRI-T2 in boys with Duchenne muscular dystrophy: effects of age and disease progression. Neuromuscul Disord 2014;24(5):393–401.

42. Gaeta M, Messina S, Mileto A, et al. Muscle fat-fraction and mapping in Duchenne muscular dystrophy: evaluation of disease distribution and correlation with clinical assessments. Preliminary experience. Skeletal Radiol 2012;41(8):955–61.

43. Bonati U, Hafner P, Schadelin S, et al. Quantitative muscle MRI: a powerful surrogate outcome measure in Duchenne muscular dystrophy. Neuromuscul Disord 2015;25(9):679–85.

44. Wary C, Azzabou N, Giraudeau C, et al. Quantitative NMRI and NMRS identify augmented disease progression after loss of ambulation in forearms of boys with Duchenne muscular dystrophy. NMR Biomed 2015;28(9):1150–62.

45. Dixon WT. Simple proton spectroscopic imaging. Radiology 1984;153(1):189–94.
46. Filli L, Ulbrich EJ, Guggenberger R, et al. Effect of Gd-DOTA on fat quantification in skeletal muscle using two-point Dixon technique - preliminary data. Eur J Radiol 2016;85(1):131–5.
47. Wokke BH, Bos C, Reijnierse M, et al. Comparison of dixon and T1-weighted MR methods to assess the degree of fat infiltration in Duchenne muscular dystrophy patients. J Magn Reson Imaging 2013; 38(3):619–24.
48. Arpan I, Forbes SC, Lott DJ, et al. T(2) mapping provides multiple approaches for the characterization of muscle involvement in neuromuscular diseases: a cross-sectional study of lower leg muscles in 5-15-year-old boys with Duchenne muscular dystrophy. NMR Biomed 2013;26(3):320–8.
49. Kim HK, Laor T, Horn PS, et al. T2 mapping in Duchenne muscular dystrophy: distribution of disease activity and correlation with clinical assessments. Radiology 2010;255(3):899–908.
50. Marden FA, Connolly AM, Siegel MJ, et al. Compositional analysis of muscle in boys with Duchenne muscular dystrophy using MR imaging. Skeletal Radiol 2005;34(3):140–8.
51. Mathur S, Lott DJ, Senesac C, et al. Age-related differences in lower-limb muscle cross-sectional area and torque production in boys with Duchenne muscular dystrophy. Arch Phys Med Rehabil 2010; 91(7):1051–8.
52. Mavrogeni S, Papavasiliou A, Douskou M, et al. Effect of deflazacort on cardiac and sternocleidomastoid muscles in Duchenne muscular dystrophy: a magnetic resonance imaging study. Eur J paediatric Neurol 2009;13(1):34–40.
53. Arpan I, Willcocks RJ, Forbes SC, et al. Examination of effects of corticosteroids on skeletal muscles of boys with DMD using MRI and MRS. Neurology 2014;83(11):974–80.
54. Willcocks RJ, Rooney WD, Triplett WT, et al. Multicenter prospective longitudinal study of magnetic resonance biomarkers in a large Duchenne muscular dystrophy cohort. Ann Neurol 2016;79(4): 535–47.
55. Polavarapu K, Manjunath M, Preethish-Kumar V, et al. Muscle MRI in Duchenne muscular dystrophy: evidence of a distinctive pattern. Neuromuscul Disord 2016;26(11):768–74.
56. Tasca G, Iannaccone E, Monforte M, et al. Muscle MRI in Becker muscular dystrophy. Neuromuscul Disord 2012;22(Suppl 2):S100–6.
57. Faridian-Aragh N, Wagner KR, Leung DG, et al. Magnetic resonance imaging phenotyping of Becker muscular dystrophy. Muscle Nerve 2014; 50(6):962–7.
58. Fischer D, Hafner P, Rubino D, et al. The 6-minute walk test, motor function measure and quantitative thigh muscle MRI in Becker muscular dystrophy: a cross-sectional study. Neuromuscul Disord 2016; 26(7):414–22.
59. Wagner KR, Fleckenstein JL, Amato AA, et al. A phase I/II trial of MYO-029 in adult subjects with muscular dystrophy. Ann Neurol 2008;63(5):561–71.
60. Mercuri E, Bushby K, Ricci E, et al. Muscle MRI findings in patients with limb girdle muscular dystrophy with calpain 3 deficiency (LGMD2A) and early contractures. Neuromuscul Disord 2005;15(2):164–71.
61. Fischer D, Walter MC, Kesper K, et al. Diagnostic value of muscle MRI in differentiating LGMD2I from other LGMDs. J Neurol 2005;252(5):538–47.
62. Wattjes MP, Kley RA, Fischer D. Neuromuscular imaging in inherited muscle diseases. Eur Radiol 2010;20(10):2447–60.
63. Hicks D, Sarkozy A, Muelas N, et al. A founder mutation in Anoctamin 5 is a major cause of limb-girdle muscular dystrophy. Brain 2011; 134(Pt 1):171–82.
64. Kesper K, Kornblum C, Reimann J, et al. Pattern of skeletal muscle involvement in primary dysferlinopathies: a whole-body 3.0-T magnetic resonance imaging study. Acta Neurol Scand 2009;120(2):111–8.
65. Sarkozy A, Deschauer M, Carlier RY, et al. Muscle MRI findings in limb girdle muscular dystrophy type 2L. Neuromuscul Disord 2012;22(Suppl 2): S122–9.
66. Brummer D, Walter MC, Palmbach M, et al. Long-term MRI and clinical follow-up of symptomatic and presymptomatic carriers of dysferlin gene mutations. Acta Myol 2005;24(1):6–16.
67. Kornblum C, Lutterbey GG, Czermin B, et al. Whole-body high-field MRI shows no skeletal muscle degeneration in young patients with recessive myotonia congenita. Acta Neurol Scand 2010; 121(2):131–5.
68. Day JW, Ricker K, Jacobsen JF, et al. Myotonic dystrophy type 2: molecular, diagnostic and clinical spectrum. Neurology 2003;60(4):657–64.
69. Fleckenstein JL. MRI of neuromuscular disease: the basics. Semin Musculoskelet Radiol 2000;4(4): 393–419.
70. Jungbluth H, Davis MR, Muller C, et al. Magnetic resonance imaging of muscle in congenital myopathies associated with RYR1 mutations. Neuromuscul Disord 2004;14(12):785–90.
71. Klein A, Jungbluth H, Clement E, et al. Muscle magnetic resonance imaging in congenital myopathies due to ryanodine receptor type 1 gene mutations. Arch Neurol 2011;68(9):1171–9.
72. Quijano-Roy S, Carlier RY, Fischer D. Muscle imaging in congenital myopathies. Semin Pediatr Neurol 2011;18(4):221–9.
73. Raynaud JS, Duteil S, Vaughan JT, et al. Determination of skeletal muscle perfusion using arterial spin labeling NMRI: validation by comparison with

venous occlusion plethysmography. Magn Reson Med 2001;46(2):305–11.

74. Andreisek G, White LM, Sussman MS, et al. T2*-weighted and arterial spin labeling MRI of calf muscles in healthy volunteers and patients with chronic exertional compartment syndrome: preliminary experience. AJR Am J Roentgenol 2009;193(4): W327–33.

75. Partovi S, Karimi S, Jacobi B, et al. Clinical implications of skeletal muscle blood-oxygenation-level-dependent (BOLD) MRI. Magma 2012;25(4): 251–61.

76. Ledermann HP, Heidecker HG, Schulte AC, et al. Calf muscles imaged at BOLD MR: correlation with TcPO2 and flowmetry measurements during ischemia and reactive hyperemia–initial experience. Radiology 2006;241(2):477–84.

77. Meyer RA, Towse TF, Reid RW, et al. BOLD MRI mapping of transient hyperemia in skeletal muscle after single contractions. NMR Biomed 2004;17(6): 392–8.

78. Jacobi B, Bongartz G, Partovi S, et al. Skeletal muscle BOLD MRI: from underlying physiological concepts to its usefulness in clinical conditions. J Magn Reson Imaging 2012;35(6):1253–65.

79. Partovi S, Schulte AC, Aschwanden M, et al. Impaired skeletal muscle microcirculation in systemic sclerosis. Arthritis Res Ther 2012;14(5):R209.

80. Qi J, Olsen NJ, Price RR, et al. Diffusion-weighted imaging of inflammatory myopathies: polymyositis and dermatomyositis. J Magn Reson Imaging 2008;27(1):212–7.

81. Ai T, Yu K, Gao L, et al. Diffusion tensor imaging in evaluation of thigh muscles in patients with polymyositis and dermatomyositis. Br J Radiol 2014; 87(1043):20140261.

82. Filli L, Piccirelli M, Kenkel D, et al. Simultaneous multislice echo planar imaging with blipped controlled aliasing in parallel imaging results in higher acceleration: a promising technique for accelerated diffusion tensor imaging of skeletal muscle. Invest Radiol 2015;50(7):456–63.

83. Ponrartana S, Ramos-Platt L, Wren TA, et al. Effectiveness of diffusion tensor imaging in assessing disease severity in Duchenne muscular dystrophy: preliminary study. Pediatr Radiol 2015;45(4):582–9.

84. Le Bihan D, Breton E, Lallemand D, et al. MR imaging of intravoxel incoherent motions: application to diffusion and perfusion in neurologic disorders. Radiology 1986;161(2):401–7.

85. Filli L, Boss A, Wurnig MC, et al. Dynamic intravoxel incoherent motion imaging of skeletal muscle at rest and after exercise. NMR Biomed 2015;28(2):240–6.

86. Torriani M, Townsend E, Thomas BJ, et al. Lower leg muscle involvement in Duchenne muscular dystrophy: an MR imaging and spectroscopy study. Skeletal Radiol 2012;41(4):437–45.

87. Kan HE, Klomp DW, Wong CS, et al. In vivo 31P MRS detection of an alkaline inorganic phosphate pool with short T1 in human resting skeletal muscle. NMR Biomed 2010;23(8):995–1000.

88. Amarteifio E, Nagel AM, Kauczor HU, et al. Functional imaging in muscular diseases. Insights Imaging 2011;2(5):609–19.

89. Okuma H, Kurita D, Ohnuki T, et al. Muscle metabolism in patients with polymyositis simultaneously evaluated by using 31P-magnetic resonance spectroscopy and near-infrared spectroscopy. Int J Clin Pract 2007;61(4):684–9.

90. Park JH, Olsen NJ, King L Jr, et al. Use of magnetic resonance imaging and P-31 magnetic resonance spectroscopy to detect and quantify muscle dysfunction in the amyopathic and myopathic variants of dermatomyositis. Arthritis Rheum 1995; 38(1):68–77.

91. Hsieh TJ, Jaw TS, Chuang HY, et al. Muscle metabolism in Duchenne muscular dystrophy assessed by in vivo proton magnetic resonance spectroscopy. J Comput Assist Tomogr 2009;33(1):150–4.

92. McCullough MB, Domire ZJ, Reed AM, et al. Evaluation of muscles affected by myositis using magnetic resonance elastography. Muscle Nerve 2011; 43(4):585–90.

93. West J, Dahlqvist Leinhard O, Romu T, et al. Feasibility of MR-based body composition analysis in large scale population studies. PLoS One 2016; 11(9):e0163332.

94. Karlsson A, Rosander J, Romu T, et al. Automatic and quantitative assessment of regional muscle volume by multi-atlas segmentation using whole-body water-fat MRI. J Magn Reson Imaging 2015;41(6): 1558–69.

95. Crawford RJ, Filli L, Elliott JM, et al. Age- and level-dependence of fatty infiltration in lumbar paravertebral muscles of healthy volunteers. AJNR Am J Neuroradiol 2016;37(4):742–8.

Imaging of Juvenile Idiopathic Arthritis

Dimitriou Christos, MD[a],*, Boitsios Grammatina, MD[a], Phu-Quoc Lê, MD[b],
Laurence Goffin, MD[b], Badot Valérie, MD, PhD[c], Paolo Simoni, MD, PhD, MBA[a]

KEYWORDS

- Juvenile idiopathic arthritis • Juvenile spondyloarthropathies • Radiography • Ultrasound
- MR imaging • MR imaging scoring system

KEY POINTS

- Multimodal imaging analysis plays a key role in the diagnosis and treatment monitoring of juvenile idiopathic arthritis (JIA).
- A concrete knowledge of normal joint anatomy throughout pediatric age groups is important.
- A reproducible, accurate, and established scoring system for use in international routine clinical care for monitoring and predicting long-term response to therapeutic interventions is still to be developed for any joints on MR imaging.

INTRODUCTION

JIA is an umbrella term covering several distinct categories that share common features.[1]

The term JIA replaced, in the 1990s, the older terms, juvenile rheumatoid arthritis (used commonly in the United States) and juvenile chronic arthritis (preferred in Europe). As defined by the International League of Associations for Rheumatology (ILAR), JIA diagnosis relies on the presence of arthritis that persists for at least 6 weeks, begins before the age of 16 years, and is of unknown origin.[2] The classification, established in Durban in 1997 and revised in Edmonton in 2001, defines different subtypes characterized by their clinical, demographic, and genetic features, translating into different responses to treatment (Box 1).

Modern multimodal imaging, including conventional radiographs (CRs), ultrasound (US), and MR imaging, plays a key role in the diagnosis, follow-up, and treatment monitoring of JIA. Unlike imaging of rheumatoid arthritis and other inflammatory joint conditions in adults, extensively studied in the past 2 decades, the available literature for JIA is more limited, and consensus articles about the role of imaging of the different manifestations of JIA have been published only recently.

The European League Against Rheumatism and the Pediatric Rheumatology European Society have recently published a consensus article with recommendations to guide radiologists and clinicians in choosing the best imaging technique for each particular clinical setting.[3] Specific scoring system for each joint may contribute to make the staging and the follow–up more reproducible.

EPIDEMIOLOGY OF JUVENILE IDIOPATHIC ARTHRITIS

Based on the current classification established by the ILAR in 2001, the incidence of JIA in European children is approximately 3 to 15 individuals per

Disclosure Statement: The authors have nothing to disclose.
[a] Radiology Department, Hôpital Universitaire des Enfants Reine Fabilola, Avenue Jean Joseph Crocq 15, Brussels 1020, Belgium; [b] Pediatric Rheumatology Department, Hôpital Universitaire des Enfants Reine Fabilola, Avenue Jean Joseph Crocq 15, Brussels 1020, Belgium; [c] Service de Rhumatologie et Médecine Physique Rhumatologie Adulte et Pédiatrique, Hôpital Erasme, 808 Route de Lennik, Brussels 1070, Belgium
* Corresponding author.
E-mail address: dchristosd@gmail.com

HLA-B27, other associations have been described for both HLA or non-HLA susceptibility loci with some JIA categories, in particular, *HLA-DRB1:01* and *PTPN22* or *STAT4* variants with oligoarticular or RF-negative polyarticular JIA, shared epitope encoding *HLA-DRB1* with RF-positive polyarticular JIA. Some alleles that predispose to the risk of category might be also protective against another JIA category.[9]

In combination with genetic factors, environmental triggers are also described as involved in the pathogenesis of JIA. Infectious viral or bacterial agents are mainly considered potential triggers. It has been reported an interaction between the immune system and microbiome which may play a role in the autoimmunity or contributing in the development of JIA.[10]

JIA is an immune-mediated disease. In a majority of JIA subset, errors of adaptive immunity (mistakes by antigen-specific T and B cells) initiates an inflammatory response because a defect in normal self-inhibitory mechanisms. Conversely, systemic JIA could be considered an autoinflammatory disorder involving pathways associated with innate immunity. Several cells types, including monocytes/macrophages, T lymphocytes or B lymphocytes, or specific cytokines, such as tumor necrosis factor (TNF)-α, interleukin-6, and interleukin-1, play an important role in the pathophysiology of JIA. Therapeutic advances with biologics agents are known to be efficient for specific categories of JIA, suggesting a specific role of these cells or cytokines in the disease with a different way. Polyarticular and oligoarticular JIA are better responders to TNF-α blocking agents compared with systemic JIA, where anti–IL-6 or anti–IL-1 blocking agent is more efficient. Further insights into the disease pathogenesis will be provided by the continuous advances in understanding of mechanisms related to the immune response and inflammatory process implicated in JIA.

100,000 individuals younger than 16 years.[4] Chronic arthritis seems worldwide in distribution, but the reported incidence and prevalence vary considerably throughout the world. Ethnic differences have been reported to have a significant influence on JIA epidemiology, whites being more affected than African American and Asian individuals.[5,6]

Age at disease onset and gender ratio depends on clinical subset. In most published series of patients with JIA, the female/male ratio is of 2/1 to 3/1, although equal gender ratios have been reported in certain ethnic groups, such as Indian and black South African children.[5] JIA onset occurs at approximately 6 years of age in patients with polyarticular disease in both genders, whereas young patients with oligoarticular disease have a mean age of approximately 4 years in girls and 10 years in boys.[7] Gender has a high influence in determining some features of JIA. As an example, oligoarticular JIA has a female preponderance as high as 8:1 in children younger than 8 years, mainly in a subset of patient with antinuclear antibodies positivity and associated iridocyclitis.[8]

PATHOGENESIS

The etiology and pathogenesis of JIA are unclear but thought to be the result of a combination of genetics and environmental factors. Twin and family studies suggest a role of genetic factors in the predisposition to JIA. Numerous associations between HLA alleles and JIA categories have been reported in multiple populations. Although the juvenile spondyloarthopathies or enthesitis-related arthritis (ERA) is strongly associated with the

CURRENT CLASSIFICATION

1. The most frequent clinical subtype of patients with JIA is oligoarthritis (27%–60%).[4] By definition, the oligoarthritis subtype involves fewer than 4 joints within the 6 months of onset of the disease. It occurs typically in very young girls and is often associated with the presence of antinuclear antibodies. The patients of this subtype are at increased risk of asymptomatic uveitis and should be monitored closely to detect it early. Most patients in this group are first referred for an episode of arthritis of the knee. The second most frequent clinical

presentation in this group of patients is an inflamed ankle (up to 40% of patients). Ankle involvement often occur in girls ages less than age 5 years.[11] Some patients develop a polyarticular involvement after the first 6 months and are considered as having extended oligoarthritis.

2. The subset of patients with a polyarticular presentation (≥5 joints affected within the first 6 months after the onset) and negative rheumatoid factor (RF) accounts for 11% to 28% of all JIA patients.[4,12] In this subgroup, girls are more frequently affected than boys (2:1). Two age peaks can be observed: an early peak between 2 years and 4 years and a later peak between 6 years and 12 years.[4] Small joints are symmetrically involved, but large joints can also be affected in the early stage of the disease.

3. Patients with a polyarticular presentation (≥5 joints affected within the first 6 months after the onset) and positive RF account for only 2% to 7% of all patients with JIA. Girls are more affected than boys.[4] Almost all patients in this group develop bone erosions during the first 5 years after the onset, leading to joint damage. Hand and wrist are typical locations. Uveitis, lung, and aortic involvement are rarely observed in this subgroup of patients.

4. Psoriatic arthritis is a form of JIA found in 2% to 11% of patients with JIA.[4] Arthritis is associated with psoriasis or with a familial history of psoriasis. Dactylitis, nail pitting, and psoriasis are specific features of this subset of patients. In 50% of this subgroup, arthritis occurs before the skin changes, whereas skin and joint are simultaneously affected in only 10% of patients. In patients with psoriatic arthritis, both large and small joints may be involved. At the early stage, the involvement is mostly oligoarticular but a symmetric polyarticular evolution may eventually occur. Sternoclavicular joint inflammation has been reported as typical in these patients.[13]

5. Patients with ERA account for only 3% to 11% of all patients with JIA. It occurs mostly in boy aged more than 10 years, which will develop first peripheral arthritis and entesopathies, and probably evolve to spondylarthritis with axial involvement. They are often HLA-B27 positive. Up to one-third of these patients develop an inflammation of sacroiliac (SI) joints. Patients with fewer than 4 joints involved usually have a better prognosis.

6. Systemic arthritis is the most severe form and refers to Still disease of adults. Arthritis is accompanied by prolonged high fever associated with a typical rash, adenopathies, hepatosplenomegaly, or serositis. This subtype is classified as an autoinflammatory syndrome and has a different pattern of response to biologics. This subtype includes only 4% to 17% of patients with JIA.[4] Life-threatening acute complications can occur as macrophage activation syndrome (5%–10% of cases). Amyloidosis can be observed as a late complication due to chronic uncontrolled inflammation.

7. The undifferentiated subtype includes those patients (11%–21%) who do not match the criteria to be included in the subsets (discussed previously) of patients or who could be included in more than 1 of the previous 6 subtypes.[4]

IMAGING IN JUVENILE IDIOPATHIC ARTHRITIS: GENERAL FEATURES

JIA shares the same imaging findings of inflammatory joint disease in adults, including soft tissue swelling, joint effusion, periarticular osteopenia, erosions, synovitis, and bone edema.

Because of the specific lesions of bone and joints in children, some additional pathologic features can be revealed by imaging in JIA not present in adults, including epiphyseal growth disturbances, premature physeal fusion, limb length inequality, and abarticular periosteal reaction.

Due to the heterogeneity of imaging findings in JIA, there is not a stand-alone imaging modality to asses all the different features of JIA.

CR, US, and MR imaging are the current imaging modalities used in clinical and are analyzed later.

Other techniques, such as PET and scintigraphy, have been proposed in the past but are not currently performed in clinical settings. CT is used but is limited by the high radiation dose (although it might be helpful in the evaluation of facet joints in cervical spine as well cone-beam CT evaluates bony changes in temporomandibular joints [TMJs]).

After the discussion of each imaging modality, recommendations for the use of imaging in JIA are summarized based on expert consensus literature.

Conventional Radiology

CRs in the early stages of JIA are often normal.[14–16] The first radiographic changes consist of soft tissue swelling, joint effusion, periarticular osteopenia, epiphyseal remodeling–widening, periostitis, and osseous overgrowth. A CR of the knee may be the first examination requested by clinicians facing an asymmetric inflammatory swelling.

On CR, persistent inflammation and synovial hypertrophy will result in destruction of epiphyseal cartilage and plate, and the erosive changes after significant cartilage loss will be apparent. Higher prevalence of the bony erosions as also progressive joint destruction[17] is observed[18] in children) with polyarticular than oligoarticular JIA.

Periostitis resulting in an enlarged squared-off appearance more commonly involves phalanges, metacarpal, and metatarsal bones and less frequently any long bone (**Figs. 1–4**).

Carpal crowding and squaring of the carpal bones and "balloon-like" epiphyses of the lower extremities are more observed in JIA.

Periarticular osteopenia is most commonly observed in the systemic subtype and is due to bone hyperemia.

CR also allows visualizing late complications of JIA like ankylosis, joint misalignment, enlarged epiphysis due to bone growth disturbance, premature physeal fusion causing limb length inequality, and spine deformities (**Fig. 5**).

CRs are of limited use in some conditions.

On CR, TMJ involvement may be overlooked. As another example, periarticular swelling is particularly difficult to detect on CR at the level of metacarpal/metacarpophalangeal joints.

Anatomic variations may be misinterpreted as bone erosions on CR, especially in the wrist joint, because of the large number and variation of the vascular channels, cortical irregularities, and recent ossified bones at the level of secondary ossification centers.[19–21]

Periosteal apposition observed on CR also occurs in children, in the bone adjacent to an inflammatory joint. This feature is characteristic in children and is not found in inflammatory chronic diseases of adults, such as rheumatoid arthritis. This finding can be speculated in children because they present a much high bone turnover reconstruction.

Pathologic fractures depending on treatment must be ruled out.[18,22–24]

Severe muscular atrophy can be also observed on CR on the latest stage of the disease as a complication of chronic functional joint impairment.

Recently, Ravelli and Martini[4] adapted the Sharp/van der Heijde system for JIA to evaluate the modification in erosions and joint space narrowing scores.

Ultrasound

US as a cost-effective, easily accessible and non-irradiating modality and plays a significant role in the evaluation of JIA. In addition, US allows a dynamic evaluation and makes easily possible a comparison with the contralateral side without supplementary irradiation.

US evaluates the presence of synovial thickening, synovitis, joint effusion, tenosynovitis, enthesitis and bone erosions (**Fig. 6**).[25] Synovial thickening and synovitis can be seen during the ultrasonographic examination as a solid, non-compressible, abnormally hypoechoic tissue associated with joint lines or surrounding tendons.

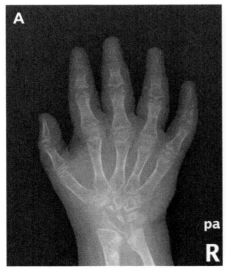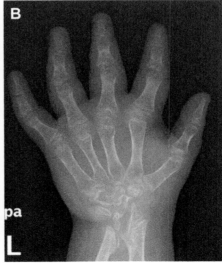

Fig. 1. (*A, B*) CRs of the hand of a young girl with severe periarticular osteopenia, diffuse space loss with erosions, and bony destructions. Epiphyseal remodeling carpal crowding and squaring of the carpal bones is a characteristic feature of chronic JIA due to periostitis.

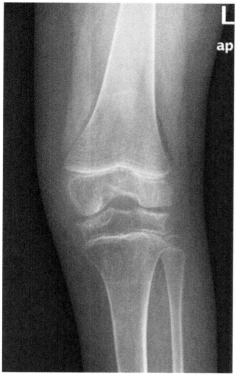

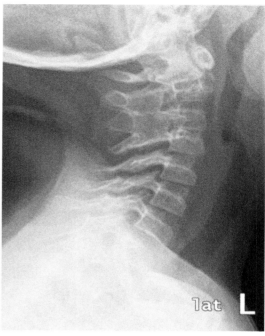

Fig. 4. Ankylosis of the posterior elements of C2-C4 visible in the lateral view radiograph of the cervical spine in a young child with JIA.

Fig. 2. Epiphyseal remodeling and marked periarticular osteopenia on an anteroposterior knee CR of a young child with JIA.

In young children, where synovial tissue may be difficult to distinguish from adjacent hypoechoic epiphyseal cartilage, evaluation of the synovium is difficult. A better visualization of the synovial

thickening when associated with a similar echogenicity of joint effusion is acquired after a bit of pressure through the transducer, which displaces the effusion. Color and power Doppler US techniques show a superiority to gray-scale US in observing active disease. Doppler US analyzes synovial blood flow, suggestive of active disease. A potential pitfall can be the physiologically synovial vascularization of the in healthy children.[26,27]

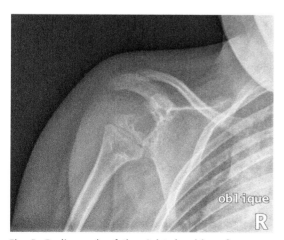

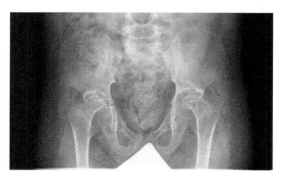

Fig. 3. Radiograph of the right shoulder of a young girl with chronic features of JIA, such as the pronounced epiphyseal remodeling–widening, severe bony destruction of epiphyseal cartilage, and periarticular osteopenia.

Fig. 5. Chronic radiographic changes of JIA. Radiograph of the pelvis in a child with long-lasting JIA, showing the bilateral hip joint chronic changes with severe bony destruction and marked epiphyseal remodeling. Bilateral widening of SI joints suggesting their involvement.

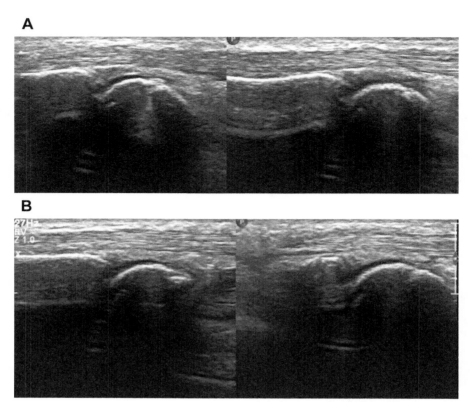

Fig. 6. (*A, B*) Mode B US of the right knee of a 6-year-old girl showing a bony erosion on the distal epiphysis of the tibia. Comparative image with the left nonaffected knee is seen on the right picture.

A joint effusion is described as an abnormal intra-articular finding, which is hypoechoic or anechoic (relative to subdermal fat) or in some cases isoechoic or hyperechoic, intra-articular material that is displaceable and compressible but does not exhibit Doppler signal. Physiologic fluid is common in children, and differentiation between normal amounts of joint fluid from a joint effusion is sometimes subtle.[28]

Epiphyseal cartilage shows a relative hypoechogenicity and it might be misinterpreted as a joint effusion in unexperienced pediatric ultrasonographers.

Tenosynovitis can be demonstrated as anechoic or hypoechoic thickened tissue with or without fluid in the tendon sheath, which may show Doppler signal and it must be observed in 2 orthogonal planes to eliminate the possible artifact of anisotropy. Tenosynovitis in children is most frequently seen along the extensor tendons of the wrist and along the ankle joint.[29]

Enthesitis is observed as an abnormally hypoechoic or thickened tendon or ligament, associated with a loss of the expected fibrillary architecture, at the tendinous or ligamentous insertion at its bony attachment that is seen in 2 perpendicular planes. This finding may contain foci of calcification and

may show abnormal Doppler signal or bony modifications like enthesophytes, erosions, or cortical irregularities, even though these associated findings are seen less commonly in children. US is found to have a high false-negative rate in detection of subtalar disease.[30,31]

A bone erosion is defined as a discontinuity of the bony cortex visible in 2 orthogonal planes. Identifying an erosive change in a child is challenging, because there are physiologic irregularities in recently ossified bone that can be mistaken as cortical erosions.[6]

The reliability of US in detecting bone erosion compared with CR has not been made in JIA although these techniques are considered equivalent in large meta-analysis performed in adult patients of rheumatoid arthritis.

US evaluates epiphyseal cartilage integrity and detect cartilage erosion and thinning as obliteration and blurring of the normally well-defined margins of its surface. Epiphyseal cartilage changes from anechoic to hypoechogenic and thickens with maturation. A recent study established the age-related and gender-related normal reference standards for cartilage thickness of the knee, ankle, wrist, and metacarpophalangeal and proximal interphalangeal joints for children between the ages of 7 years and 16 years. This work was further evaluated by showing good agreement between MR imaging and US for the measurement of cartilage thickness in healthy children. JIA patients has a thinner cartilage when compared with age-matched and gender-matched controls, although interestingly this finding is observed in both clinically affected and nonaffected joints.

US as a more sensitive diagnostic tool than clinical examination differentiates synovitis from tenosynovitis with evident classification and therapeutic implication.[29,32–34] Additionally, subclinical enthesitis can be detected by Doppler US.[35]

The differentiation between joint effusion (and its modification in volume) with inflamed synovium (and its size and distribution changes) is useful for monitoring the disease.[30,36–39]

Color Doppler also evaluates/differentiates the degree of disease activity by the assessment of synovial vascularity.[18]

Contrast-enhanced US has been shown to improve detection and evaluation of the synovial vascularity.[40–42]

A special help of US imaging is the possibility of guiding precisely the joint aspiration or injection of anti-inflammatory agents. Thus avoid complications of extra-articular diffusion of these agents (eg, soft tissues calcifications).

Ultrasound Limitations

To be able to perform the correct diagnosis, an ultrasonographer should be familiar with the changes occurring in a healthy developing joint; for example, modification of the thickness of epiphyseal cartilage should be compared with a healthy child of the same gender and age.[43,44]

Another limitation of US, Color Doppler, CEUS is the non-documentation by research of the normal appearance of the entheses and tendons changes of the developing skeleton through age and sex which is essential to compare to patients with JIA.[45,46]

Notwithstanding the inherent limitation of US, namely the low inter and intra observer reproducibility in evaluations the synovial thickening as a semi quantitative score was proposed for JIA, but it has not been validated yet.[47]

Evaluation of bone marrow edema, TMJ, and SI joints and active subtalar disease is limited by US.[24,30,31]

MR Imaging

MR imaging examination accesses and evaluates the inflammatory process in regions where US cannot reach.

The standard MR imaging protocol includes a T1 spin-echo (SE) sequence, T2 fat-suppressed sequence or short tau inversion recovery (STIR), and T1 fat-suppressed sequence precontrast and postcontrast. The DIXON fat-suppression sequence is being used more frequent than STIR as it allows a very good evaluation of the joint and with a better signal-to-noise ratio.[48]

MR imaging is the only modality that allows the study of all relevant structures in JIA.

The joint can be easily examined in all possible plans with the multiplanar reconstructions and, with its excellent contrast resolution of bone and soft tissues, it is considered the most sensitive imaging technique when contrast-enhanced sequences are performed for detecting synovitis[43] (Figs. 7–9).

MR imaging is the only modality which can objective bone marrow edema (so called in the case pre-erosive osteitis)[49–51] (Fig. 10), which is probably a possible predictor of future erosions in adults.

Bone marrow edema (especially when it involves the epiphysis, when it is located in the areas of synovial reflection, and when it is more diffused) is an indication for treatment to avoid permanent joint destruction.[43] Longitudinal studies need to be done and distinguish the bone marrow edema seen in healthy children compared to the bone marrow edema which is going to evolve to erosions in JIA patients.[26,51]

MR imaging is a more sensitive modality which it allows to detects double the number of erosions at the wrist and even more at the SI joint.[45,52] Detection of erosions is also done earlier and with more confidence than US or radiographic examinations.[45]

Weirdly these late complications of a prolonged JIA pathology do occur in chronic recurrent multifocal osteomyelitis where inflammatory modifications are observed around the metaphysis and growing cartilage.

Cartilage and bone damages also are seen and evaluated by MR imaging.

MR Imaging Limitations

An important limitation of MR imaging is the need for sedation for children younger than 4 years to 6 years old for a correct examination. The low availability and the high costs of this examination should also be taken in consideration. During one MR imaging examination, just 1 joint can be examined with all the requested sequences (contrast-enhanced sequences that raise the potential for allergic reaction and stressful conditions for the children). As in all the other imaging modalities,

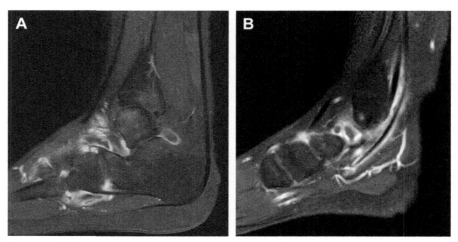

Fig. 7. (A, B) Sagittal T1 fat-suppressed sequence after contrast enhancement of an ankle with a long-standing arthritis showing on the left picture an inhomogeneous, patchy synovial enhancement indicating fibrotic and active synovitis and, on the right, tenosynovitis of the tibias posterior and flexor digitorum tendon.

MR imaging is limited in distinguishing the normal findings in a developing joint from pathology.

CURRENT OPINIONS ON IMAGING ROLE IN CLINICAL MANAGEMENT OF JUVENILE IDIOPATHIC ARTHRITIS: AN UPDATE

Many efforts have been made by several groups worldwide to improve MR imaging of JIA.

In JIA, TMJ joint inflammation is detected mostly by MR imaging with contrast medium injection. Patients younger than 4 years old are at higher risk developing TMJ lesions.[53,54] Active inflammation of TMJ is characterized by joint effusion, synovial enhancement, and bone marrow edema. Guidance treatment is usually done by CT of fluoroscopy but some studies have been conducted using MR imaging.[55,56]

The TMJ joint monitoring damages are better done by MR imaging than US because MR imaging detects 25% of lesions whereas US detect only 17%.[53] MR imaging with gadolinium is superior in detecting TMJ inflammation than US (35.7% vs 86.7%, respectively).[57] The joints that are preferentially damaged in the earlier and in the late changes are the wrist and the hip.

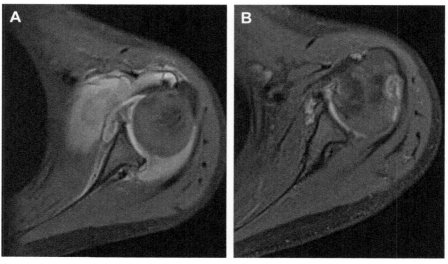

Fig. 8. (A, B) Synovial enhancement, joint effusion, marginal and central erosions, and bone marrow edema are seen at the images of a child with JIA on these MR imaging axial plane images acquired with STIR sequence and T1 fat-suppressed sequence with contrast.

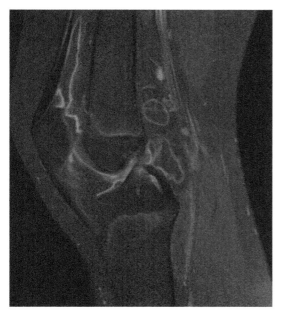

Fig. 9. Sagittal T1 SE fat-suppressed with contrast enhancement of a 15-year-old boy knee shows synovial enhancement evocative of synovitis of the anterior and the posterior compartment.

Cervical Spine

Cervical spine MR imaging is more useful than 2clinical examination in the detection of joint damage.[58] According to Tzaribachev and colleagues,[59] although only 20% of patients

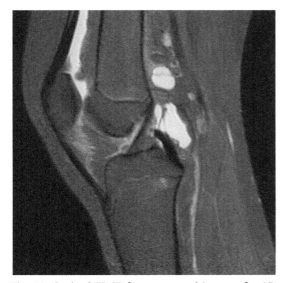

Fig. 10. Sagittal T2 SE fat-suppressed image of a 15-year-old boy knee reveals joint effusion with synovial thickening. Hoffa fat its infiltrated and bone marrow edema is slightly visible in the proximal metaphysis of the tibia.

presented clinical symptoms, such as pain or movement limitation, 87% of the MR imaging examinations showed abnormalities, which suggests that cervical spine involvement is usually silent.

Sacroiliac Joint

SI joint inflammation is seen in 30% of patients with the ERA subtype of JIA, especially men with a later age onset of the disease, acute anterior uveitis, and bone marrow edema, all of which indicate active inflammation of the disease. SI joint inflammation is detected better by MR imaging than clinical examination[60,61]; 5 years to 10 years after the onset of symptoms, SI joint abnormalities can be seen.[52,62] MR imaging detects 80% of acute inflammation damages whereas CR cannot.[63]

The evaluation of disease activity and differentiation of active synovitis to fibrotic changes is done by the aspect and characteristics of synovial enhancement. Dynamic contrast-enhanced (DCE) MR imaging sequences and the quantification of permeability values could be supportive tools in treatment decisions and disease management.[64–66] A pixel-by-pixel DCE–MR imaging time intensity curves analysis method can distinguish clinically active disease with asymptomatic patients. Recent studies showed that DCE MR analysis correlate well with the rheumatoid arthritis MR imaging scoring system.[67,68]

T2 relaxation time mapping as a recent MR imaging technique gives more information about the joint cartilage.

The pathological changes induced by JIA such as an increased permeability of the cartilage matrix, increased water content, water distribution in inflammatory tissues, results in a higher T1 and T2 relaxation times. These early changes after inflammatory process of JIA can evaluate the microstructural and reversible modification of the cartilage, allowing an early and more aggressive plan of treatment.[69,70]

In addition to a contrast-enhanced acquisitions, diffusion-weighted imaging could be helpful in differentiating synovitis for joint effusion.[71]

Whole-body MR imaging evaluates not only the activity but also the extent of the disease in the same examination (**Fig. 11**).

What is needed for a precise monitoring and treatment response is a standard validated and feasible scoring system for the use of MR imaging in JIA (even for knee arthritis[27,72,73]). The existing Juvenile Arthritis MRI Scoring system which assesses the synovial enhancement can differentiate JIA patients from asymptomatic control at group level, but needs extra adaptions to distinguish synovitis to synovial enhancement in unaffected

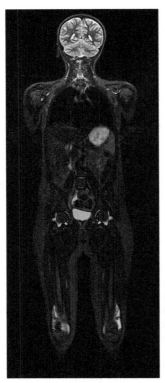

Fig. 11. Whole-body MR imaging, STIR sequence in the coronal plane demonstrates joint effusion in the both shoulders, hips, and knees. Synovial thickening is also seen in both knees. The shoulders and hips involvement in the disease was revealed by imaging and not by the clinical examination.

children. A potential pitfall, mild enhancement of synovium in asymptomatic children, can eventually be eliminated with the standardized acquisition of contrast.

New studies have showed that the diagnosis and synovitis grading by contrast enhancement are influenced by time of postcontrast acquisition used for the grading, a reason why an MR imaging scoring system should be based on a standardized protocol of 1 joint at a time with a standard interval between intravenous contrast injection and postcontrast acquisition.[71]

For differentiation of synovial enhancement an improved MRI scoring with a standardize protocol for MRI acquisition and a consensus on imaging interpretation is still needed to further establish MRI as an accurate monitoring tool for JIA disease activity.

For the wrist, there are already some proposed MR imaging scoring systems,[43] but they are not yet clinically accepted.

Nusman and colleagues[74] proposed an MR imaging protocol of the wrist after the recommendations from the Outcome Measures in Rheumatology Clinical Trials (OMERACT) MR imaging in JIA Working Group and the Health-e-Child project.[75]

ROLE IN PROGNOSIS AND MONITORING

In JIA, CR is useful for predicting further joint damage. In terms of prognosis, persistent inflammation on US or MR imaging is a prediction of subsequent joint damage. CR is useful for the prediction of progression: at 5 years with a wrist CR baseline with a Sharp/van der Heijde score greater than 1, patients with erosions and joint space narrowing in the first 6 months of the study spent more time with clinically active disease and were less likely to achieve clinical remission or medication.[74]

US and MR imaging are useful in monitoring disease activity. MR imaging is superior in detecting knee inflammation than US.[36,76,77] They also are better making the differential diagnosis between pannus and effusion.

ROLE IN TREATMENT AND REMISSION

The treatment guidance of intra-articular injection is usually done by US. US allows accurate assessment of the needle placement during intra-articular injection of medication.[78] According to Parra and colleagues,[56] verified by CT an accurate intra articular placement of the needle under US guidance in 91% of patients. According to Sauremann and colleagues,[79] TMJ injections guided by MR imaging confirmed that 65% of injections were accurately placed. A similar study confirmed that 100% of injections were accurate in the treatment of SI joints.[80]

US and MR imaging are useful in the follow up of asymptomatic patients during remission periods to rule out subclinical inflammation. Synovitis is seen in US B mode in patients with clinical remission in up to 84.1% of joints and power Doppler activity in up to 48.6% of joints.[40]

Examination of clinically inactive joints can reveal on MR imaging a knee inflammation in 50% of patients and bone marrow edema in 33.3%.[81,82]

In recent studies, asymptomatic patients with a positive MRI and signs of inflammation at US are more likely to develop an active disease or show a disease progression at 6-month follow–up.[82]

SUMMARY

Multimodal imaging contributes to diagnosis and treatment monitoring of JIA.

The importance of an early diagnosis and adjustment of the treatment are critical to avoid joint deformities and ankylosis.

A thorough knowledge of normal joint anatomy throughout pediatric age groups is important. Based to this knowledge, an imaging scoring system could be created, as it exists for adults suffering from RA. An imaging scoring systems could be created that can be used as a powerful tool in clinical trials for new therapies monitoring. Standard MR imaging protocols and scoring systems should be validated in the near future for a reliable evaluation of drug effects and clinical course in clinical trials. In addition these protocols and scoring systems should be tailored for each joint.

REFERENCES

1. Prakken B, Albani S, Martini A. Juvenile idiopathic arthritis. Lancet 2011;377(9783):2138–49.
2. Sheybani EF, Khanna G, White AJ, et al. Imaging of juvenile idiopathic arthritis: a multimodality approach. Radiographics 2013;33(5):1253–73.
3. Colebatch-Bourn AN, Edwards CJ, Collado P, et al. EULAR-PReS points to consider for the use of imaging in the diagnosis and management of juvenile idiopathic arthritis in clinical practice. Ann Rheum Dis 2015;74(11):1946–57.
4. Ravelli A, Martini A. Juvenile idiopathic arthritis. Lancet 2007;369(9563):767–78.
5. Haffejee IE, Raga J, Coovadia HM. Juvenile chronic arthritis in black and Indian South African children. S Afr Med J 1984;65(13):510–4.
6. Lawrence RC, Helmick CG, Arnett FC, et al. Estimates of the prevalence of arthritis and selected musculoskeletal disorders in the United States. Arthritis Rheum 1998;41(5):778–99.
7. Schaller JG. Juvenile rheumatoid arthritis: Series 1. Arthritis Rheum 1977;20(2 Suppl):165–70.
8. Cassidy JT, Sullivan DB, Petty RE. Clinical patterns of chronic iridocyclitis in children with juvenile rheumatoid arthritis. Arthritis Rheum 1977;20(2 Suppl):224–7.
9. Hersh AO, Prahalad S. Immunogenetics of juvenile idiopathic arthritis: a comprehensive review. J Autoimmun 2015;64:113–24.
10. Verwoerd A, Ter Haar NM, de Roock S, et al. The human microbiome and juvenile idiopathic arthritis. Pediatr Rheumatol Online J 2016;14(1):55.
11. Davidson J. Juvenile idiopathic arthritis: a clinical overview. Eur J Radiol 2000;33(2):128–34.
12. Ravelli A, Martini A. Early predictors of outcome in juvenile idiopathic arthritis. Clin Exp Rheumatol 2003;21(5 Suppl 31):S89–93.
13. Sudoł-Szopińska I, Matuszewska G, Gietka P, et al. Imaging of juvenile idiopathic arthritis. Part I: clinical classifications and radiographs. J Ultrason 2016; 16(66):225–36.
14. Johnson K, Gardner-Medwin J. Childhood arthritis: classification and radiology. Clin Radiol 2002;57(1): 47–58.
15. Pettersson H, Rydholm U. Radiologic classification of knee joint destruction in juvenile chronic arthritis. Pediatr Radiol 1984;14(6):419–21.
16. Ansell BM, Kent PA. Radiological changes in juvenile chronic polyarthritis. Skeletal Radiol 1977;1(3):129–44.
17. Mason T, Reed AM, Nelson AM, et al. Frequency of abnormal hand and wrist radiographs at time of diagnosis of polyarticular juvenile rheumatoid arthritis. J Rheumatol 2002;29(10):2214–8.
18. Johnson K. Imaging of juvenile idiopathic arthritis. Pediatr Radiol 2006;36(8):743–58.
19. Avenarius DM, Ording Müller LS, Eldevik P, et al. The paediatric wrist revisited—findings of bony depressions in healthy children on radiographs compared to MRI. Pediatr Radiol 2012;42(7):791–8.
20. Rossi F, Di Dia F, Galipò O, et al. Use of the sharp and larsen scoring methods in the assessment of radiographic progression in juvenile idiopathic arthritis. Arthritis Care Res 2006;55(5):717–23.
21. Poznanski AK, Hernandez RJ, Guire KE, et al. Carpal length in children—a useful measurement in the diagnosis of rheumatoid arthritis and some congenital malformation syndromes. Radiology 1978;129(3):661–8.
22. Restrepo R, Lee EY. Epidemiology, pathogenesis, and imaging of arthritis in children. Orthop Clin North Am 2012;43(2):213–25, vi.
23. Azouz EM. Juvenile idiopathic arthritis: how can the radiologist help the clinician? Pediatr Radiol 2008; 38(Suppl 3):S403–8.
24. Cohen PA, Job-Deslandre CH, Lalande G, et al. Overview of the radiology of juvenile idiopathic arthritis (JIA). Eur J Radiol 2000;33(2):94–101.
25. Grassi W, Filippucci E, Farina A, et al. Ultrasonography in the evaluation of bone erosions. Ann Rheum Dis 2001;60(2):98–103.
26. Magni-Manzoni S, Malattia C, Lanni S, et al. Advances and challenges in imaging in juvenile idiopathic arthritis. Nat Rev Rheumatol 2012;8(6): 329–36.
27. Nusman CM, Ording Muller L-S, Hemke R, et al. Current Status of efforts on standardizing magnetic resonance imaging of juvenile idiopathic arthritis: report from the OMERACT MRI in JIA working group and health-e-child. J Rheumatol 2016;43(1):239–44.
28. Moroldo MB, Tague BL, Shear ES, et al. Juvenile rheumatoid arthritis in affected sibpairs. Arthritis Rheum 1997;40(11):1962–6.
29. Fujikawa S, Okuni M. Clinical analysis of 570 cases with juvenile rheumatoid arthritis: results of a nationwide retrospective survey in Japan. Acta Paediatr Jpn 1997;39(2):245–9.
30. Petty RE, Southwood TR, Manners P, et al. International League of Associations for Rheumatology

classification of juvenile idiopathic arthritis: second revision, Edmonton, 2001. J Rheumatol 2004;31(2):390–2.

31. Janow GL, Panghaal V, Trinh A, et al. Detection of active disease in juvenile idiopathic arthritis: sensitivity and specificity of the physical examination vs ultrasound. J Rheumatol 2011;38(12):2671–4.

32. Pascoli L, Wright S, McAllister C, et al. Prospective evaluation of clinical and ultrasound findings in ankle disease in juvenile idiopathic arthritis: importance of ankle ultrasound. J Rheumatol 2010;37(11):2409–14.

33. Rooney ME, McAllister C, Burns JFT. Ankle disease in juvenile idiopathic arthritis: ultrasound findings in clinically swollen ankles. J Rheumatol 2009;36(8):1725–9.

34. Laurell L, Court-Payen M, Nielsen S, et al. Ultrasonography and color doppler in juvenile idiopathic arthritis: diagnosis and follow-up of ultrasound-guided steroid injection in the wrist region. A descriptive interventional study. Pediatr Rheumatol Online J 2012;10:11.

35. Jousse-Joulin S, Breton S, Cangemi C, et al. Ultrasonography for detecting enthesitis in juvenile idiopathic arthritis. Arthritis Care Res 2011;63(6):849–55.

36. El-Miedany YM, Housny IH, Mansour HM, et al. Ultrasound versus MRI in the evaluation of juvenile idiopathic arthritis of the knee. Joint Bone Spine 2001;68(3):222–30.

37. Sureda D, Quiroga S, Arnal C, et al. Juvenile rheumatoid arthritis of the knee: evaluation with US. Radiology 1994;190(2):403–6.

38. Fedrizzi MS, Ronchezel MV, Hilario MO, et al. Ultrasonography in the early diagnosis of hip joint involvement in juvenile rheumatoid arthritis. J Rheumatol 1997;24(9):1820–5.

39. Cellerini M, Salti S, Trapani S, et al. Correlation between clinical and ultrasound assessment of the knee in children with mono-articular or pauci-articular juvenile rheumatoid arthritis. Pediatr Radiol 1999;29(2):117–23.

40. Doria AS, Kiss MH, Lotito AP, et al. Juvenile rheumatoid arthritis of the knee: evaluation with contrast-enhanced color doppler ultrasound. Pediatr Radiol 2001;31(7):524–31.

41. Newman JS, Laing TJ, McCarthy CJ, et al. Power Doppler sonography of synovitis: assessment of therapeutic response–preliminary observations. Radiology 1996;198(2):582–4.

42. Mouterde G, Carotti M, D'Agostino MA. Échographie de contraste et pathologie ostéo-articulaire. J Radiol 2009;90(1, Part 2):148–55.

43. Damasio MB, Malattia C, Martini A, et al. Synovial and inflammatory diseases in childhood: role of new imaging modalities in the assessment of patients with juvenile idiopathic arthritis. Pediatr Radiol 2010;40(6):985–98.

44. Chauvin NA, Ho-Fung V, Jaramillo D, et al. Ultrasound of the joints and entheses in healthy children. Pediatr Radiol 2015;45(9):1344–54.

45. Malattia C, Damasio MB, Magnaguagno F, et al. Magnetic resonance imaging, ultrasonography, and conventional radiography in the assessment of bone erosions in juvenile idiopathic arthritis. Arthritis Rheum 2008;59(12):1764–72.

46. Larché MJ, Roth J. Toward standardized ultrasound measurements of cartilage thickness in children. J Rheumatol 2010;37(12):2445–7.

47. Mandl P, Naredo E, Wakefield RJ, et al. A systematic literature review analysis of ultrasound joint count and scoring systems to assess synovitis in rheumatoid arthritis according to the OMERACT Filter. J Rheumatol 2011;38(9):2055–62.

48. Del Grande F, Santini F, Herzka DA, et al. Fat-suppression techniques for 3-T MR imaging of the musculoskeletal system. Radiographics 2014;34(1):217–33.

49. McQueen FM, Benton N, Perry D, et al. Bone edema scored on magnetic resonance imaging scans of the dominant carpus at presentation predicts radiographic joint damage of the hands and feet six years later in patients with rheumatoid arthritis. Arthritis Rheum 2003;48(7):1814–27.

50. Ording Muller L-S, Humphries P, Rosendahl K. The joints in juvenile idiopathic arthritis. Insights Imaging 2015;6(3):275–84.

51. Müller LS, Avenarius D, Damasio B, et al. The paediatric wrist revisited: redefining MR findings in healthy children. Ann Rheum Dis 2011;70(4):605–10.

52. Bollow M, Braun J, Biedermann T, et al. Use of contrast-enhanced MR imaging to detect sacroiliitis in children. Skeletal Radiol 1998;27(11):606–16.

53. Müller L, Kellenberger CJ, Cannizzaro E, et al. Early diagnosis of temporomandibular joint involvement in juvenile idiopathic arthritis: a pilot study comparing clinical examination and ultrasound to magnetic resonance imaging. Rheumatology (Oxford) 2009;48(6):680–5.

54. Argyropoulou MI, Margariti PN, Karali A, et al. Temporomandibular joint involvement in juvenile idiopathic arthritis: clinical predictors of magnetic resonance imaging signs. Eur Radiol 2009;19(3):693–700.

55. Fritz J, Thomas C, Tzaribachev N, et al. MRI-guided injection procedures of the temporomandibular joints in children and adults: technique, accuracy, and safety. AJR Am J Roentgenol 2009;193(4):1148–54.

56. Parra DA, Chan M, Krishnamurthy G, et al. Use and accuracy of US guidance for image-guided injections of the temporomandibular joints in children with arthritis. Pediatr Radiol 2010;40(9):1498–504.

57. Küseler A, Pedersen TK, Herlin T, et al. Contrast enhanced magnetic resonance imaging as a method to diagnose early inflammatory changes in

the temporomandibular joint in children with juvenile chronic arthritis. J Rheumatol 1998;25(7):1406–12.

58. Oren B, Oren H, Osma E, et al. Juvenile rheumatoid arthritis: cervical spine involvement and MRI in early diagnosis. Turk J Pediatr 1996;38(2):189–94.

59. Tzaribachev N, Tzaribachev C, Koos B. High Prevalence of Cervical Spine and Temporomandibular Joint Involvement in Patients with Juvenile Idiopathic Arthritis. [abstract]. Arthritis Rheum 2012;2012:2026.

60. Lin C, MacKenzie JD, Courtier JL, et al. Magnetic resonance imaging findings in juvenile spondyloarthropathy and effects of treatment observed on subsequent imaging. Pediatr Rheumatol Online J 2014;12:25.

61. Burgos-Vargas R, Vázquez-Mellado J, Cassis N, et al. Genuine ankylosing spondylitis in children: a case-control study of patients with early definite disease according to adult onset criteria. J Rheumatol 1996;23(12):2140–7.

62. Bollow M, Braun J, Hamm B, et al. Early sacroiliitis in patients with spondyloarthropathy: evaluation with dynamic gadolinium-enhanced MR imaging. Radiology 1995;194(2):529–36.

63. Pagnini I, Savelli S, Matucci-Cerinic M, et al. Early predictors of juvenile sacroiliitis in enthesitis-related arthritis. J Rheumatol 2010;37(11):2395–401.

64. Graham TB, Laor T, Dardzinski BJ. Quantitative magnetic resonance imaging of the hands and wrists of children with juvenile rheumatoid arthritis. J Rheumatol 2005;32(9):1811–20.

65. Malattia C, Damasio MB, Basso C, et al. Dynamic contrast-enhanced magnetic resonance imaging in the assessment of disease activity in patients with juvenile idiopathic arthritis. Rheumatology (Oxford) 2010;49(1):178–85.

66. Workie DW, Dardzinski BJ, Graham TB, et al. Quantification of dynamic contrast-enhanced MR imaging of the knee in children with juvenile rheumatoid arthritis based on pharmacokinetic modeling. Magn Reson Imaging 2004;22(9):1201–10.

67. Boesen M, Kubassova O, Bouert R, et al. Correlation between computer-aided dynamic gadolinium-enhanced MRI assessment of inflammation and semi-quantitative synovitis and bone marrow oedema scores of the wrist in patients with rheumatoid arthritis—a cohort study. Rheumatology 2012;51(1):134–43.

68. Orguc S, Tikiz C, Aslanalp Z, et al. Comparison of OMERACT-RAMRIS scores and computer-aided dynamic magnetic resonance imaging findings of hand and wrist as a measure of activity in rheumatoid arthritis. Rheumatol Int 2013;33(7):1837–44.

69. Kim HK, Laor T, Graham TB, et al. T2 relaxation time changes in distal femoral articular cartilage in children with juvenile idiopathic arthritis: a 3-year longitudinal study. AJR Am J Roentgenol 2010;195(4):1021–5.

70. Kight AC, Dardzinski BJ, Laor T, et al. Magnetic resonance imaging evaluation of the effects of juvenile rheumatoid arthritis on distal femoral weight-bearing cartilage. Arthritis Rheum 2004;50(3):901–5.

71. Barendregt AM, Nusman CM, Hemke R, et al. Feasibility of diffusion-weighted magnetic resonance imaging in patients with juvenile idiopathic arthritis on 1.0-T open-bore MRI. Skeletal Radiol 2015;44(12):1805–11.

72. Hemke R, van Rossum MA, van Veenendaal M, et al. Reliability and responsiveness of the Juvenile Arthritis MRI Scoring (JAMRIS) system for the knee. Eur Radiol 2013;23(4):1075–83.

73. Rieter JF, de Horatio LT, Nusman CM, et al. The many shades of enhancement: timing of post-gadolinium images strongly influences the scoring of juvenile idiopathic arthritis wrist involvement on MRI. Pediatr Radiol 2016;46(11):1562–7.

74. Nusman CM, Rosendahl K, Maas M. MRI protocol for the assessment of juvenile idiopathic arthritis of the wrist: recommendations from the OMERACT MRI in JIA working group and health-e-child. J Rheumatol 2016;43(6):1257–8.

75. Ringold S, Seidel KD, Koepsell TD, et al. Inactive disease in polyarticular juvenile idiopathic arthritis: current patterns and associations. Rheumatology (Oxford) 2009;48(8):972–7.

76. Eich GF, Hallé F, Hodler J, et al. Juvenile chronic arthritis: Imaging of the knees and hips before and after intraarticular steroid injection. Pediatr Radiol 1994;24(8):558–63.

77. Pascoli L, Napier NJ, Wray M, et al. THU0318 A prospective comparative study of three methods of assessment of the knee joint in juvenile idiopathic arthritis: clinical examination, ultrasound and MRI. (a newly developed knee MRI scoring system). Ann Rheum Dis 2013;71(Suppl 3):263.

78. Young CM, Shiels WE, Coley BD, et al. Ultrasound-guided corticosteroid injection therapy for juvenile idiopathic arthritis: 12-year care experience. Pediatr Radiol 2012;42(12):1481–9.

79. 2015 ACR/ARHP annual meeting abstract supplement. Arthritis Rheumatol 2015;67(Suppl 10):1–4046. http://dx.doi.org/10.1002/art.39448.

80. Fritz J, Tzaribachev N, Thomas C, et al. Evaluation of MR imaging guided steroid injection of the sacroiliac joints for the treatment of children with refractory enthesitis-related arthritis. Eur Radiol 2011;21(5):1050–7.

81. Hemke R, Maas M, van Veenendaal M, et al. Contrast-enhanced MRI compared with the physical examination in the evaluation of disease activity in juvenile idiopathic arthritis. Eur Radiol 2014;24(2):327–34.

82. van Veenendaal M, Hemke R, Bos M, et al. MRI evaluation of clinical remission in juvenile idiopathic arthritis. Pediatr Rheumatol Online J 2011;9(Suppl 1):P114.

Imaging in Osteoarthritis

Daichi Hayashi, MD, PhD[a,b], Frank W. Roemer, MD[a,c],
Mohamed Jarraya, MD[a,d], Ali Guermazi, MD, PhD[a],*

KEYWORDS

- Osteoarthritis • Imaging • MR imaging • Cartilage • Meniscus • Bone marrow • Knee
- Radiography

KEY POINTS

- Radiography remains the most commonly used imaging technique for establishing an imaging-based diagnosis of osteoarthritis.
- Major limitations of radiography are inability to visualize most tissues of the joint other than bone and its lack of association with clinical symptoms.
- In osteoarthritis research, MR imaging has played an important role in understanding the natural history of the disease and in the search for new therapies.
- Clinical relevance of MR imaging findings related to osteoarthritic joints remains unclear due to high prevalence in asymptomatic persons.
- Ultrasound may be a useful imaging technique for osteoarthritis, particularly of small joints of the hand.

INTRODUCTION

Osteoarthritis (OA) is a joint disorder that primarily affects the elderly population worldwide and is a major public health concern. For instance, almost 10% of the US population lives with symptomatic knee OA by age 60.[1] The annual health care expenditures related to OA have been estimated at $US186 billion.[2] Arthroplasty is an effective therapy for late-stage disease, and there is an on-going research effort exploring effective nonsurgical therapies, including disease-modifying drugs of OA. The increasing importance of imaging in OA for diagnosis, prognostication, and follow-up is well recognized. Conventional radiography remains the gold-standard imaging technique for the evaluation of OA in both clinical practice and research, but it has limitations, which were demonstrated by large MR imaging–based OA studies in recent years.[3,4] Traditionally, cartilage has been thought to be the central feature of OA and the primary target for intervention. However, nowadays OA is considered a disease of the whole joint, involving osseous and nonosseous articular and periarticular tissues. Only MR imaging can assess all structures of the joint, including cartilage, meniscus, ligaments, muscle, subchondral bone marrow, and synovium and is able to visualize the joint in a 3-dimensional (3D) fashion without the projectional limitations of radiography.[5] Moreover, MR imaging enables the assessment of 3D cartilage morphology and biochemical composition. This article describes the roles and limitations of different imaging

Disclosure Statement: A. Guermazi is the president of Boston Imaging Core Lab, LLC (BICL), Boston, MA, a company providing radiological image assessment services. He is a consultant to AstraZeneca, Genzyme, MerckSerono, OrthoTrophix, and TissueGene. F.W. Roemer is a shareholder of BICL. None of the other authors have declared any possible conflict of interest.
^a Department of Radiology, Quantitative Imaging Center, Boston University School of Medicine, 820 Harrison Avenue, FGH Building, 3rd Floor, Boston, MA 02118, USA; ^b Department of Radiology, Yale New Haven Health at Bridgeport Hospital, 267 Grant Street, Bridgeport, CT 06610, USA; ^c Department of Radiology, University of Erlangen-Nuremburg, Maximiliansplatz 2, 91054 Erlangen, Germany; ^d Department of Radiology, Mercy Catholic Medical Center, 1500 Lansdowne Avenue, Darby, PA 19023, USA
* Corresponding author.
E-mail address: guermazi@bu.edu

Radiol Clin N Am 55 (2017) 1085–1102
http://dx.doi.org/10.1016/j.rcl.2017.04.012
0033-8389/17/© 2017 Elsevier Inc. All rights reserved.

modalities and discusses the optimum imaging protocol, imaging diagnostic criteria of OA, differential diagnoses, and what the referring physician needs to know.

ANATOMIC STRUCTURES RELEVANT TO OSTEOARTHRITIS

OA can affect articular and periarticular structures, including osteochondral and nonosteochondral tissues. Traditionally, OA was thought to be primarily a degenerative disease of articular cartilage, but recent research studies have revealed OA is a whole-joint process. Affected tissues include hyaline cartilage, subchondral bone and bone marrow, menisci in the knee, labrum in the shoulder and hip, periarticular ligaments and tendons, periarticular bursae, synovium-lined joint capsule, intervertebral discs in the spine, and triangular fibrocartilage complex (TFCC) in the wrist. Imaging features of each OA-affected tissues/lesions are described later in this article.

IMAGING TECHNIQUES FOR OSTEOARTHRITIS AND RELEVANT REVIEW OF LITERATURE
Conventional Radiography

Radiography is an inexpensive and most commonly used modality for imaging of OA. It allows detection of OA-associated bony features, such as osteophytes, subchondral sclerosis, and cysts.[6] Radiography can also determine joint space width (JSW), which is a surrogate marker for cartilage thickness and meniscal integrity in knees, but direct visualization of these articular structures is impossible using radiographic techniques. Despite this limitation, slowing of radiographically detected joint space narrowing (JSN) remains the only structural end point currently approved by the US Food and Drug Administration to demonstrate efficacy of disease-modifying OA drugs in phase 3 clinical trials. OA is radiographically defined by the presence of marginal osteophytes.[7] Worsening of JSN is the most commonly used criterion for the assessment of structural OA progression, and the total loss of JSW is one of the structural indicators for arthroplasty.

In the knee joint, JSN is caused not only by cartilage loss but also by changes in the meniscus, such as meniscal extrusion and meniscal substance loss.[8] The lack of sensitivity and specificity of radiography for the detection of most of OA-associated articular tissue damage, and its poor sensitivity to change over time, are other limitations of radiography.[9] Changes in joint positioning

can also be problematic in longitudinal studies and can affect the quantitative measurement of various radiographic parameters, including JSW.[10] Despite these limitations, radiography remains the gold standard for establishing an imaging-based diagnosis of OA and for assessment of structural modification in clinical trials of OA.

Semiquantitative analysis
The severity of radiographic OA can be assessed with semiquantitative scoring systems. The Kellgren and Lawrence (KL) grading system[11] (Box 1) is a widely accepted method for defining radiographic OA based on the presence of a definite osteophyte (= grade 2). However, KL grading has its limitations; in particular, KL grade 3 includes all degrees of JSN, regardless of the actual extent (Fig. 1). Recently, the so-called atrophic phenotype of knee OA, characterized by definite

---

Box 1
Diagnostic criteria

Radiography-based criteria: simplified KL grade

- Radiographic OA if grade 2 or above
- Grade 0 = no feature of OA
- Grade 1 = equivocal osteophytes
- Grade 2 = definite osteophytes
- Grade 3 = JSN
- Grade 4 = bone-on-bone appearance

MR imaging–based criteria: proposed by the OARSI OA Imaging Working Group

A *definition of tibiofemoral OA on MR imaging* = the presence of both group [A] features or one group [A] feature and 2 or more group [B] features.

Group [A] after exclusion of joint trauma within the last 6 months (by history) and exclusion of inflammatory arthritis (by radiographs, history, and laboratory parameters): (i) definite osteophyte formation, (ii) full-thickness cartilage loss.

Group [B]: (i) subchondral BML or cyst not associated with meniscal or ligamentous attachments, (ii) meniscal subluxation, maceration, or degenerative (horizontal) tear, (iii) partial-thickness cartilage loss (where full-thickness loss is not present), (iv) bone attrition.

A *definition of patellofemoral OA* requires all of the following involving the patella and/or anterior femur: (i) definite osteophyte formation, (ii) partial- or full-thickness cartilage loss.

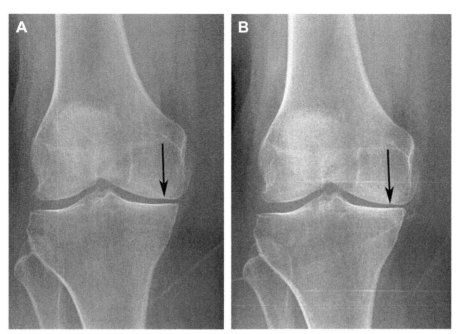

Fig. 1. Insensitivity of semiquantitative assessment of radiographic JSN. (*A*) Anteroposterior (AP) radiograph of the knee shows definite JSN of the medial tibiofemoral compartment (*arrow*). This represents grade 3 tibiofemoral OA according to the KL grading scheme. (*B*) Two years later, there is definite worsening in JSN (*arrow*), but still no bone-to-bone contact. This still will be coded as grade 3 according to KL grading scheme. Semiquantitative scoring has only limited capacities in assessing progression in KL grade 3 OA.

JSN without concomitant osteophyte formation (**Fig. 2**), has gained increasing attention as a potential risk factor for more rapid progressive OA, which may be considered a potential adverse event in anti–nerve growth factor drug trials, a class of new antianalgesic compounds currently under investigation.[12] Although this phenotype is rare, it needs special attention in the research community because it potentially also is a reflection of more rapid disease progression.[13]

The revised OA Research Society International (OARSI) atlas[6] provides image examples for grades for specific features of OA rather than assigning global scores for a whole joint according to definitions like the KL grading system. The atlas grades tibiofemoral JSW and osteophytes separately for each compartment of the knee (medial tibiofemoral, lateral tibiofemoral, and patellofemoral). A study using data from the OA Initiative and the OARSI atlas for semiquantitative grading

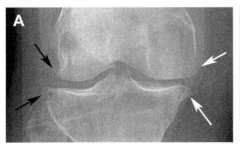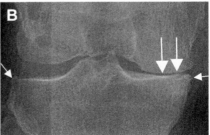

Fig. 2. Radiographic manifestations of OA. (*A*) AP radiograph of the knee shows large marginal osteophytes of the medial (*white arrows*) and lateral (*black arrows*) tibiofemoral compartments. Note additional JSN of the medial compartment. Image represents the hypertrophic phenotype of tibiofemoral OA with severe osteophyte formation and comparatively discrete JSN. (*B*) Atrophic phenotype of OA. AP radiograph of the knee shows severe JSN of the medial compartment (*large arrows*). Only tiny osteophytes are seen at the medial and lateral (*small arrows*) joint margins.

of JSN showed centralized radiographic reading is important because even expert readers seem to apply different thresholds for JSN grading.[14]

Quantitative analysis

JSW is the distance between the projected femoral and tibial margins on the anteroposterior radiograph. Measurements can be performed manually or semiautomatically using computer software. Quantification using image processing software requires a digital image, that is, digitized plain films or images acquired using computed radiography or digital radiography. Minimum JSW is the standard metric, but the use of location-specific JSW has also been reported.[15] Using software analysis of digital knee radiographs, measures of location-specific JSW were shown to be comparable with MR imaging for detection of OA progression.[16] A recent study reported that fixed-location JSW predicts surgical knee replacement more strongly than minimum JSW, whereas MR imaging predicted knee replacement with similar accuracy to radiographic JSW.[17] Various degrees of responsiveness have been observed depending on the degree of OA severity, length of the follow-up period, and the knee-positioning protocol.[15,16] Measurements of JSW obtained from knee radiographs have been found to be reliable, especially when the study lasted longer than 2 years and when the radiographs were obtained with the knee in a standardized flexed position.[18]

The role of malalignment in the OA disease process has been described in the literature. A clinical trial showed that varus malalignment negated the slowing of structural progression of medial JSN by doxycycline.[19] Valgus malalignment of the lower limb was shown to increase the risk of disease progression in knees with radiographic lateral knee OA.[20] Malalignment might be a target for prevention of radiographic knee OA as determined by JSN in overweight and obese women.[21]

Other radiography-based techniques

Tomosynthesis and bone texture analysis are radiography-based techniques that can be applied to imaging of OA. Tomosynthesis generates an arbitrary number of cross-sectional images from a single pass of the x-ray tube. A recent study showed that tomosynthesis is more sensitive than radiography in the detection of osteophytes and subchondral cysts, using 3-T MR imaging as the reference warranting further exploration of this technique in OA studies.[22] Moreover, tomosynthesis was shown to offer excellent intrareader reliability regardless of the reader experience.[23] Quantification of JSW using tomosynthesis has

also been reported.[24] Bone texture analysis extracts from conventional radiographs information on 2-dimensional trabecular bone texture that relates directly to 3D bone structure. It has been shown that bone texture may be a predictor of progression of tibiofemoral OA.[25]

MR Imaging

MR imaging has become the most important imaging tool for OA research in recent years[26–29] thanks to its ability to assess abnormality of structures not visualized by radiography including but not limited to articular cartilage, menisci, ligaments, synovium, capsular structures, fluid collections, and bone marrow.[4,30–35] MR imaging–based diagnostic criteria of knee OA have been proposed (see **Box 1**). Using MR imaging, the joint can be evaluated as a whole organ and multiple tissue changes can be monitored simultaneously; pathologic changes of preradiographic OA can be detected, and biochemical changes within joint tissues such as cartilage can be assessed before morphologic changes become evident. An MR imaging–based definition of OA has been proposed.[36] In addition, with MR imaging, OA can be classified into hypertrophic and atrophic phenotypes, according to the size of osteophytes and concomitant presence or absence of JSN.[13] Importantly, the use of MR imaging has led to improved understanding of clinical manifestations of disease with structural findings such as bone marrow lesions (BMLs)[37] and synovitis,[38] with implications for future OA clinical trials. For example, the observation of fluctuation of features on MR imaging (**Fig. 3**) that are associated with pain in the same direction has shifted the focus of potential treatment targets from cartilage to bone marrow and inflammatory disease manifestations.[37]

Investigators need to choose appropriate MR pulse sequence protocols for the purpose of each study (**Table 1**). For example, focal cartilage defects and BMLs are best assessed using fluid-sensitive fast spin-echo sequences (eg, T2-weighted, proton density-weighted, or intermediate-weighted) with fat suppression.[26,27,30,31] **Fig. 4** shows an example of superior conspicuity of fast spin-echo sequences for BML and focal cartilage defect detection compared with 3D high-resolution gradient echo sequences, such as fast low angle shot (FLASH), dual echo steady state (DESS), spoiled gradient echo (SPGR), or Fast Field Echo (FFE). Moreover, MR imaging may sometimes be affected by artifacts that mimic pathologic findings. For example, susceptibility artifacts can be misinterpreted as

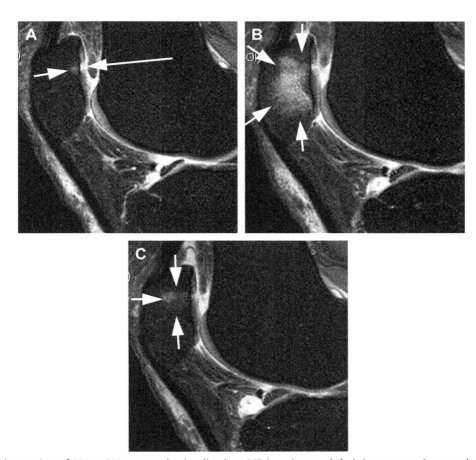

Fig. 3. Fluctuation of BMLs. BMLs are only visualized on MR imaging, and their importance in regard to clinical disease manifestations has been recognized in recent years. As BMLs exhibit a fluctuating character over time, are associated with disease progression, and are potentially reversible, these have become a potential treatment target. (A) Baseline sagittal intermediate-weighted fat-suppressed (IW FS) MR imaging shows a small subchondral BML (*short arrow*) adjacent to a focal full-thickness cartilage defect (*long arrow*). (B) Follow-up image 1 year later depicts marked increase in BML size (*arrows*). (C) Two years after baseline, marked regression is seen with only minor BML observed in the same location (*arrows*). Note that associated cartilage defect did not show increase in size over time.

cartilage loss or meniscal tear (**Fig. 5**). Gradient recalled-echo sequences are known to be particularly prone to susceptibility.[39]

Semiquantitative MR imaging analysis of knee osteoarthritis

A detailed review of semiquantitative MR imaging assessment of OA has been published.[28] In addition to the 3 well-established scoring systems, the Whole Organ Magnetic Resonance Imaging Score (WORMS),[40] the Knee Osteoarthritis Scoring System,[41] and the Boston Leeds Osteoarthritis Knee Score (BLOKS),[42] a new scoring system called the MR Imaging Osteoarthritis Knee Score (MOAKS)[43] was most recently published. Of the 3 systems, WORMS and BLOKS have been widely disseminated and used, but these

scoring systems have both strengths and weaknesses. MOAKS provides a refined scoring tool for cross-sectional and longitudinal semiquantitative MR imaging assessment of knee OA. MOAKS enables semiquantitative scoring of OA features such as BMLs, subchondral cysts, articular cartilage, osteophytes, Hoffa synovitis and synovitis-effusion, meniscus, tendons and ligaments, and periarticular features, including cysts and bursitides (**Fig. 6**).

The use of within-grade changes for longitudinal assessment is commonly applied in OA research using semiquantitative MR imaging approaches.[44] Within-grade scoring describes progression or improvement of a lesion that does not meet the criteria of a full-grade change but does represent a definite visual change in comparison to the

Table 1
Non-contrast-enhanced MR imaging sequences for assessment of knee osteoarthritis features

Osteoarthritis Features	Imaging Planes	Suggested Sequences (without Contrast)
Articular cartilage	Variable	3D high-resolution GRE sequences (eg, FLASH, DESS, SPGR) *and* T2w, IW, or PDw TSE (FS or non-FS depending on the specific question)
Meniscus	Sagittal/coronal	T1w, T2w, or PDw FS
BMLs	Axial/sagittal/coronal	T2w, IW, or PDw FS TSE/FSE, or STIR
Subchondral cysts	Axial/sagittal/coronal	T2w, IW, or PDw FS TSE/FSE, or STIR
Osteophytes	Axial/sagittal/coronal	3D high-resolution GRE sequences (eg, FLASH, DESS, SPGR) *and* Non-FS short TE-weighted (preferably T1 over PD, and non-FS over FS)
Hoffa synovitis	Mid slices of the sagittal plane	T2w, IW, or PDw FS
Effusion synovitis	Axial	T2w, IW, or PDw TSE (FS or non-FS depending on the specific question)
Ligaments	Axial/sagittal/coronal	IW or PDw FS TSE
Periarticular cysts, bursitides, and loose bodies	Axial	T2w or PDw

Abbreviations: GRE, gradient echo; PDw, proton density-weighted; STIR, short-tau inversion recovery; T1w, T1-weighted; T2w, T2-weighted; TE, time of echo; TSE/FSE, turbo spin echo/fast spin echo.

previous time point. A recent study demonstrated that within-grade changes in semiquantitative MR imaging assessment of cartilage and BMLs are valid, and their use increases the sensitivity of semiquantitative readings for detecting longitudinal changes in these structures.[45]

Synovitis is increasingly recognized as an important feature of OA and is associated with pain.[38] Although synovitis can be evaluated with non-contrast-enhanced MR imaging by using the presence of signal changes in the Hoffa fat pad or joint effusion as an indirect marker of synovitis, only contrast-enhanced MR imaging can reveal the true extent of synovial inflammation.[45] Detailed scoring systems of synovitis taking into account anatomic intraarticular location based on contrast-enhanced MR imaging have been published,[38] and these could potentially be used in clinical trials of new OA drugs that target synovitis. **Fig. 7** shows an example of synovitis evaluation using contrast-enhanced MR imaging.

Other available semiquantitative MR imaging scoring systems related to knee OA include Cartilage Repair Osteoarthritis Knee Score[46] and Anterior Cruciate Ligament Osteoarthritis Score,[47] which can be applied to research studies focusing on these structures. Specifically for imaging of cartilage repair tissue, MRI Observation Cartilage Repair Tissue (MOCART) scoring has been developed and applied to research studies involving cartilage repair surgery.[48]

Semiquantitative MR imaging analysis of hand osteoarthritis

Radiography is still the primary imaging modality for hand OA evaluation in a clinical setting, but the use of more sensitive imaging techniques such as ultrasound and MR imaging is becoming increasingly common in OA research.[49] A semiquantitative MR imaging scoring system for hand OA called the OMERACT Hand Osteoarthritis Magnetic Resonance Scoring System (HOAMRIS) has been developed and appears to offer high reliability and responsiveness.[50] Scored OA features include synovitis, erosions, cysts, osteophytes, JSN, malalignment, and BMLs. Using this scoring system, Haugen and colleagues[51] showed that MR imaging could detect approximately twice as many joints with erosions and osteophytes as conventional radiography ($P<.001$) and that moderate/severe synovitis, BMLs, erosions, and osteophytes were associated with joint tenderness independently of each other.[52] These studies demonstrated that some of the semiquantitatively assessed MR imaging features of hand OA can be targeted for therapeutic interventions.

Semiquantitative MR imaging analysis of hip osteoarthritis

The hip joint has a spherical structure, and its very thin covering of articular cartilage makes MR imaging assessment of the hip more difficult than the knee or the hand. A whole-organ semiquantitative multifeature scoring system called the Hip

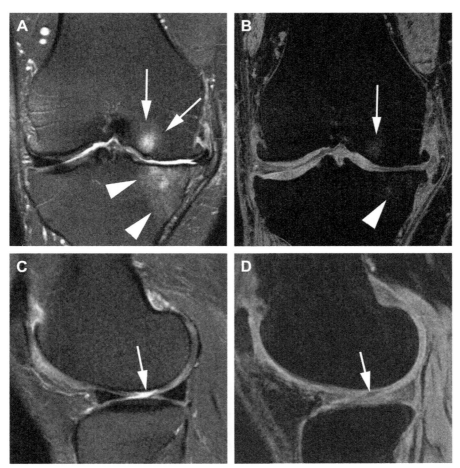

Fig. 4. Relevance of sequence selection for MR imaging assessment of different OA features. (*A*) Coronal IW FS turbo spin-echo MR image shows subchondral BMLs in the medial femur (*arrows*) and tibia (*arrowheads*). (*B*) Corresponding coronal FLASH image, commonly used for cartilage segmentation, barely depicts femoral BML (*arrow*) and shows tibial BML only to minimal extent (*arrowhead*). Note in addition marked femoral and tibial cartilage loss, marginal osteophytes and severe meniscal extrusion. (*C*) Sagittal IW FS image shows focal full-thickness cartilage damage (*arrow*). This finding cannot be depicted by radiography because JSW will not be affected by such subtle changes. (*D*) Sagittal FLASH image of same defect exemplifies that not all MR imaging sequences are suited to visualize cartilage changes in the same manner. FLASH is a high-resolution 3D gradient echo sequence that is commonly used for cartilage segmentation because of its high signal and contrast-to-noise ratio between cartilage and the subchondral bone. However, the focal defect that was easily recognizable on IW FS is not visualized on FLASH image. Only a circumscribed area of low signal (*arrow*) is shown that may likely be mistaken as an intrachondral calcification and not a defect.

Osteoarthritis MRI Scoring System (HOAMS) is available for use in observational studies and clinical trials of hip joints.[53] In HOAMS, 14 articular features are assessed: cartilage morphology, subchondral BMLs, subchondral cysts, osteophytes, acetabular labrum, synovitis (scored only when contrast-enhanced sequences are available), joint effusion, loose bodies, attrition, dysplasia, trochanteric bursitis/insertional tendonitis of the greater trochanter, labral hypertrophy, paralabral cysts, and herniation pits at the superolateral femoral neck. HOAMS showed satisfactory reliability and good agreement concerning intraobserver and interobserver assessment. Recently, another semiquantitative scoring system called Scoring Hip Osteoarthritis with MRI (SHOMRI) was introduced.[54] Direct comparison of HOAMS and SHOMRI has not been performed to date.

Quantitative MR imaging analysis of cartilage and other tissues

Quantitative analysis of cartilage morphology involves segmenting the cartilage and exploits the 3D nature of MR imaging data sets to evaluate

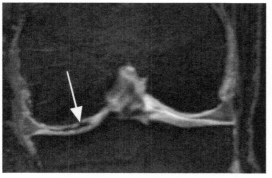

Fig. 5. Artifacts on MR imaging. Coronal DESS image shows a hypointense linear finding in the medial tibiofemoral joint space. So-called vacuum phenomenon is responsible for this artifact, which must not be mistaken as a solid structure. Assessment of the articular surface is impaired and signal loss with the cartilaginous contour must not be mistaken as a surface lesion (*arrow*).

tissue dimensions (such as thickness and volume) or signal as continuous variables. Examples of nomenclature for MR imaging–based cartilage measures and strategies for efficient analysis of

longitudinal changes in subregional cartilage thickness have been proposed.[55,56] Quantitative cartilage morphometry has been widely applied in OA studies.[57,58] Quantitative measures of articular cartilage structure, such as cartilage thickness loss and denuded areas of subchondral bone, have been shown to predict knee replacement surgery.[57] Quantitative MR imaging analysis can also be applied to evaluate noncartilage tissues in the joint, including menisci,[59] BMLs,[60] synovitis,[61] and joint effusion.[62] However, using segmentation approaches for ill-defined lesions such as BMLs is more challenging than segmentation of clearly delineated structures, such as cartilage, menisci, and effusion.

Compositional MR imaging

Compositional MR imaging enables visualization of the biochemical properties of different joint tissues. It may be sensitive to early, premorphologic changes that cannot be visualized on conventional MR imaging. Compositional MR imaging has been mostly applied for ultrastructural assessment of cartilage, although these techniques can also be used to assess other tissues such as the menisci

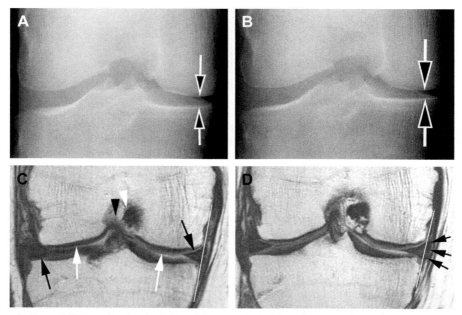

Fig. 6. Superiority or MR imaging in depicting OA as a whole-joint disease. (*A*) Baseline AP radiograph shows normal medial tibio-femoral JSW (*arrows*). (*B*) At 3 years follow-up, definite JSN is depicted (*arrows*). Soft tissues are not assessable on the radiograph. (*C*) Baseline MR imaging of same knee shows multiple tissues relevant to OA not depicted by the radiograph: Cartilage is visualized in a direct fashion as a structure of intermediate signal intensity in this IW coronal MR image (*white arrows*). The anterior (*white arrowhead*) and posterior (*black arrowhead*) cruciate ligaments are clearly depicted as hypointense structures. In addition, the menisci are visualized as hypointense triangular structures in the medial and lateral joint space (*black arrows*). Note that the medial meniscus is aligned with the medial joint margin (*white line*). (*D*) At 3-years follow-up, the MR imaging shows incident meniscal extrusion of the medial meniscal body, responsible for the radiographic JSN (*arrowheads* and *white line*). No cartilage loss is observed during the follow-up interval.

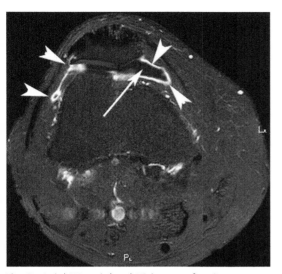

Fig. 7. Axial T1-weighted FS image after intravenous contrast administration. Synovitis is depicted as hyperintense linear thickening along the joint cavity (*arrowheads*). Joint effusion is visualized as intraarticular hypointensity (*arrow*). Only contrast-enhanced images are able to differentiate between joint effusion and synovitis.

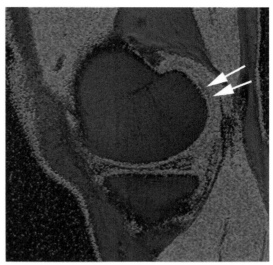

Fig. 8. Sagittal multi-echo spin echo sequence used for T2 relaxometry ("mapping") of the articular cartilage of the medial tibiofemoral joint. After color-coding, the posterior femoral condyle shows an increase in T2 time (*arrow*) reflecting early intrachondral degeneration without associated articular surface damage.

or ligaments. Detailed reviews on this topic and its potential role in OA research have been published recently.[63,64] Compositional MR imaging of cartilage matrix changes can be performed using advanced MR imaging techniques such as delayed gadolinium-enhanced MR imaging of cartilage (dGEMRIC), T1 rho, and T2 mapping (Fig. 8).[65] Of these, the first 2 take advantage of the concentration of highly negatively charged glycosaminoglycans (GAGs) in healthy hyaline cartilage; loss of these GAGs in focal areas affected by possible early disease can be visualized. Both dGEMRIC and T1 rho focus on charge density in cartilage. In contrast, T2 concentrations are affected by a complex combination of collagen orientation and hydration of cartilage.

Compositional MR imaging techniques are currently considered research tools that, besides T2 mapping techniques that are part of the routine on most clinical MR imaging systems, are available only at a limited number of institutions, but they have been applied in clinical trials and observational studies. A recent placebo-controlled double-blind pilot study of collagen hydrolysate for mild knee OA demonstrated that the dGEMRIC index increased (meaning higher GAG content and better cartilage status) in tibial cartilage regions of interest in patients receiving collagen hydrolysate and decreased in the placebo group, with a significant difference being observed at 24 weeks.[66] A decrease in dGEMRIC indices has been shown to be associated with an increase in cartilage thickness in the medial compartment of the knee, suggesting that an increase in cartilage thickness might also be related to a decrease in proteoglycan concentration.[67] Another study[68] demonstrated that acute loading of the knee joint resulted in a significant decrease in T1 rho and T2 relaxation times in the medial tibiofemoral compartment and especially in cartilage regions with small focal defects, suggesting that changes of T1 rho values under mechanical loading may be related to the biomechanical and structural properties of cartilage. Light exercise was associated with low cartilage T2 values but moderate and strenuous exercise was associated with high T2 values in women, suggesting that activity levels can affect cartilage composition.[69] An interventional study assessing the effect of weight loss on articular cartilage demonstrated improved cartilage quality was reflected as an increase in the dGEMRIC index over 1 year for the medial but not the lateral compartment,[70] highlighting the role of weight loss in possible clinical and structural improvement.

Newer compositional MR imaging techniques are being explored, including in vivo diffusion tensor imaging,[71] T2* mapping,[72] ultrashort echo time-enhanced T2* mapping,[73] and sodium imaging.[74] These techniques show promise but require further research and validation.

Ultrasound

Ultrasound enables real-time, dynamic, multiplanar imaging. It offers reliable assessment of OA-associated features, including inflammatory and structural abnormalities, without contrast administration or exposure to radiation.[75] Ultrasound equipment is portable and thus can be used in various locations including outpatient clinics. Limitations of ultrasound include operator-dependency and limited ability to assess deep articular structures and the subchondral bone, which is shown in exemplary fashion in **Fig. 9**.

Ultrasound is useful for evaluation of cortical erosive changes and synovitis in inflammatory arthritis. In OA, the major advantage of ultrasound over radiography is the ability to detect synovial abnormality. Current generation ultrasound technology can detect synovial hypertrophy, increased vascularity, and the presence of synovial fluid in OA-affected joints.[75]

A preliminary ultrasound scoring system for hand OA was published in 2008[76] and included evaluation of gray-scale synovitis and power Doppler signal in 15 joints of the hand. These features were assessed for their presence/absence, and if present, were scored semiquantitatively using a 1 to 3 scale. Overall, moderate to good intrareader and interreader reliability has been demonstrated. This publication showed that an ultrasound outcome measure suitable for multicenter trials assessing hand OA is feasible and likely to be reliable and has provided a foundation for further development.

Ultrasound has been increasingly used for evaluation of hand OA. Kortekaas and colleagues[77] showed that ultrasound-detected osteophytes and JSN of the interphalangeal joints are associated with pain. The same group of investigators also demonstrated that ultrasound-detected signs of inflammation are associated with development of erosions in hand OA, implicating inflammation

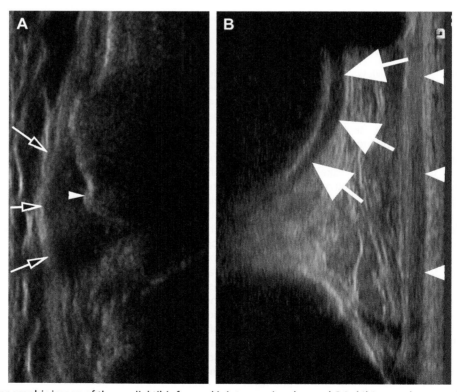

Fig. 9. Sonographic image of the medial tibiofemoral joint space in advanced OA. (*A*) Image shows marked extrusion of the body of the medial meniscus (*arrows*). In addition, a small femoral osteophyte is depicted (*arrowhead*). Note that there is sound extinction toward the more central parts of the joint (right side in image), which does not allow for assessment of the cartilage surface and the ligaments in these areas of the joint. (*B*) Anterior patellofemoral joint as depicted by ultrasound. The patellar tendon is visualized as a hypoechoic linear structure (*arrowheads*). Femoral cartilage is shown as a hypoechoic structure at the anterior femoral condyle (*arrows*). Note sound extinction distally to probe due to cartilage-bone interface (black area in upper left part of image).

plays a role in its pathogenesis and could be a therapeutic target.[78] Ultrasound can be used to evaluate the therapeutic efficacy. A reduction in pain correlated with a decrease in synovial thickening and power Doppler ultrasound markers before and after weekly ultrasound-guided intraarticular injections of hyaluronic acid.[79] Real-time fusion of ultrasound and MR imaging in hand and wrist OA have been attempted and was found to have a high concordance of the bony profile visualization at the level of osteophytes.[49]

Ultrasound has also been used to evaluate features of knee OA and hip OA. A cross-sectional, multicenter European study analyzed 600 patients with painful knee OA and found ultrasound-detected synovitis correlated with advanced radiographic OA and clinical symptoms and signs suggestive of an inflammatory "flare."[80] Ultrasound-detected inflammatory features were positively and linearly associated with knee pain in motion in patients with equal radiographic grades of knee OA in both knees,[81] supporting the association between synovitis and knee pain. An advantage of ultrasound over MR imaging in regard to meniscal extrusion measurements in the knee is the possibility to carry out weight-bearing examinations.[82]

Computed Tomography

Computed tomography (CT) is excellent for depicting cortical bone and soft tissue calcifications and helps detailed evaluation of bony structures of the upper and lower extremity joints, such as subchondral bone sclerosis, subchondral cysts, and osteophytes (Fig. 10). 3D CT is of particular help for orthopedic planning of joint arthroplasty. However, ionizing radiation and limited ability for soft tissue evaluation restrict the routine use of CT in clinical imaging of OA.

Computed Tomography and Magnetic Resonance Arthrography

CT or MR arthrography enables multiplanar evaluation of cartilage damage with high anatomic resolution.[83–85] CT arthrography is currently the most accurate method for evaluating superficial and focal cartilage defects, offering high spatial resolution and high contrast between the low-attenuating cartilage and high-attenuating superficial (contrast material filling the joint space) and deep (subchondral bone) boundaries.[83] For subchondral changes, MR arthrography allows delineation of subchondral BMLs on fluid-sensitive sequences.[83] Both techniques enable visualization of central osteophytes, which are associated with more severe changes of OA than marginal osteophytes.[86] Because of the invasive nature and potential risks, albeit low, associated with intraarticular injection of contrast, arthrographic examinations are rarely used in large-scale clinical or epidemiologic OA studies.

Nuclear Medicine

Nuclear medicine imaging with radiotracers enables imaging of active metabolism and visualization of bone turnover changes seen with osteophyte formation, subchondral sclerosis, subchondral cyst formation, and BMLs as well as sites of synovitis.[87] Scintigraphy with 99mTc-hydroxymethane diphosphonate and PET with 2-^{18}F-fluoro-2-deoxy–D-glucose ([18]FDG) or 18F-fluoride

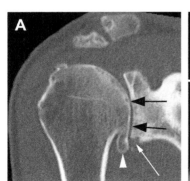
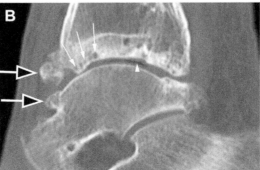

Fig. 10. CT. (A) Coronal CT image of the shoulder in advanced posttraumatic instability OA (grade 3 according to the Samilson-Prieto classification). There is severe JSN of the glenohumeral joint (short arrows). In addition, a large inferior humeral osteophyte is depicted (arrowhead), and a small subchondral cyst in the inferior glenoid is shown (long arrow). (B) Sagittal CT image of posttraumatic ankle OA. Large anterior osteophytes are depicted at the tibiotalar joint margin (large arrows). In addition, anterior JSN and small subchondral cyst are observed (small arrows). Note intraarticular vacuum phenomenon (arrowhead) visualized as a hypodense intraarticular line, a common finding in osteoarthritic joints.

(18-F⁻) have been used to assess OA. Bone scintigraphy can provide a full-body survey that helps to discriminate between soft tissues and bone origin of pain and to locate the site of pain in patients with complex symptoms.[81] 18-FDG-PET can demonstrate the site of synovitis and BMLs associated with OA as exemplified in **Fig. 11**.[88] In addition, there have been increasing research efforts to apply single-photon emission computed tomography/CT for imaging of OA.[89] A major limitation of radioisotope methods is poor anatomic resolution that may be overcome by the increasing application of hybrid technologies, such as PET-CT and PET-MR imaging that combine functional imaging with high-resolution anatomic imaging. However, nuclear medicine imaging is not commonly applied to imaging of OA in a routine clinical setting.

Imaging Findings/Pathology

Cartilage damage
Articular cartilage is one of the main tissues involved in OA disease process. Because cartilage cannot be directly visualized on radiography, MR imaging is the modality of choice for morphologic assessment of cartilage and its lesions. As described earlier, choice of appropriate pulse sequence is essential for accurate assessment of cartilage damage.[27] In the early stage of the OA disease process before development of thinning of focal defects, one may observe intrasubstance T2 hyperintensity, although clinical significance of this signal abnormality remains unclear. Once morphologic changes develop, fluid signal fills the focal defects or diffusely thinned portion of the cartilage. In advanced OA, diffuse full-thickness cartilage loss can be seen, giving bone-on-bone appearance on radiography.

Meniscal lesions
Menisci are 2 semicircular fibrocartilage structures positioned between the joint surfaces of the femur and tibia in the medial and lateral knee joint compartments. MR imaging is the preferred imaging method for menisci, which has many functions in the knee, including load bearing, shock absorption, stability enhancement, and lubrication. Degenerative meniscal lesions, such as horizontal cleavages, oblique or complex tears, can be appreciated on MR imaging because linear or complex T2 hyperintensity that reaches the joint surface is associated with old age. Meniscal extrusion and meniscal root tears are also relevant to OA disease process.[90]

Bone marrow lesions
BMLs, or bone marrow edema-like lesions, are defined on MR imaging as noncystic subchondral areas of ill-defined hyperintensity on fluid-sensitive sequences and areas of hypointensity on T1-weighted spin-echo images. Differential diagnoses for BMLs are broad and summarized in **Box 2**. Degenerative BMLs in association with OA are frequently detected in conjunction with cartilage damage in the same region. BMLs in OA are associated with pain, are known to

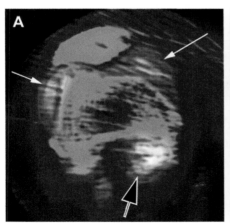
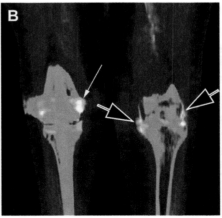

Fig. 11. FDG-PET. (*A*) Axial fusion images of CT and FDG-PET of the knee joint in a patient with OA shows marked synovial glucose accumulation reflecting an inflammatory flare. Typical anatomic locations of synovitis in knee OA are the peripatellar recesses (*small arrows*) and the region posterior to the posterior cruciate ligament (*large arrow*). (*B*) Coronal fusion images show perimeniscal synovitis in the right knee (*large arrows*) and synovitic glucose accumulation in the perifemoral region in the left knee (*small arrow*) that shows a status post total knee arthroplasty. Soft tissue assessment in joints with arthroplasty metal hardware is impaired using MR imaging, and FDG-PET is a valid alternative in these cases.

Box 2
Differential diagnosis of bone marrow lesions

Traumatic BMLs

- Bone contusions, fractures, stress reaction

Nontraumatic BMLs

- Avascular necrosis
- Spontaneous osteonecrosis of the knee (SONK, or SPONK)
- Bone marrow edema syndrome (including transient osteoporosis of the hip, regional migratory osteoporosis, complex regional pain syndrome, reflex sympathetic dystrophy)
- Inflammatory BMLs (such as chronic polyarthritis, reactive arthritis, rheumatoid arthritis, bacterial arthritis)
- Malignancy (lymphoma, myeloma, leukemia)
- Benign tumors (Langerhans cell histiocytosis, chondroblastoma, osteoid osteoma, osteoblastoma)

---

fluctuate over time,[37] and are associated with worsening rates of radiographic JSN.[91]

Subchondral cysts

Subchondral cysts, or subchondral cystlike lesions, are a common finding in OA. On MR imaging, these lesions demonstrate well-defined rounded areas of fluidlike signal intensity on nonenhanced imaging. Subchondral cysts are commonly present alongside with BMLs in the same subregion of the joint and may develop within the areas of BMLs.

Osteophytes

Osteophytes are osteocartilaginous protrusions growing at the margins of OA joints from a process that involves endochondral ossification. It is well established that osteophytes are a hallmark feature of OA, that is, its presence on radiography defines radiographic OA in the KL grading system.[11] Osteophytes can be detected by conventional radiography, but small ones may only be visualized in tomographic imaging such as tomosynthesis, CT, and MR imaging.[22]

Joint effusion and synovitis

Effusion and synovitis are frequently present in OA. As in the case of synovitis in rheumatoid arthritis, synovitis in OA is best evaluated using contrast-enhanced MR imaging, which enables differentiation between thickened enhancing synovium and nonenhancing synovial fluid (= effusion).[92] Recent studies using contrast-enhanced

MR imaging showed the association of increasing synovitis with knee cartilage deterioration[93] and incident joint tenderness in hand OA.[94] When contrast-enhanced MR imaging is not available, non-contrast-enhanced MR imaging can still be used to evaluate synovitis by using a surrogate marker, that is, signal changes in Hoffa fat pad. This abnormality is described as diffuse hyperintense signal on fluid-sensitive MR imaging sequences within the Hoffa fat pad and can be referred to as "Hoffa synovitis."[43] Large effusions may be associated with pain and stiffness in OA.[95] It should be kept in mind that "effusion" on noncontrast MR imaging includes synovitis and effusion. Thus, this imaging feature should preferably be referred to as "effusion-synovitis."[43]

Ligaments

Tear of intraarticular and periarticular ligaments can lead to OA of the affected joint. In the case of knee joint, anterior and posterior cruciate ligaments as well as collateral ligaments can be involved. These ligamentous structures are best evaluated using MR imaging, which demonstrates the presence of abnormal intrasubstance T2 hyperintensities with or without fibrous discontinuity.

Periarticular cysts, bursitis, and loose bodies

A wide spectrum of periarticular cysts and bursitides may be seen in OA. Most cystic lesions are encapsulated fluid collections exhibiting low T1 signal and high T2 signal. Details of each of these cysts and bursitides have been published elsewhere.[96] Loose bodies are often seen in conjunction with OA, particularly in advanced stage. Chondral fragments, detached osteophytes, and fragments of meniscus or labrum, for example, may give rise to loose bodies in OA. A differential diagnosis would include synovial osteochondromatosis (**Box 3**).

Subchondral attrition

Subchondral attrition is defined as flattening or depression of the subchondral osseous surface unrelated to gross fracture. It can be evaluated using radiography and is usually present in advanced knee OA, although it may also appear in knees with mild OA without JSN. Precise pathogenesis of this OA feature is unknown, but subchondral microfracture and remodeling due to changes in mechanical loading may explain development of bone attrition in OA. Its association with knee pain has been demonstrated.[97]

Other joint-specific lesions

In the hip and shoulder joints, the acetabular or glenoidal labrum can be torn secondary to

---

Box 3
Differential diagnosis of osteoarthritis

Spontaneous osteonecrosis of the knee (SONK or SPONK)

- Common in elderly women, occurs following minor trauma with severe pain; common in medial tibiofemoral compartment of the knee.

Rheumatoid arthritis

- Unlike OA, associated with marked erosive changes and affects both medial and lateral tibiofemoral compartments equally.

Calcium pyrophosphate dehydrate deposition disease

- The clinical manifestation is called pseudogout. If OA-like changes are seen in locations that are uncommon for primary OA, identification of calcifications (eg, meniscus in the knee, TFCC in the wrist, and symphysis pubis in the pelvis) helps differentiate from OA.

Synovial osteochondromatosis

- Numerous intraarticular loose bodies are present. Loose bodies in OA are usually limited in number.

Box 4
Pearls, pitfalls, and variants of osteoarthritis imaging

Pearls:

- JSW of the knee joint on radiography reflects the status of not only cartilage but also menisci.
- MR imaging enables visualization of nonosteochondral OA features that are not visible on radiography.
- Synovitis is best evaluated using contrast-enhanced MR imaging sequence.

Pitfalls:

- On radiography, patient positioning can be variable, and meaningful comparison of JSW on standing knee radiographs with 2 or more time points may be problematic.
- On MR imaging, focal cartilage defects and BMLs will be underestimated or even missed when evaluated using gradient recalled-echo sequences.
- On MR imaging, gradient recalled-echo sequences are known to be particularly prone to susceptibility artifacts, which can be misinterpreted as cartilage loss or meniscal tear.

Variants:

- OA does not usually show osseous erosion, but in erosive OA of the hand, central erosion at interphalangeal joints can be seen demonstrating a "gull wing" sign on radiography.

---

degenerative processes. Likewise, in the wrist joint, TFCC may be torn as OA disease process progresses. In the spine, degenerative changes can affect structures such as intervertebral discs and ligamentum flavum. These joint-specific nonosseous lesions are best evaluated using MR imaging.

SUMMARY

Boxes 4 and 5 summarize the key messages from this article. Despite known limitations, radiography is still the most commonly used modality for semiquantitative and quantitative evaluation of OA in the upper and lower extremities. MR imaging is becoming an increasingly more important imaging modality for OA research, and available assessment options include semiquantitative, quantitative, and compositional techniques. Ultrasound is commonly used particularly in hand OA studies and is especially useful for evaluation of synovitis and for guidance of joint-related procedures. Nuclear medicine, CT, and CT-MR arthrography have limited roles compared with radiography, MR imaging, and ultrasound. Imaging of OA has helped investigators to understand risk factors for disease onset and progression and the interactions between

---

Box 5
What the referring physician needs to know

- OA is considered a disease of the whole joint.
- In clinical practice, radiography remains the main imaging modality for OA assessment due to cost and relative simplicity of evaluation.
- MR imaging has added much to the understanding of all the joint tissues involved in OA disease process and their significance explain pain and structural progression.
- In the clinical evaluation of OA, the main role of MR imaging is to help rule out other arthropathies.
- The use of appropriate MR imaging pulse sequences is crucial for accurate assessment and quantification of OA features.
- Contrast-enhanced MR imaging should be considered in the assessment of synovitis in OA.

different joint tissues and periarticular tissue changes.

REFERENCES

1. Losina E, Weinstein AM, Reichmann WM, et al. Lifetime risk and age at diagnosis of symptomatic knee osteoarthritis in the US. Arthritis Care Res (Hoboken) 2013;65:703–11.
2. Kotlarz H, Gunnarsson CL, Fang H, et al. Insurer and out-of-pocket costs of osteoarthritis in the US: evidence from national survey data. Arthritis Rheum 2009;60:3546–53.
3. Guermazi A, Hayashi D, Roemer F, et al. Severe radiographic knee osteoarthritis – does Kellgren and Lawrence grade 4 represent end stage disease? – the MOST study. Osteoarthritis Cartilage 2015;23:1499–505.
4. Guermazi A, Niu J, Hayashi D, et al. Prevalence of abnormalities in knees detected by MRI in adults without knee osteoarthritis: population based observational study (Framingham Osteoarthritis Study). BMJ 2012;345:e5339.
5. Guermazi A, Roemer FW, Crema MD, et al. Imaging of non-osteochondral tissues in osteoarthritis. Osteoarthritis Cartilage 2014;22:1590–605.
6. Altman RD, Gold GE. Atlas of individual radiographic features in osteoarthritis, revised. Osteoarthritis Cartilage 2007;15(Suppl A):A1–56.
7. Altman R, Asch E, Bloch D, et al. Development of criteria for the classification and reporting of osteoarthritis. Classification of osteoarthritis of the knee. Diagnostic and Therapeutic Criteria Committee of the American Rheumatism Association. Arthritis Rheum 1986;29:1039–49.
8. Hunter DJ, Zhang YQ, Tu X, et al. Change in joint space width: hyaline articular cartilage loss or alteration in meniscus? Arthritis Rheum 2006;54:2488–95.
9. Guermazi A, Roemer FW, Burstein D, et al. Why radiography should no longer be considered a surrogate outcome measure for longitudinal assessment of cartilage in knee osteoarthritis. Arthritis Res Ther 2011;13:247.
10. Guermazi A, Eckstein F, Hayashi D, et al. Baseline radiographic osteoarthritis and semi-quantitatively assessed meniscal damage and extrusion and cartilage damage on MRI is related to quantitatively defined cartilage thickness loss in knee osteoarthritis: the Multicenter Osteoarthritis Study. Osteoarthritis Cartilage 2015;23:2191–8.
11. Kellgren JH, Lawrence JS. Radiological assessment of osteo-arthrosis. Ann Rheum Dis 1957;16:494–502.
12. Roemer FW, Hayes CW, Miller CG, et al. Imaging atlas for eligibility and on-study safety of potential knee adverse events in anti-NGF studies (Part 1). Osteoarthritis Cartilage 2015;23(Suppl 1):S22–42.
13. Roemer FW, Guermazi A, Niu J, et al. Prevalence of magnetic resonance imaging-defined atrophic and hypertrophic phenotypes of knee osteoarthritis in a population-based cohort. Arthritis Rheum 2012;64:429–37.
14. Guermazi A, Hunter DJ, Li L, et al. Different thresholds for detecting osteophytes and joint space narrowing exist between the site investigators and the centralized reader in a multicenter knee osteoarthritis study–data from the Osteoarthritis Initiative. Skeletal Radiol 2012;41:179–86.
15. Nevitt MC, Peterfy C, Guermazi A, et al. Longitudinal performance evaluation and validation of fixed-flexion radiography of the knee for detection of joint space loss. Arthritis Rheum 2007;56:1512–20.
16. Duryea J, Neumann G, Niu J, et al. Comparison of radiographic joint space width with magnetic resonance imaging cartilage morphometry: analysis of longitudinal data from the Osteoarthritis Initiative. Arthritis Care Res (Hoboken) 2010;62:932–7.
17. Eckstein F, Boudreau R, Wang Z, et al. Comparison of radiographic joint space width and magnetic resonance imaging for prediction of knee replacement: a longitudinal case-control study from the Osteoarthritis Initiative. Eur Radiol 2016;26:1942–51.
18. Reichmann WM, Maillefert JF, Hunter DJ, et al. Responsiveness to change and reliability of measurement of radiographic joint space width in osteoarthritis of the knee: a systematic review. Osteoarthritis Cartilage 2011;19:550–6.
19. Mazzuca SA, Brandt KD, Chakr R, et al. Varus malalignment negates the structure-modifying benefits of doxycycline in obese women with knee osteoarthritis. Osteoarthritis Cartilage 2010;18:1008–11.
20. Felson DT, Niu J, Gross KD, et al. Valgus malalignment is a risk factor for lateral knee osteoarthritis incidence and progression: findings from MOST and the osteoarthritis initiative. Arthritis Rheum 2013;65:355–62.
21. Runhaar J, van Middelkoop M, Reijman M, et al. Malalignment: a possible target for prevention of incident knee osteoarthritis in overweight and obese women. Rheumatology (Oxford) 2014;53:1618–24.
22. Hayashi D, Xu L, Roemer FW, et al. Detection of osteophytes and subchondral cysts in the knee with use of tomosynthesis. Radiology 2012;263:206–15.
23. Hayashi D, Xu L, Gusenburg J, et al. Reliability of semiquantitative assessment of osteophytes and subchondral cysts on tomosynthesis images by radiologists with different levels of expertise. Diagn Interv Radiol 2014;20:353–9.
24. Kalinosky B, Sabol JM, Piacsek K, et al. Quantifying the tibiofemoral joint space using x-ray tomosynthesis. Med Phys 2011;38:6672–82.
25. Woloszynski T, Podsiadlo P, Stachowiak GW, et al. Prediction of progression of radiographic knee

osteoarthritis using tibial trabecular bone texture. Arthritis Rheum 2012;64:688–95.

26. Hayashi D, Guermazi A, Roemer FW. MRI of osteoarthritis: the challenges of definition and quantification. Semin Musculoskelet Radiol 2012;16:419–30.

27. Hayashi D, Roemer FW, Guermazi A. Choice of pulse sequences for magnetic resonance imaging-based semiquantitative assessment of cartilage defects in osteoarthritis research: comment of the article by Dore et al. Arthritis Rheum 2010;62: 3830–1.

28. Guermazi A, Roemer FW, Haugen IK, et al. MRI-based semiquantitative scoring of joint pathology in osteoarthritis. Nat Rev Rheumatol 2013;9:236–51.

29. Alizai H, Roemer FW, Hayashi D, et al. An update on risk factors for cartilage loss in knee osteoarthritis assessed using MRI-based semiquantitative grading methods. Eur Radiol 2015;25:883–93.

30. Hayashi D, Guermazi A, Kwoh CK, et al. Semiquantitative assessment of subchondral bone marrow edema-like lesions and subchondral cysts of the knee at 3T MRI: a comparison between intermediate-weighted fat-suppressed spin echo and Dual Echo Steady State sequences. BMC Musculoskelet Disord 2011;12:198.

31. Crema MD, Roemer FW, Hayashi D, et al. Comment on: Bone marrow lesions in people with knee osteoarthritis predict progression of disease and joint replacement: a longitudinal study. Rheumatology 2011;50:996–7.

32. Hayashi D, Englund M, Roemer FW, et al. Knee malalignment is associated with an increased risk for incident and enlarging bone marrow lesions in the more loaded compartments: the MOST study. Osteoarthritis Cartilage 2012;20:1227–33.

33. Roemer FW, Felson DT, Wang K, et al. Co-localisation of non-cartilaginous articular pathology increases risk of cartilage loss in the tibiofemoral joint–the MOST study. Ann Rheum Dis 2013;72: 942–8.

34. Roemer FW, Kwoh CK, Hannon MJ, et al. Risk factors for magnetic resonance imaging-detected patellofemoral and tibiofemoral cartilage loss during a six-month period: the joints on glucosamine study. Arthritis Rheum 2012;64:1888–98.

35. Roemer FW, Guermazi A, Felson DT, et al. Presence of MRI-detected joint effusion and synovitis increases the risk of cartilage loss in knees without osteoarthritis at 30-month follow-up: the MOST study. Ann Rheum Dis 2011;70:1804–9.

36. Hunter DJ, Arden N, Conaghan P, et al. Definition of osteoarthritis on MRI: results of a Delphi exercise. Osteoarthritis Cartilage 2011;19:963–9.

37. Zhang Y, Nevitt M, Niu J, et al. Fluctuation of knee pain and changes in bone marrow lesions, effusions, and synovitis on magnetic resonance imaging. Arthritis Rheum 2011;63:691–9.

38. Guermazi A, Roemer FW, Hayashi D, et al. Assessment of synovitis with contrast-enhanced MRI using a whole-joint semiquantitative scoring system in people with, or at high risk of, knee osteoarthritis: the MOST study. Ann Rheum Dis 2011;70:805–11.

39. Jarraya M, Hayashi D, Guermazi A, et al. Susceptibility artifacts detected on 3T MRI of the knee: frequency, change over time and associations with radiographic findings: data from the joints on glucosamine study. Osteoarthritis Cartilage 2014; 22:1499–503.

40. Peterfy CG, Guermazi A, Zaim S, et al. Whole-Organ Magnetic Resonance Imaging Score (WORMS) of the knee in osteoarthritis. Osteoarthritis Cartilage 2004;12:177–90.

41. Kornaat PR, Ceulemans RY, Kroon HM, et al. MRI assessment of knee osteoarthritis: Knee Osteoarthritis Scoring System (KOSS)–inter-observer and intraobserver reproducibility of a compartment-based scoring system. Skeletal Radiol 2005;34:95–102.

42. Hunter DJ, Lo GH, Gale D, et al. The reliability of a new scoring system for knee osteoarthritis MRI and the validity of bone marrow lesion assessment: BLOKS (Boston Leeds Osteoarthritis Knee Score). Ann Rheum Dis 2008;67:206–11.

43. Hunter DJ, Guermazi A, Lo GH, et al. Evolution of semi-quantitative whole joint assessment of knee OA: MOAKS (MRI Osteoarthritis Knee Score). Osteoarthritis Cartilage 2011;19:990–1002.

44. Roemer FW, Nevitt MC, Felson DT, et al. Predictive validity of within-grade scoring of longitudinal changes of MRI-based cartilage morphology and bone marrow lesion assessment in the tibiofemoral joint - the MOST Study. Osteoarthritis Cartilage 2012;20:1391–8.

45. Loeuille D, Sauliere N, Champigneulle J, et al. Comparing non-enhanced and enhanced sequences in the assessment of effusion and synovitis in knee OA: associations with clinical, macroscopic and microscopic features. Osteoarthritis Cartilage 2011;19:1433–9.

46. Roemer FW, Guermazi A, Trattnig S, et al. Whole joint MRI assessment of surgical cartilage repair of the knee: cartilage repair osteoarthritis knee score (CROAKS). Osteoarthritis Cartilage 2014;22:779–99.

47. Roemer FW, Frobel R, Lohmaner LS, et al. Anterior Cruciate Ligament OsteoArthritis Score (ACLOAS): longitudinal MRI-based whole joint assessment of anterior cruciate ligament injury. Osteoarthritis Cartilage 2014;22:668–82.

48. Welsch GH, Zak L, Mamisch TC, et al. Advanced morphological 3D magnetic resonance observation of cartilage repair tissue (MOCART) scoring using a new isotropic 3D proton-density, turbo spin echo sequence with variable flip angle distribution (3D-SPACE) compared to an isotropic 3D steady-state free precession sequence (True-FISP) and standard

2D sequences. J Magn Reson Imaging 2011;33: 180–8.

49. Iagnocco A, Perella C, D'Agostino MA, et al. Magnetic resonance and ultrasonography real-time fusion imaging of the hand and wrist in osteoarthritis and rheumatoid arthritis. Rheumatology (Oxford) 2011;50:1409–13.

50. Haugen IK, Eshed I, Gandjbakhch F, et al. The longitudinal reliability and responsiveness of the OMERACT Hand Osteoarthritis Magnetic Resonance Imaging Scoring System (HOAMRIS). J Rheumatol 2015;42:2486–91.

51. Haugen IK, Boyesen P, Slatkowsky-Christensen B, et al. Comparison of features by MRI and radiographs of the interphalangeal finger joints in patients with hand osteoarthritis. Ann Rheum Dis 2012;71: 345–50.

52. Haugen IK, Boyesen P, Slatkowsky-Christensen B, et al. Associations between MRI-defined synovitis, bone marrow lesions and structural features and measures of pain and physical function in hand osteoarthritis. Ann Rheum Dis 2012;71:899–904.

53. Roemer FW, Hunter DJ, Winterstein A, et al. Hip Osteoarthritis MRI Scoring System (HOAMS): reliability and associations with radiographic and clinical findings. Osteoarthritis Cartilage 2011;19: 946–62.

54. Lee S, Nardo L, Kumar D, et al. Scoring hip osteoarthritis with MRI (SHOMRI): a whole joint osteoarthritis evaluation system. J Magn Reson Imaging 2015;41: 1549–57.

55. Eckstein F, Ateshian G, Burgkart R, et al. Proposal for a nomenclature for magnetic resonance imaging based measures of articular cartilage in osteoarthritis. Osteoarthritis Cartilage 2006;14:974–83.

56. Wirth W, Buck R, Nevitt M, et al. MRI-based extended ordered values more efficiently differentiate cartilage loss in knees with and without joint space narrowing than region-specific approaches using MRI or radiography–data from the OA initiative. Osteoarthritis Cartilage 2011;19:689–99.

57. Eckstein F, Kwoh CK, Boudreau RM, et al. Quantitative MRI measures of cartilage predict knee replacement: a case-control study from the Osteoarthritis Initiative. Ann Rheum Dis 2013;72:707–14.

58. Eckstein F, Collins JE, Nevitt MC, et al. Cartilage thickness change as an imaging biomarker of knee osteoarthritis progression – data from the FNIH OA Biomarkers Consortium. Arthritis Rheum 2015;67: 3184–9.

59. Wenger A, Englund M, Wirth W, et al. Relationship of 3D meniscal morphology and position with knee pain in subjects with knee osteoarthritis: a pilot study. Eur Radiol 2012;22:211–20.

60. Roemer FW, Khrad H, Hayashi D, et al. Volumetric and semiquantitative assessment of MRI-detected subchondral bone marrow lesions in knee osteoarthritis: a comparison of contrast-enhanced and non-enhanced imaging. Osteoarthritis Cartilage 2010;18:1062–6.

61. Fotinos-Hoyer AK, Guermazi A, Jara H, et al. Assessment of synovitis in the osteoarthritic knee: comparison between manual segmentation, semi-automated segmentation and semiquantitative assessment using contrast-enhanced fat-suppressed T1-weighted MRI. Magn Reson Med 2010; 64:604–9.

62. Habib S, Guermazi A, Ozonoff A, et al. MRI-based volumetric assessment of joint effusion in knee osteoarthritis using proton density-weighted fat-suppressed and T1-weighted contrast-enhanced fat-suppressed sequences. Skeletal Radiol 2011;40: 1581–5.

63. Guermazi A, Roemer FW, Alizai H, et al. State of the art: MR imaging after knee cartilage repair surgery. Radiology 2015;277:23–43.

64. Guermazi A, Alizai H, Crema MD, et al. Compositional MRI techniques for evaluation of cartilage degeneration in osteoarthritis. Osteoarthritis Cartilage 2015;23:1639–53.

65. Burstein D, Gray M, Mosher T, et al. Measures of molecular composition and structure in osteoarthritis. Radiol Clin North Am 2009;47:675–86.

66. McAlindon TE, Nuite M, Krishnan N, et al. Change in knee osteoarthritis cartilage detected by delayed gadolinium enhanced magnetic resonance imaging following treatment with collagen hydrolysate: a pilot randomized controlled trial. Osteoarthritis Cartilage 2011;19:399–405.

67. Crema MD, Hunter DJ, Burstein D, et al. Association of changes in delayed gadolinium-enhanced MRI of cartilage (dGEMRIC) with changes in cartilage thickness in the medial tibiofemoral compartment of the knee: a 2 year follow-up study using 3.0T MRI. Ann Rheum Dis 2014;73:1935–41.

68. Souza RB, Stehling C, Wyman BT, et al. The effects of acute loading on T1rho and T2 relaxation times of tibiofemoral articular cartilage. Osteoarthritis Cartilage 2010;18:1557–63.

69. Hovis KK, Stehling C, Souza RB, et al. Physical activity is associated with magnetic resonance imaging-based knee cartilage T2 measurements in asymptomatic subjects with and those without osteoarthritis risk factors. Arthritis Rheum 2011;63:2248–56.

70. Anandacoomarasamy A, Leibman S, Smith G, et al. Weight loss in obese people has structure-modifying effects on medial but not on lateral knee articular cartilage. Ann Rheum Dis 2012;71:26–32.

71. Raya JG, Horng A, Dietrich O, et al. Articular cartilage: in vivo diffusion-tensor imaging. Radiology 2012;262:550–9.

72. Newbould RD, Miller SR, Toms LD, et al. T2* measurement of the knee articular cartilage in osteoarthritis at 3T. J Magn Reson Imaging 2012;35:1422–9.

73. Wiliams A, Qian Y, Golla S, et al. UTE-T2* mapping detects sub-clinical meniscus injury after anterior cruciate ligament tear. Osteoarthritis Cartilage 2012;20:486–94.

74. Madelin G, Babb J, Xia D, et al. Articular cartilage: evaluation with fluid-suppressed 7.0T sodium MR imaging in subjects with and subjects without osteoarthritis. Radiology 2013;268:481–91.

75. Keen HI, Conaghan PG. Ultrasonography in osteoarthritis. Radiol Clin North Am 2009;47:581–94.

76. Keen HI, Lavie F, Wakefield RJ, et al. The development of a preliminary ultrasonographic scoring system for features of hand osteoarthritis. Ann Rheum Dis 2008;67:651–5.

77. Kortekaas MC, Kwok WY, Reijnierse M, et al. Osteophytes and joint space narrowing are independently associated with pain in finger joints in hand osteoarthritis. Ann Rheum Dis 2011;70:1835–7.

78. Kortekaas MC, Kwok WY, Reijnierse M, et al. Association of inflammation with development of erosions in patients with hand osteoarthritis: a prospective ultrasonography study. Arthritis Rheum 2016;68:392–7.

79. Klauser AS, Faschingbauer R, Kupferthaler K, et al. Sonographic criteria for therapy follow-up in the course of ultrasound-guided intra-articular injections of hyaluronic acid in hand osteoarthritis. Eur J Radiol 2012;81:1607–11.

80. Conaghan PG, D'Agostino MA, Le Bars M, et al. Clinical and ultrasonographic predictors of joint replacement for knee osteoarthritis: results from a large, 3-year, prospective EULAR study. Ann Rheum Dis 2010;69:644–7.

81. Wu PT, Shao CJ, Wu KC, et al. Pain in patients with equal radiographic grades of osteoarthritis in both knees: the value of gray scale ultrasound. Osteoarthritis Cartilage 2012;20:1507–13.

82. Nogueira-Barbosa MH, Gregio-Junior E, Lorenzato MM, et al. Ultrasound assessment of medial meniscal extrusion: a validation study using MRI as reference standard. AJR Am J Roentgenol 2015;204:584–8.

83. Omoumi P, Mercier GA, Lecouvet F, et al. CT arthrography, MR arthrography, PET and scintigraphy in osteoarthritis. Radiol Clin North Am 2009;47:595–615.

84. Omoumi P, Michoux N, Thienpont E, et al. Anatomical distribution of areas of preserved cartilage in advanced femorotibial osteoarthritis using CT arthrography (Part 1). Osteoarthritis Cartilage 2015;23:83–7.

85. Omoumi P, Michoux N, Roemer FW, et al. Cartilage thickness at the posterior medial femoral condyle is increased in femorotibial knee osteoarthritis: a

86. cross-sectional CT arthrography study (Part 2). Osteoarthritis Cartilage 2015;23:224–31.

86. McCauley TR, Kornaat PR, Jee WH. Central osteophytes in the knee: prevalence and association with cartilage defects on MR imaging. AJR Am J Roentgenol 2001;176:359–64.

87. Etchebehere EC, Etchebehere M, Gamba R, et al. Orthopedic pathology of the lower extremities: scintigraphic evaluation in the thigh, knee and leg. Semin Nucl Med 1998;28:41–61.

88. Nakamura H, Masuko K, Yudoh K, et al. Positron emission tomography with 18F-FDG in osteoarthritic knee. Osteoarthritis Cartilage 2007;15:673–81.

89. Maas O, Joseph GB, Sommer G, et al. Association between cartilage degeneration and subchondral bone remodeling in patients with knee osteoarthritis comparing MRI and (99m)Tc-DPD-SPECT/CT. Osteoarthritis Cartilage 2015;23:1713–20.

90. Guermazi A, Hayashi D, Jarraya M, et al. Medial posterior meniscal root tears are associated with development or worsening of medial tibiofemoral cartilage damage: the multicenter osteoarthritis study. Radiology 2013;268:814–21.

91. Edwards MH, Parsons C, Bruyere O, et al. High Kellgren-Lawrence grade and bone marrow lesions predict worsening rates of radiographic joint space narrowing: the SEKOIA study. J Rheumatol 2016; 43:657–65.

92. Hayashi D, Roemer FW, Katur A, et al. Imaging of synovitis in osteoarthritis: current status and outlook. Semin Arthritis Rheum 2011;41:116–30.

93. De Lange-Brokaar BJ, Ioan-Facsinay A, Yusuf E, et al. Evolution of synovitis in osteoarthritic knees and its association with clinical features. Osteoarthritis Cartilage 2016;24(11):1867–74.

94. Haugen IK, Slatkowsky Christensen B, Boyesen P, et al. Increasing synovitis and bone marrow lesions are associated with incident joint tenderness in hand osteoarthritis. Ann Rheum Dis 2016;75(4):702–8.

95. Hill CL, Gale DG, Chaisson CE, et al. Knee effusions, popliteal cysts, and synovial thickening: association with knee pain in osteoarthritis. J Rheumatol 2001;28:1330–7.

96. Hayashi D, Roemer FW, Dhina Z, et al. Longitudinal assessment of cyst-like lesions of the knee and their relation to radiographic osteoarthritis and MRI-detected effusion and synovitis in patients with knee pain. Arthritis Res Ther 2010;12:R172.

97. Torres L, Dunlop DD, Peterfy C, et al. The relationship between specific tissue lesions and pain severity in persons with knee osteoarthritis. Osteoarthritis Cartilage 2006;14:1033–40.

Interventions and Therapy in Rheumatology

Mario Muto, MD[a], Francesco Giurazza, MD, PhD[b],*, Giulia Frauenfelder, MD[b],
Stefano Marcia, MD[c], Salvatore Masala, MD[d], Gianluigi Guarnieri, MD[a]

KEYWORDS

- Rheumatology • Glucocorticosteroids • Secondary osteoporosis • Vertebroplasty
- Magnetic Resonance

KEY POINTS

- Patients affected by rheumatic conditions present frequently with secondary osteoporosis caused by long-term oral glucocorticosteroid therapy with consequent loss of trabecular bone.
- Patients with secondary osteoporosis from oral steroid therapy may be affected by vertebral fractures amenable to percutaneous vertebroplasty.
- Patient selection for vertebroplasty is based on both clinical (pain and timing of symptoms) and imaging criteria: hypointensity in T1-weighted and hyperintensity in short tau-inversion recovery or magnetic resonance sequences or increased uptake at technetium-99m scintigraphy bone scan, without computed tomography signs of bone sclerosis.
- Even if in the short time vertebroplasty significantly reduces pain and improves the quality of life, patients should be informed of the procedural outcomes in the long term, underlying the risk of re-fracture because of the ongoing of the osteoporosis and the possible need for reintervention.
- Vertebroplasty represents the symptomatic treatment of the fracture pain, so patients must always be included into a specific therapeutic workup of the rheumatic condition.

INTRODUCTION

In patients affected by rheumatic conditions, spine degeneration has a higher incidence than in the general population; this is because of the early involvement of disco-somatic units. In this scenario, vertebral compression fractures (VCF) are frequently observed and not only in elderly populations; they are certainly related to the disease itself but even more to the medical therapies, especially glucocorticosteroids (GCs).[1]

Since their introduction in the 1950s, GCs have been widely used in a variety of inflammatory diseases, and they are key drugs of therapeutic regimens in most autoimmune rheumatic conditions because of their effectiveness, versatility, and low cost.[2] Early data shortly after the introduction of GCs suggested potential slowing of radiographic progression in rheumatoid arthritis.[3]

However, even at low doses ($\leq$7.5 mg of prednisolone or equivalent), GCs rapidly induce bone loss,[4,5] more marked in the trabecular bone. This bone loss leads to GC-induced osteoporosis (GIO) and consequent increased risk of bone fractures, particularly elevated for vertebral fractures (2–5 times, depending on the daily dosage) that already occurs 3 months after treatment has

The authors have nothing to disclose.

[a] Neuroradiology Department, Ospedale Cardarelli, Via Antonio Cardarelli 9, Naples 80100, Italy; [b] Radiology Department, Università Campus Bio-Medico, Via Alvaro Del Portillo 200, Rome 00100, Italy; [c] Radiology Department, Ospedale Santissima Trinità, Via Is Mirrionis 92, Cagliari 09121, Italy; [d] Musculoskeletal Interventional Radiology Department, Università Tor Vergata, Via di Tor Vergata, Rome 00100, Italy
* Corresponding author.
E-mail address: francescogiurazza@hotmail.it

radiologic.theclinics.com

started.[6] Besides bone loss, the risk of fracture is also increased by a reduced bone quality.[7] Higher dose and longer duration of GC use are strongly associated with the risk of VCF,[8,9] but a threshold dose or duration has not been well described, as wide individual variation is seen. Therefore, GC therapy is the most common cause of secondary osteoporosis.[4]

Various guidelines for GIO stress the importance of initiating an anti–osteoporosis prophylaxis[10,11] in terms of bisphosphonates and teriparatide assumption. However, many patients do not receive such treatment,[10–12] and despite efforts to prevent GIO, patients may still present with VCF,[13] requiring pharmacologic pain control (eg, acetaminophen, nonsteroidal anti-inflammatory drugs, or narcotic analgesics) and protracted immobilization; this finally induces worsening of the quality of life and causes secondary complications such as atelectasis, pneumonia, or pulmonary embolus.

In this clinical scenario, a mini-invasive approach provided by interventional radiology techniques, especially vertebroplasty (VP), plays a relevant role in the pain management of these patients. For approximately 20 years,[13] cases of GIO in rheumatology patients with VCF have been described in which VP offered a unique method for pain management.

The pathogenesis of spine pain in these patients is related to the stretching of periosteal nervous fibers caused by micromovements[14]; therefore, the goal of intravertebral cement, poly(methyl methacrylate) (PMMA), injection is the stabilization of those microfractures.[15]

So, patients with secondary osteoporosis from oral steroid therapy may present with VCF amenable to percutaneous VP; this report describes patient selection criteria, technique, and outcomes of VP in patients affected by rheumatic disease and GIO.

PATIENT SELECTION CRITERIA

Based on clinical and radiologic criteria (**Fig. 1**), it is essential to correctly select the patients suffering from GIO fractures amenable to VP to avoid harm.

First, asymptomatic patients are excluded. Clinical inclusion criteria (**Table 1**) include symptomatic patients without neurologic complications and with intractable pain not responding to conservative therapy, namely refractory after at least 3 weeks of analgesic assumption and/or decreased daily living activities.[14–16]

In addition to clinics, radiologic imaging clearly plays a pivotal role in patient selection. A vertebral collapse is typically detected with radiographs or computed tomography (CT) scan, but these data need to be verified by magnetic resonance (MR) imaging or scintigraphy bone scan, because fractures amenable to VP are those in the acute/subacute phase.[15] MR imaging (**Fig. 2**) shows marrow edema using spin-echo T1-weighted, T2-weighted, and short tau-inversion recovery sequences (STIR). It presents nuanced hypointensity in T1 and marked hyperintensity in STIR. Additionally the rim fracture can be appreciated in T1 as a linear hypointensity. Technetium-99 m scintigraphy bone scan detects an increased uptake.

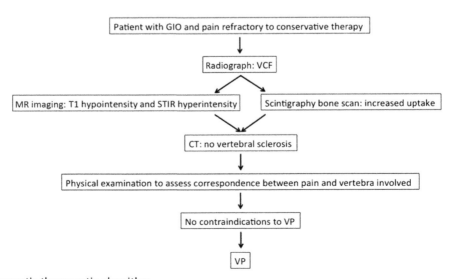

Fig. 1. Diagnostic-therapeutic algorithm.

Table 1
Inclusion and exclusion criteria for vertebroplasty

	Inclusion Criteria	Exclusion Criteria
Clinical	Pain Failure of conservative therapies	Asymptomatic Neurologic complications
Radiologic	Radiograph: vertebral collapse MR imaging: T1 hypointensity, STIR hyperintensity Scintigraphy: increased uptake	CT: vertebral sclerosis
Technical	Patient able to tolerate the procedure	Untreatable coagulopathies Allergy to PMMA Vertebral infections

Furthermore, no sclerosis of the soma must be evident at CT (Fig. 3), otherwise this indicates that fracture is not recent and there is no way for the PMMA cement injection to stabilize the trabecular bone; usually VP is performed between 3 weeks and 4 months after the fracture occurred.[16] Then the patient must be examined to confirm that the fractured vertebrae are those responsible for the pain.

Finally, absolute procedural contraindications need to be excluded: untreatable coagulopathies, allergy to PMMA, and concomitant vertebral infections. Vertebral posterior wall involvement is a relative contraindication.[14–16] From a technical point of view, the interventionist should verify that the patient is able to lie prone for the entire procedure (at least 30 minutes) or should consider performing the procedure under general anesthesia.

TECHNICAL ASPECTS

VPs are performed under fluoroscopic guidance and mild sedation. Local anesthesia (lidocaine, or bupivacaine) are used to anesthetize the skin and soft tissues, including the periosteum over each

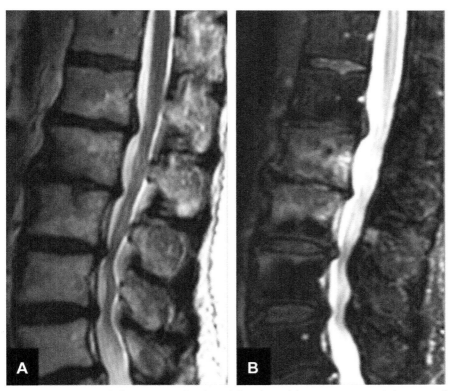

Fig. 2. MR imaging scan in sagittal plane, T2-weighted TSE (*A*) and STIR (*B*) sequences. Porotic fractures of the soma of D8 and D9 with bone edema clearly appreciable in STIR sequence. This patient underwent VP. TSE, turbo spin echo.

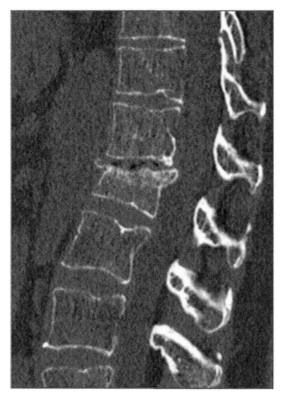

Fig. 3. CT scan in sagittal plane. Collapse of the soma of D8, with sclerosis of the upper plate. This patient is unsuitable for VP.

fractured vertebra. A 4-mm skin incision is made to allow entrance of the VP needle. An 11- or 13-gauge trocar is then advanced through the pedicle under fluoroscopy guidance into the anteriormost portion of the vertebral body.

PMMA mixed with sterile barium sulfate is injected into the vertebral body during continuous fluoroscopic screening. Bone cement is injected into the central anterior intravertebral space until adequate filling is achieved without extravasation. If cross-filling is inadequate, a bipedicular approach is then used. Ideally, the cement should distribute from the superior to the inferior end plate, from the medial cortex of the pedicle to the medial cortex of the contralateral pedicle, and from the anterior cortex of the vertebral body to the posterior third of the vertebral body.

Cement injection is always performed in the lateral screening projection with intermittent fluoroscopic checking in the anteroposterior projection (Fig. 4). If any paraspinal or intradisk leakage of cement occurs, injection is temporarily halted to allow hardening of cement and then reattempted. If any epidural extravasation occurs, the injection phase is stopped. All patients are observed in the recovery room for 2 hours and then discharged to their previous disposition. Antibiotic prophylaxis is performed as well.

Sacrum is another typical location of osteoporotic insufficiency fractures treatable with cementoplasty; those lesions present an H shape with the involvement of the sacrum wings connected by a transverse linear interruption.

PMMA cement is known to be 36 times stronger than vertebral cancellous bone,[17] and it could alter the spinal load with consequent fractures of the adjacent vertebra. Another risk factor for adjacent fractures is a leak of cement into the intradiscal space.[14–16]

Some investigators proposed to follow a relatively low-volume cement-filling technique so that less of the denser bone cement is available to crush the surrounding vertebral osteoporotic bone.[14] Another technical solution is to perform a prophylactic VP by injecting bone cement into the adjacent part of the vertebral bodies, including the caudal part of the superior adjacent vertebral body and the cephalic part of the inferior adjacent

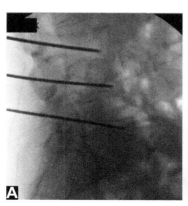
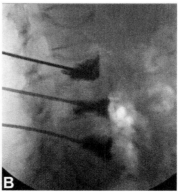
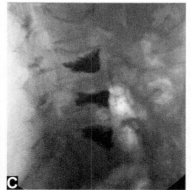

Fig. 4. Fluoroscopic images in lateral projection during the VP of L3, L4, and L5. (A) Needle positioning, (B) PMMA injection, (C) final control. L2 is collapsed as well, but the fracture is not recent and has not been treated.

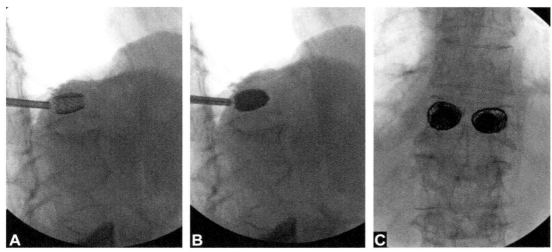

Fig. 5. Same patient of **Fig. 2**, presenting 8 months after VP with the collapse of D12. In this case, because of the consequent severe kyphotic deformity, a KP has been performed, using the Vertebral Body Stent System. The procedure of KP is performed always with a bilateral transpedicular approach. Fluoroscopic images in lateral projection show stent release (*A*) and cement filling (*B*) and final control in anteroposterior projection (*C*).

vertebral body; this procedure should prevent the propagation of vertebral fractures by significantly lowering the incidence of adjacent fractures and reducing the necessity of multiple repeated VP procedures.[14]

In this category of patients, VP is preferred over kyphoplasty (KP) because of the multiple segments frequently involved, the shorter procedural time, and the reduced expense.[18] KP was originally related to the use of balloon to restore vertebral height before cement injection; now more than 18 different KP-like devices are available on the market with the same target of original KP but using metallic stent or synthetic implant.

KP is indicated in cases of porotic fractures at thoracolumbar levels with vertebral height reduction of at least 30% to 40%; the goal of this approach is to obtain a partial or total restoration of the vertebral height and the reduction of the kyphotic deformity (**Figs. 5–7**).[14]

OUTCOMES

Adverse events are rare, and the procedure is considered safe. The most frequent adverse event is cement outflow in surrounding structures (veins, disc, epidural space) during injection, which usually is completely asymptomatic; recently, the development of new viscous cements has helped reduce these events. In 2% of the cases, epidural cement extravasation causes radiculopathy or medullary compression. Symptomatic pulmonary embolism, cement allergy, and infections are even more uncommon (1%).[16]

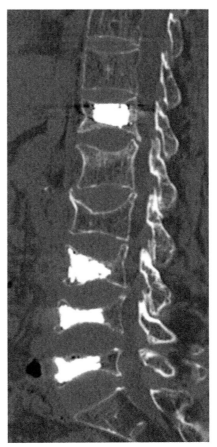

Fig. 6. CT scan in sagittal plane of the same patient of **Figs. 4** and **2**. The treatment effects are evident on the soma of D12, L3, L4, and L5 without cement outflows.

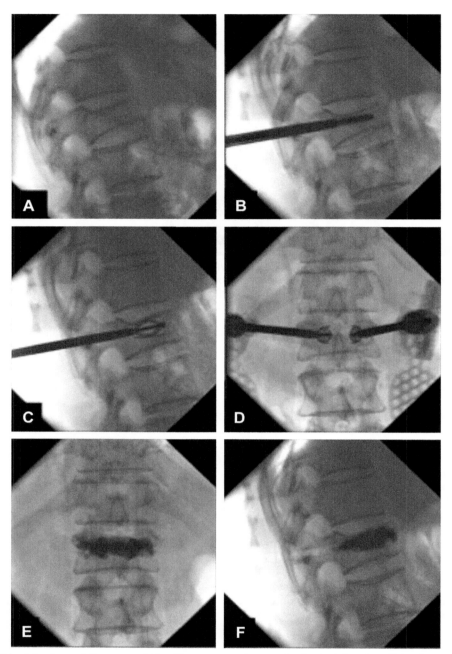

Fig. 7. Vertebral fracture of the soma of L1 with consequent severe kyphotic deformity. KP has been performed, using the Spine Jack (Vexim, Balma, France). Fluoroscopic images show the initial vertebral height, positioning of the device just below the collapsed upper plate, and release of the Spine Jack (*A–C* in lateral projection respectively). Bilateral and symmetrical release of Spine Jack, just before cement injection (*D* in anteroposterior projection). Final controls show procedural success without cement outflow and restored vertebral height (*E* and *F* in anteroposterior and lateral projections, respectively).

Relevant trials have been published in the last years with controversial results about the effectiveness of VP in managing painful osteoporotic vertebral fractures. Two blinded randomized, controlled trials published together in 2009[19–21] found no benefit of VP over placebo at any time. Both studies enrolled patients with osteoporotic fractures and back pain for up to 1 year with an average pain duration of 16 to 18 weeks[20] and 10 weeks, respectively.[21]

Additionally, in 2010, an open-label randomized, controlled trial (Vertos II)[22] compared VP in acute phase with usual care and found positivity for VP with enhanced reduction in pain and disability in the VP group at each time point up to 1 year after the intervention.[22] According to the Vertos II findings, in 2016, another trial (VAPOR)[23] found VP superior to placebo intervention for pain reduction in patients with acute osteoporotic spinal fractures. Interestingly, the researchers of Vertos II[22] and VAPOR[23] trials limited enrollment to painful fractures of less than 6 weeks' duration, whereas the 2 blinded trials[20,21] included predominantly nonacute fractures in which the bone may have already healed. Patient selection could explain the outcomes difference.

Another issue is that some data show VP as effective in reducing pain and favoring mobilization only in the short term[16]; long-term data are controversial mainly because of the risk of refracture.

Some investigators[24,25] did not find any difference between VP and conservative therapy in terms of refracture rate at 1 year, with 50% of new fractures occurring in the adjacent vertebra. Others instead[26–28] feel that there is an increased risk of new fractures in the adjacent vertebra caused by the previous VP primarily for 3 reasons[29]: increased load on adjacent vertebra related to the different stiffness of PMMA compared with the osteoporotic bone, increased pressure on the adjacent discs, and increased physical activity because of an improved quality of life.

However, just as in an untreated osteoporotic population, new fractures in patients treated with VP involve typically the dorsal-lumbar spine and the superior plate of the adjacent vertebra. Furthermore, it should be taken into account that the basilar rate of new fractures in untreated osteoporotic patients is 20% per year. Focusing on GIO, the symptomatic refracture rates after VP are higher compared with those in patients with primary osteoporosis. Patients on oral steroid therapy at the time of initial VP are almost twice as likely to have refracture than those patients with primary osteoporosis.[15]

It seems that the delayed new fractures are not caused by the VP procedure but are the result of the natural course of GIO[30–32]; rheumatologic patients receiving oral steroids are inherently predisposed to increased vertebral body instability compared with patients with primary osteoporosis and are more likely to have refracture. Some investigators propose to perform the preventive VP for the adjacent vertebral bodies as a solution to reduce the risk of adjacent fracture after VP.[33]

SUMMARY

Patients affected by rheumatic conditions present early spine degeneration because of the involvement of disco-somatic units but mainly because of the long-term medical therapies, especially glucocorticosteroids. Percutaneous VP is a safe and effective procedure for pain management in patients with vertebral compression fractures related to GIO, but selection criteria, both clinical and radiologic, must be strictly followed. It is crucial to stress that VP represents the treatment of the fracture pain and not of the GIO, so VP must always be included in a specific therapeutic workup.

REFERENCES

1. Hwang YG, Saag K. The safety of low-dose glucocorticoids in rheumatic diseases: results from observational studies. Neuroimmunomodulation 2015;22: 72–82.
2. Jacobs J, Bijlsma J, van Laar JM. Glucocorticoids in early rheumatoid arthritis:are the benefits of joint-sparing effects offset by the adverse effect of osteoporosis? the effects on bone in the utrecht study and the CAMERA-II Study. Neuroimmunomodulation 2015;22:66–71.
3. A COMPARISON of cortisone and aspirin in the treatment of early cases of rheumatoid arthritis; a report by the Joint Committee of the Medical Research Council and Nuffield Foundation on Clinical Trials of Cortisone, A.C.T.H., and Other Therapeutic Measures in Chronic Rheumatic Diseases. Br Med J 1954;1(4873):1223–7.
4. Mazzantini M, Di Munno O. Glucocorticoid-induced osteoporosis: 2013 update. Reumatismo 2014; 66(1):144–52.
5. Van Staa TP, Leufkens HG, Cooper C. The epidemiology of corticosteroid-induced osteoporosis:a meta-analysis. Osteoporos Int 2002;13:777–87.
6. Van Staa TP. The pathogenesis, epidemiology and management of glucocorticoid-induced osteoporosis. Calcif Tissue Int 2006;79:129–37.
7. Lems WF. Bisphosphonates and glucocorticoids: effects on bone quality. Arthritis Rheum 2007;56: 3518–22.
8. Van Staa TP, Laan RF, Barton IP, et al. Bone density threshold and other predictors of vertebral fracture in patients receiving oral glucocorticoid therapy. Arthritis Rheum 2003;48:3224–9.
9. Steinbuch M, Youket TE, Cohen S. Oral glucocorticoid use is associated with an increased risk of fracture. Osteoporos Int 2004;15:323–8.
10. Feldstein AC, Elmer PJ, Nichols GA, et al. Practice patterns in patients at risk for glucocorticoid-induced osteoporosis. Osteoporos Int 2005;16: 2168–74.

11. Grossman JM, Gordon R, Ranganath VK, et al. American College of Rheumatology 2010 recommendations for the prevention and treatment of glucocorticoid-induced osteoporosis. Arthritis Care Res 2010;62:1515–26.

12. Curtis JR, Westfall AO, Allison JJ, et al. Longitudinal patterns in the prevention of osteoporosis in glucocorticoid-treated patients. Arthritis Rheum 2005;52:2485–94.

13. Mathis JM, Petri M, Naff N. Percutaneous vertebroplasty treatment of steroid-induced osteoporotic compression fractures. Arthritis Rheum 1998;41: 171–5.

14. Muto M, Giurazza F, Guarnieri G, et al. What's new in vertebral cementoplasty? Br J Radiol 2016;89: 20150337.

15. Syed MI, Patel NA, Jan S, et al. Symptomatic refractures after vertebroplasty in patients with steroid-induced osteoporosis. AJNR Am J Neuroradiol 2006;27:1938–43.

16. Aubry-Rozier B, Theumann N. Les vertèbroplasties: point de vue rhumatologue. Rev Med Suisse 2009;5: 585–90.

17. Baroud G. Biomechanical explanation of adjacent fractures following vertebroplasty. Radiology 2003; 229:606–8.

18. Gonzalez-Macia J, del Pino-Montes J, Olmos JM, et al. Guías de práctica clínica en la osteoporosis posmenopáusica, glucocorticoidea y del varón. Sociedad Espanola de Investigación Ósea y del Metabolismo Mineral (3.a versión actualizada 2014). Rev Clin Esp 2015. http://dx.doi.org/10.1016/j.rce.2015.08.003.

19. Clark W, Bird P, Diamond T, et al. Vertebroplasty for acute painful osteoporotic fractures (VAPOR): study protocol for a randomized controlled trial. Trials 2015;16:159.

20. Kallmes DF, Comstock BA, Heagerty PJ, et al. A randomized trial of vertebroplasty for osteoporotic spinal fractures. N Engl J Med 2009;361(6):569–79.

21. Buchbinder R, Osborne RH, Ebeling PR, et al. A randomized trial of vertebroplasty for painful osteoporotic vertebral fractures. N Engl J Med 2009; 361(6):557–68.

22. Klazen CA, Lohle PN, de Vries J, et al. Vertebroplasty versus conservative treatment in acute osteoporotic vertebral compression fractures (Vertos II): an open-label randomised trial. Lancet 2010;376: 1085–92.

23. Clark W, Bird P, Gonski P, et al. Safety and efficacy of vertebroplasty for acute painful osteoporotic fractures (VAPOR): a multicentre, randomised, double-blind, placebo-controlled trial. Lancet 2016;1(388): 1408–16.

24. Diamond TH, Bryant C, Browne L, et al. Clinical outcomes after acute osteoporotic fractures: A 2-year non-randomised trial comparing percutaneous vertebroplasty with conservative therapy. Med J Aust 2006;184:113–7.

25. Zhang YZ, Kong LD, Cao JM, et al. Incidence of subsequent vertebral body fractures after vertebroplasty. J Clin Neurosci 2014;21(8):1292–7.

26. Uppin AA, Hirsch JA, Centenera LV. Occurrence of new vertebral body fracture after percutaneous vertebroplasty in patients with osteoporosis. Radiology 2003;226:119–24.

27. Voormolen MH, Lohle PN. The risk of new osteoporotic vertebral compression fractures in the year after percutanous vertebroplasty. J Vasc Interv Radiol 2006;17:71–6.

28. Trout AT, Kallmes DF, Kaufmann TJ. New fractures after vertebroplasty: adjacent fractures occur significantly sooner. AJNR Am J Neuroradiol 2006;27: 217–23.

29. Qing-Hua T, Chun-Gen W, Quan-Ping X, et al. Percutaneous vertebroplasty of the entire thoracic and lumbar vertebrae for vertebral compression fractures related to chronic glucocorticosteriod use: case report and review of literature. Korean J Radiol 2014;15(6):797–801.

30. Lindsay R, Silverman SL, Cooper C, et al. Risk of new vertebral fracture in the year following a fracture. JAMA 2001;285:320–3.

31. Klazen CA, Venmans A, de Vries J, et al. Percutaneous vertebroplasty is not a risk factor for new osteoporotic compression fractures: results from VERTOS II. AJNR Am J Neuroradiol 2010;31:1447–50.

32. Shi MM, Cai XZ, Lin T, et al. Is there really no benefit of vertebroplasty for osteoporotic vertebral fractures? A meta-analysis. Clin Orthop Relat Res 2012;470:2785–99.

33. Yen CH, Teng MM, Yuan WH, et al. Preventive vertebroplasty for adjacent vertebral bodies: a good solution to reduce adjacent vertebral fracture after percutaneous vertebroplasty. AJNR Am J Neuroradiol 2012;33(5):826–32.

Imaging of Posttraumatic Arthritis, Avascular Necrosis, Septic Arthritis, Complex Regional Pain Syndrome, and Cancer Mimicking Arthritis

Andrey Rupasov, DO, Usa Cain, MD, Simone Montoya, MD,
Johan G. Blickman, MD, PhD*

KEYWORDS

- Arthritis • Posttraumatic • Septic • Avascular • Necrosis • CRPS • Osteodystrophy

KEY POINTS

- Radiographic changes of posttraumatic arthritis typically reflect the underlying trauma to the joint and the resultant manifestations of osteoarthritis.
- Avascular necrosis imaging demonstrates the sequela of osseous ischemia, frequently complicated by collapse of articular surfaces and joint destruction.
- Septic arthritis should be a leading differential in acutely painful joint with effusion and increased levels of inflammatory markers; contrast MR imaging is helpful in the absence of radiographic findings.
- Several benign synovial tumors as well as malignant lesions can mimic arthritis; history is important in formulating differential diagnoses and recommending appropriate follow-up.
- Although complex regional pain syndrome remains a clinical diagnosis, bone scintigraphy may be used as a confirmatory test.

POSTTRAUMATIC ARTHRITIS

Andrey Rupasov (University of Rochester Medical Center; Rochester, New York)

Posttraumatic arthritis is a common form of secondary osteoarthritis (OA) that results from a prior insult to the joint.[1] Injuries may damage the structural integrity and change the mechanics of the joint, leading to early degenerative changes. The process is further accelerated by continued injury and factors predisposing to OA, such as excess body weight. Radiographic changes of posttraumatic arthritis typically reflect the underlying trauma to the joint and the resultant manifestations of OA. Treatment options range from conservative measures to joint arthroplasty, directed by the severity of injury, the level of physical activity, and long-term goals.

An estimated 10% to 15% of diagnosed cases of OA have a posttraumatic cause.[2] Although any joint may be involved, this condition most frequently affects weight-bearing joints, particularly the hip,

Disclosure: The authors have nothing to disclose.
Imaging Sciences, University of Rochester Medical Center, 601 Elmwood Avenue, PO Box 648, Rochester, NY 14642-0636, USA
* Corresponding author.
E-mail address: johan_blickman@urmc.rochester.edu

knee, and ankle, which are the most susceptible to trauma and to the stresses imposed by ongoing functional demands. OA of the joints rarely affected by this disease, including the wrist and the elbow, has an underlying posttraumatic cause in most cases.[1]

The inciting event initiating or accelerating joint degeneration in posttraumatic arthritis is acute structural joint injury. The injury may be in the form of fracture, cartilage damage, meniscal or ligamentous damage, or a combination of these processes. The severity of joint degeneration and speed of onset are proportionate to the damage sustained in the inciting trauma.[2] Joint surface incongruity following an intra-articular fracture often leads to established arthritic change within a year. The potential for repair in hyaline cartilage is very limited, and the fibrocartilage subsequently deposited does not possess the same longevity or resilience.[3] This limitation leads to premature wear and denuding of the articular cartilage down to subchondral bone (**Fig. 1**).

The initial injury not only disrupts the structural integrity of the tissues but results in increased expression of inflammatory mediators, cartilage-degrading proteinases, and stress response factors that lead to additional injury and death of tissues, including those beyond the area of initial impact.[4] Mechanical stress can also induce production of reactive oxygen species that lead to oxidative stress, which impairs growth factor response and has adverse effects on the survival and functionality of the resident cell populations.[5,6]

In vitro studies have shown that inhibition of reactive oxygen species decreased injury-induced chondrocyte death.[5]

Secondary injury results from chronic loading abnormalities caused by ligamentous, meniscal, and joint capsular damage, in addition to possible articular incongruity.[7] Joint instability alters the location where joint surfaces make contact, resulting in localized areas of cartilage degeneration in areas not typically loaded in the natural state.[8] Loss of anterior cruciate ligament (ACL) stability, for instance, causes increased medial femoral condyle translation on the tibial plateau, leading to altered wear patterns. Even in cases in which no surface injury or joint inflammation was appreciated following the initial injury, the existence of uncorrected ligamentous or capsule tears has resulted in posttraumatic arthritis over a period of years, likely stemming from increased joint instability.

The risk factors for arthritic initiation and progression in patients with posttraumatic OA are similar to those for idiopathic OA, suggesting that the systemic host factors and local biomechanical factors interact and compound. Obesity, female gender, and preexisting early-stage OA contribute significantly to adverse radiographic and clinical outcomes.[9] Additional patient risk factors include proprioceptive defects, calcium crystal deposition disease, and other disease states that may lead to disruption of normal joint structures or mechanics.

The symptoms of posttraumatic arthritis are joint pain, swelling, and decreased tolerance for

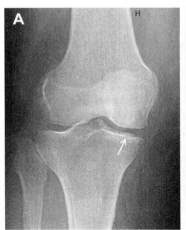
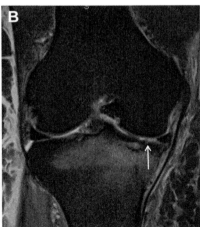
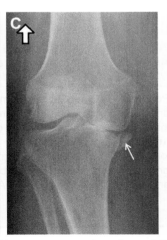

Fig. 1. (A) Anteroposterior (AP) radiograph of the right knee in a 60-year-old woman presenting after a fall shows subtle cortical irregularity along the medial tibial plateau (*arrow*). (B) Coronal long-recovery-time fat-saturated (FS) MR image confirms a nondisplaced fracture of the medial tibial plateau, with intra-articular extension and disruption of cartilage at the arrow. (C) AP radiograph of the right knee less than 2 years later shows severe joint space narrowing and subchondral sclerosis at the medial compartment, along with sequelae of the medial plateau fracture that include a displaced osseous fragment (*small arrow*).

activities that stress the joint. Classically, it is an indolent but progressive monoarthritis with a history of remote articular injury, which is vital to creating the clinical context for proper diagnosis. The major differential considerations are pigmented villonodular synovitis, synovial osteochondromatosis, or monoarticular involvement with crystalline arthropathies or Charcot arthropathy.

Radiography is the imaging modality primarily used to detect the onset and progression of joint degeneration following trauma, although the development of radiographic features of OA may take decades to occur. The imaging hallmarks are the same as those of OA, and include joint space narrowing, sclerosis, and osteophytosis.[10] If all 3 of these findings are not present, another diagnosis should be considered. The asymmetry of joint wear typically reflects the original injury pattern (**Fig. 2**). Sclerotic changes tend to occur at joint margins, and are a reliable finding, unless the patient is severely osteoporotic.

Radiographic changes of posttraumatic arthritis typically show the sequelae of underlying trauma to the joint.[11] Evidence of malunion or articular incongruity can be observed on plain radiographs. Residual articular step-off on imaging and the quality of fracture reduction seem to be important predictors of subsequent development of posttraumatic arthritis, and have been reported to correlate with patient outcomes.[12] Although

computed tomography (CT) is more sensitive than plain radiographs for gaps and step-offs associated with intra-articular fractures, radiographs are able to detect nonanatomic reductions, and a strong association between final radiographic outcome and clinical outcome has been shown.[13] Depending on the pattern of injury, osseous resorption, and remodeling, posttraumatic changes may mimic erosive changes of inflammatory arthritides (**Fig. 3**).

CT arthrography with intra-articular contrast has been used to evaluate patients following acute knee trauma and has been shown to have high sensitivity for detecting various features of joint degeneration, including cartilage loss, meniscal damage, and subchondral cysts and sclerosis. Furthermore, CT arthrography may be used to assess and quantify the thickness of articular cartilage. The disadvantage of CT arthrography is that it is an invasive procedure and involves significant radiation expose, which limits its use in screening or in longitudinal studies.[14]

MR imaging is a noninvasive modality that is sensitive for detection of early cartilage degeneration, and can evaluate other joint structures, including the menisci, bone marrow, tendons, and ligaments, given its excellent soft tissue contrast. To assess the collagen and proteoglycan content in the knee cartilage matrix, compositional assessment techniques such as T2 mapping, delayed gadolinium-enhanced MR imaging of cartilage, sodium imaging, and diffusion-weighted imaging have been used in research and clinical settings.[15] The availability and cost of MR limit its longitudinal utility; additionally, implanted orthopedic hardware has the potential to interfere with joint imaging.

Quantitative assessment of knee radiographs using standardized views has been found to be comparable with MR imaging for detecting OA progression, and is a well-suited modality for longitudinal assessment of cartilage degeneration.[16] However, unlike MR, radiography is unable to determine spatial distribution of tibiofemoral cartilage loss, and has poor sensitivity for detecting early cartilage degeneration. Meniscal and ACL injuries represent the greatest proportion of traumatic knee injuries, each greatly increasing susceptibility to OA, and may be assessed with MR. Increased degrees of instability following partial or complete ACL tear have been shown to correlate directly with the development of articular cartilage damage.[17]

As many as 1 in 4 patients develop early OA after fractures of the acetabulum.[18] Protrusio acetabuli is a hip deformity characterized by bulging of the femoral head and medial acetabular wall into the

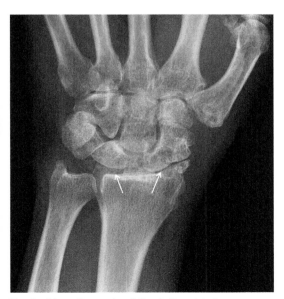

Fig. 2. PA radiograph of the left wrist shows severe posttraumatic arthritis of the radioscaphoid joint, with subchondral cyst formation and osteophytosis. Marked joint space asymmetry is observed at the radiocarpal articulation (*arrows*). Prior basal joint arthroplasty is evident.

pelvis. Secondary protrusio deformity is much more common, and unilateral cases are highly suspicious for being the sequelae of prior trauma (Fig. 4). This deformity may result in overgrowth of the superior acetabulum, which in turn provides a pincer mechanism for femoral acetabular impingement. The radiographic hallmarks include medialization of the medial wall of the acetabulum past the ilioischial line (Kohler line), and center-edge angle (angle of Wiberg) greater than 40° on anteroposterior (AP) projection.[19]

Patients with protrusio acetabuli typically have decreased active and passive range of motion of the hip and may develop a fixed flexion contracture. Secondary protrusio deformity usually does not cause significant pain until degenerative changes have occurred.[20] For this reason, arthroplasty is usually the surgical procedure of choice for the symptomatic adult hip with medial protrusion.

Idiopathic OA of the ankle is rare, and, in the individuals diagnosed with ankle OA, prior trauma is the most common cause (Fig. 5). More than 50% of patients with fractures of the distal tibial articular surface develop early OA. Osteoarthritic changes, as well as possible malunion, incongruity, and intra-articular loose bodies, can be observed on

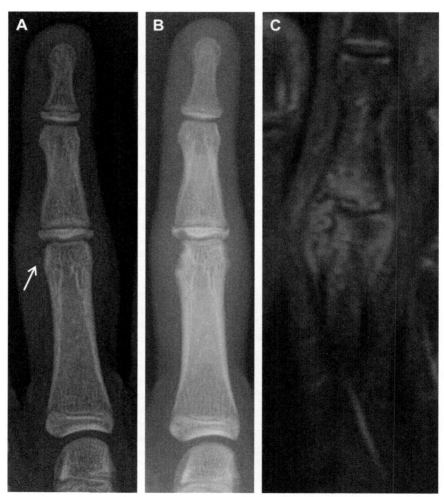

Fig. 3. (A) Posteroanterior (PA) radiograph of the right third digit in a 13-year-old girl after a jamming injury shows pronounced soft tissue swelling surrounding the proximal interphalangeal joint. A faint linear density is present at the radial aspect of the head of the proximal phalanx (*arrow*), consistent with a small avulsion fracture. (B) Follow-up radiograph 6 months later reveals juxta-articular erosive changes, evoking the possibility of juvenile idiopathic arthritis. (C) Contrast-enhanced T1 FS image of the finger shows mild marrow edema adjacent to the erosive changes, and only mild enhancement of the synovium. Concurrent bloodwork revealed normal erythrocyte sedimentation rate (ESR) and C-reactive protein (CRP) level. Findings were most consistent with posttraumatic arthritis.

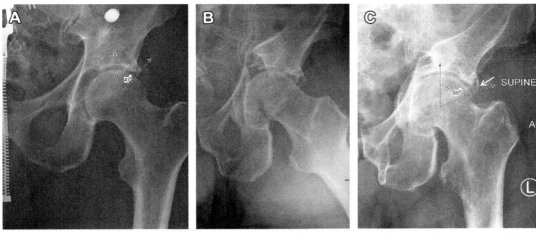

Fig. 4. (A) AP radiograph of the left hip in a 66-year-old man shows moderate degenerative changes, with angle of Wiberg at the upper limits of normal. (B) AP radiograph obtained following a fall, showing a comminuted fracture involving the medial wall of the left acetabulum. (C) AP radiograph obtained 1 year later shows progression of degenerative changes in the left hip joint with relative overgrowth of the superior acetabulum (*white arrow*), as well as acetabular protrusio deformity and increased angle of Wiberg.

plain radiographs and CT.[21] Concurrent existence of medial or lateral ligamentous injury may also lead to articular wear and progressive arthritis in the posttraumatic ankle.

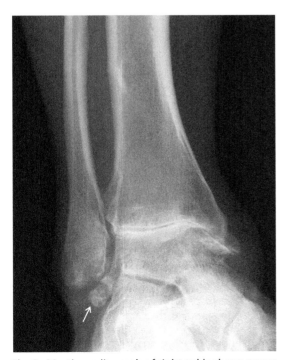

Fig. 5. Mortise radiograph of right ankle shows severe posttraumatic arthritic changes, with asymmetric loss of joint space, subchondral cyst formation, and sclerosis. Multiple osseous loose bodies are present in the posterolateral joint space (*arrow*).

Idiopathic OA of the elbow is also uncommon, and prior trauma underlies most cases. Plain radiographs typically reveal osteophytes along the anterior and posterior aspects of the joint, best appreciated on lateral projections, whereas the AP projection may reveal osteophytes in the olecranon fossa.[11] Underlying malunion, incongruency of the ulnohumeral or radiocapitellar joints, loose bodies, and bone loss or heterotopic bone formation may be seen, and CT may be helpful to further evaluate these findings. MR has a limited role in evaluation of the elbow, except in evaluation of subtle posttraumatic instability.

Posttraumatic glenohumeral arthritis may arise from chondral damage or fracture of either the glenoid or the humeral head. Plain radiographs typically show attendant degenerative changes, including asymmetric loss of joint space and inferior humeral head osteophyte. The degree of malunion and integrity of the rotator cuff are important prognostic and treatment considerations, especially when considering a patient for shoulder arthroplasty, and may be assessed with MR.[22]

The treatment of posttraumatic arthritis is broadly classified as conservative or surgical measures. Conservative measures begin with weight loss and low-impact exercise. Nonsteroidal antiinflammatory medicine is frequently used for symptom control, and arthritic joints may be injected with cortisone or hyaluronic acid; however, these measures neither halt nor reverse the articular damage.[23] At present, surgical therapies remain the only means of correcting the structural and mechanical abnormalities caused by joint injury, and include debridement, reconstruction, and arthroplasty of the worn-out joint surface.[24] Partial joint resurfacing and minimally invasive joint-unloading implants have recently emerged to address the concerns of prosthesis durability in young patients.

A significant number of patients still progress to clinical OA even with the best surgical care of the initial joint injuries.[25] The clear precipitating event presents a unique window of opportunity to intervene early in the acute posttraumatic period. Among trialed therapies for early posttraumatic intervention are caspase inhibitors, which have been shown to reduce chondrocyte apoptosis; and cytokine inhibitors, namely interleukin-1 inhibitors, which have shown antifibrotic and symptom-modifying activity in early patient trials. Growth factors and stem cell therapy have shown articular cartilage regeneration and increased tissue repair, and are currently in clinical evaluation.[26]

AVASCULAR NECROSIS
Andrey Rupasov (University of Rochester Medical Center; Rochester, New York)

Avascular necrosis (AVN), also known as ischemic necrosis, osteonecrosis, and aseptic necrosis, is a disease of impaired osseous blood flow, leading to cellular death and subsequent osseous collapse. AVN has multiple underlying causes and associations, the most frequent of which are trauma, corticosteroid use, and alcohol abuse.[27] The imaging features on plain film radiographs provide the basis for classification and staging of the disease. Treatment options range from conservative measures to joint arthroplasty, directed by location and extent of disease, level of physical activity, and patient age.

The exact prevalence of AVN is not known, and depends on the site involved. The disease commonly affects patients between the third and fifth decades of life and occurs more commonly in men in almost all cases, except for cases associated with systemic lupus erythematosus.[28] By some estimates, AVN of the hip has a male to female predominance of 4:1.[29] No clear racial predilection exists, except for cases associated with sickle cell disease, which occurs in people of African and Mediterranean descent.

AVN has an association with traumatic and nontraumatic conditions. A definitive causal role has been established for some of the associations, based on longitudinal studies and meta-analyses. For example, in patients with direct damage to the vasculature, as with displaced fractures, or direct injury to the bone or marrow elements, as with radiation injury, the cause is clearly identifiable. The causal roles and mechanisms for most associations are less definable, and they are considered risk factors, with the final common pathway of interrupted osseous blood flow.[30]

Traumatic causes of AVN include fracture and dislocation, most commonly involving the hip. The duration of dislocation seems to be a risk factor for progression to necrosis, occurring twice more often in cases in which more than 12 hours have passed before the reduction. Displaced fractures of the femoral neck have been associated with a 15% to 50% prevalence of femoral head necrosis, depending on fracture type, time until reduction, and accuracy of reduction.[31]

The most common nontraumatic cause is use of corticosteroids, which are often used to treat underlying diseases such as systemic lupus erythematosus and rheumatoid arthritis. The incidence of developing AVN as a consequence of these medications is 21% to 37%, and it is estimated to be causative in approximately 30% to 40% of cases in the hip.[32] Patients treated with prolonged high doses of corticosteroids seem to be at the greatest risk of developing AVN; however, these patients often have multiple other risk factors. In many cases, it is difficult to separate the effects on bone of corticosteroids from those of the underlying diseases, such as mineralization defects and osteoporosis associated with renal and liver failure, and vasculitis associated with systemic lupus erythematosus.

Excessive alcohol intake has been identified as an causal factor in osteonecrosis, but difficulties have been encountered in defining the term excessive. A dose-response relationship has been noted, with an intake of more than 400 mL of alcohol per week increasing the risk 10-fold.[33] Alcohol has been considered an associated risk factor in up to 31% of the patients with AVN evaluated; the true prevalence has been difficult to determine because most reports are cross-sectional.

Other disorders associated with AVN include sickle cell disease, Gaucher disease, caisson disease, human immunodeficiency virus (HIV), pancreatitis, and liver and kidney disease. Because AVN eventually develops in only a small percentage of patients with any of these conditions, understanding the cause has been a challenge.[34] Attention has been focused on understanding underlying predispositions to the development of AVN, including genetic mutations leading to hypercoagulability, when challenged by environmental factors. The pathophysiology of all aforementioned nontraumatic causes has the generally agreed-on common pathway of interrupted blood flow, likely occurring by way of intravascular coagulation and/or microcirculatory thrombosis.

Although it can affect any bone, AVN primarily affects the epiphyses of long bones, classically the shoulder, hip, and knee.[30] The most common site is the anterolateral femoral head; other common sites include the femoral condyles, humeral head, proximal tibia, vertebrae, and small bones of the hand and foot. Approximately half of cases show multiple sites of damage, thus, in patients who present with AVN of the knee, shoulder, or other nonhip joint, evaluation of the hips is recommended.

The most common presenting symptom is pain that increases over time.[35] Groin pain that may be referred to the thigh is the usual presentation in patients with femoral head disease. The presence of marrow edema on imaging is highly correlated with degree of pain. Development of fracture or collapse may acutely exacerbate the clinical picture, and findings of limited range of motion or clicking of a joint suggests established collapse of the necrotic fragment. Early diagnosis may provide the opportunity to prevent collapse; because most patients present late in the course of disease, a high index of suspicion is necessary for those with known risk factors.

The imaging of AVN provides the basis for classification and staging systems, such as the Ficat and Arlet classification (Table 1), which is most commonly used by radiologists.[36,37] Although early stages of the disease may not show any radiographic changes, plain films should still be the first step in the diagnostic evaluation. The earliest findings are mild density changes as the surrounding living bone becomes resorbed secondary to reactive hyperemia. This stage is followed by patchy sclerosis along the necrotic trabecula, secondary to new bone formation. Microfractures of the subchondral bone accumulate, creating a crescentic subchondral lucency termed crescent sign (Fig. 6), and eventually leading to articular surface collapse.[38] The size of the infarct is variable, ranging from a small focus to the entire epiphysis, and is associated with higher risk of articular surface collapse.

Evaluation of the hips should begin with AP and frog-leg lateral radiographs. Lateral projection is necessary to evaluate the superior portion of the femoral head, in which subchondral abnormalities are often seen. Advanced findings in the femoral head include subchondral crescent sign signifying impending fracture, loss of sphericity of the femoral head following articular surface collapse, and ultimately joint space narrowing and other degenerative changes of the hip joint (Fig. 7).

CT scans can further characterize the collapse of the femoral head, but provide little additional information and are seldom used, although infrequent asymptomatic cases of AVN are sometimes incidentally discovered. Technetium-99 bone scans were previously used for high-risk patients who had a negative radiographic examination. Increased bone turnover at the junction of dead and reactive bone results in increased uptake surrounding a cold area; this has been called the doughnut sign. Recent studies have shown that bone scans have limited value and are often misleading because they are false-negative in 25% to 45% of cases that have been confirmed by MR imaging.[39] Sensitivity was lowest in patients with early-stage lesions.

MR imaging has become the standard for diagnosing aseptic necrosis, with a sensitivity of 97% and specificity of 98%. In addition, changes may be detected early in the course of the disease, preceding positive findings on other modalities. Any MR protocol for the evaluation of hip pain should include at least 1 sequence that images the opposite hip, preferably a T1-weighted and/or a short tau inversion recovery (STIR) coronal sequence, for the purposes of comparison and detection of asymptomatic disease (Fig. 8). Contrast should be given, if feasible, to better delineate nonviable segments.

Table 1
Ficat and Arlet 4-stage radiologic classification of osteonecrosis of the femoral head

Type of Necrosis	Stages	Joint Line	Femoral Head Contour	Trabeculae
Simple	I	Normal	Normal	Normal or very slight osteoporosis
	II	Normal	Normal	Osteoporosis/mixed sclerosis/porosis
Complicated by collapse	III	Normal	Flattened, subchondral infraction, collapse	Sequestrum formation
	IV	Narrowed	Collapsed	Destruction of superior pole

Data from Jawad MU, Haleem AA, Scully SP. In brief: Ficat classification: avascular necrosis of the femoral head. Clin Orthop Relat Res 2012;470(9):2636–9.

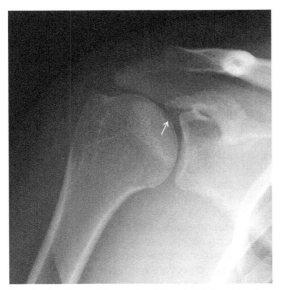

Fig. 6. Grashey radiograph of the right shoulder in a 20-year-old woman on chronic corticosteroids. Sclerosis of the medial humeral head and crescentic subchondral lucency (*arrow*) consistent with avascular necrosis with impending subchondral collapse. (*Case contributed by* Dr Scott Schiffman, University of Rochester Medical Center.)

Early MR findings show nonspecific bone marrow edema, characterized by decreased T1 signal and increased signal on fluid-sensitive sequences.[40] This appearance is nonspecific and has a broad differential; time and evidence of progression are often needed before diagnosis becomes apparent. Characteristic MR changes do not appear until the healing process begins, which may take more than a month. A serpentine line of decreased signal, termed the reactive interface

line and representing sclerosis, appears at the margin of the infarct. Advancing granulation tissue at the inner edge of the sclerotic line is seen as a bright line on T2-weighted sequences, and together they represent the double-line sign, which is a pathognomonic finding (Fig. 9).[41]

It is important to differentiate AVN of the hip from a similarly presenting disorder known as transient osteoporosis of the hip, also known as bone marrow edema syndrome. Transient osteoporosis is most commonly seen in middle-aged men and pregnant women in the third trimester of pregnancy, and is differentiated on MR by increased signal throughout the femoral head and neck Fig. 10. This finding is in contrast with AVN, which appears as a discrete lesion in the femoral head on an MR imaging scan. Transient osteoporosis is self-limiting and is treated conservatively, whereas AVN often requires surgical treatment.[42]

The ultimate goal of treating AVN in any bone is preservation of the joint. Although several therapeutic approaches, ranging from conservative measures to arthroplasty, have been used, nonoperative management has generally been ineffective at halting the progression of disease. These measures include bed rest; partial weight bearing with crutches; and use of analgesics, bisphosphonates, and anticoagulants. Reports suggest that adequate clinical results are attained in only 20% of patients.[43]

Total joint replacement is performed in the shoulders, hips, and knees in cases of collapse with significant osteoarthritis; in cases of collapse without osteoarthritis, a hemiarthroplasty may be performed. Typically, joint replacement is performed only when symptoms justify the surgery. Among the joint-preserving procedures, core decompression is currently the most common, used in early stages of AVN, predominantly in the femoral head and humeral head.[31] Stem cell–based therapies are currently in clinical evaluation.

SEPTIC ARTHRITIS
Usa Cain (University of Rochester Medical Center; Rochester, New York)

In general terms, septic arthritis refers to a joint infection, typically by bacteria, which results in an acute inflammatory process that leads to destructive changes within the joint. The classic definition of a septic arthritis requires clinical signs of an infected joint, usually an erythematous, tender, swollen joint with restricted movement. These clinical signs are seen in combination with positive blood cultures, organisms isolated from the joint, and/or radiologic findings consistent with septic arthritis. Septic arthritis can also be caused by

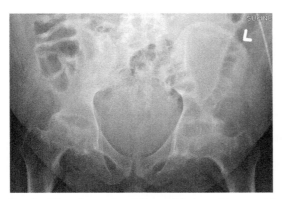

Fig. 7. AP radiograph of the pelvis in a 51-year-old man with alcoholism, presenting after inability to ambulate for several weeks because of bilateral hip pain. Bilateral avascular necrosis of the hips with marked flattening of the femoral heads and severe degenerative disease of bilateral hips.

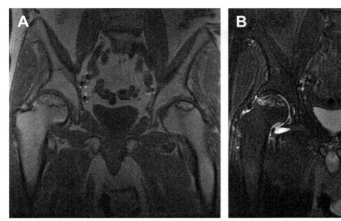

Fig. 8. Coronal T1 (*A*) and coronal T2 FS (*B*) MR images show serpiginous bands of abnormal signal surrounding a geographic focus of bone marrow replacement in the weight-bearing aspect of the femoral heads, consistent with bilateral avascular necrosis. (*Case contributed by* Dr Scott Schiffman, University of Rochester Medical Center.)

infection by fungi, mycobacteria, and spirochetes, which tend to have a more indolent course.[44,45] Predisposing factors include prosthetic joint; intravenous drug use; recent procedure or surgery; age greater than 80 years; and immunocompromised states, such as diabetes, HIV, and rheumatoid arthritis. The primary mode of inoculation is via hematogenous spread, which has been estimated to occur in approximately 72% of cases.[45] The most commonly affected joints include knees, hips, ankles, and wrists. Diagnosis is obtained by synovial fluid aspiration, which is generally purulent with the leukocyte count greater than 50,000/mL. Gram stain and culture may or may not be positive. Blood cultures and serum inflammatory markers,

including C-reactive protein (CRP) and erythrocyte sedimentation rate (ESR) may also be obtained. Inflammatory markers are useful for monitoring treatment response. Procalcitonin is a new serum marker, which has increasing use. Increased procalcitonin levels may be helpful in ruling in septic arthritis but may not be sensitive enough to rule out septic arthritis; cutoff values for diagnosis vary between 0.2 and 0.5 ng/mL.[46]

Treatment is by joint drainage and antibiotics. The joint may be aspirated to dryness as often as needed. Arthroscopy or arthrotomy may be needed for large joints. The most common nongonococcal pathogen is *Staphylococcus aureus*, but streptococci can also be seen. Gram-negative bacilli are

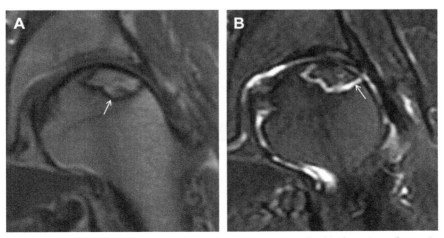

Fig. 9. Coronal T1 and coronal T2 FS MR images show the characteristic double-line sign of aseptic necrosis. (*A*) The T1-hypointense outer dark line (*arrow*) represents sclerosis at the border between the infarcted and normal bone. (*B*) The T2-bright inner line (*arrow*) is created by the advancing granulation tissue/inflammatory response. (*Case contributed by* Dr Scott Schiffman, University of Rochester Medical Center.)

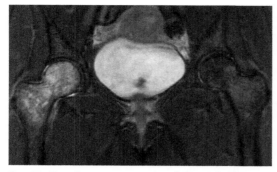

Fig. 10. Transient osteoporosis of the right hip in a 33-year-old woman. Coronal inversion recovery sequence shows diffusely increased marrow signal throughout the proximal right femur, in a more diffuse pattern than is present in osteonecrosis and without a discrete fracture.

typically seen in immunocompromised patients, intravenous (IV) drug users, and in the setting of trauma.

Empiric treatment is with intravenous antibiotics: common treatment regimens include vancomycin for gram-positive cocci; ceftriaxone for gram-negative cocci; azithromycin for chlamydia coverage; and ceftazidime, cefepime, piperacillin-tazobactam, or a carbapenem for gram-negative rods. If the Gram stain is negative, consider vancomycin in combination with ceftriaxone or cefepime. There is no role for intra-articular therapy because parenteral and oral therapy are sufficient to produce therapeutic levels of drug within synovial fluid. The use of corticosteroids is controversial; however, it may improve the recovery rate of septic arthritis in children.

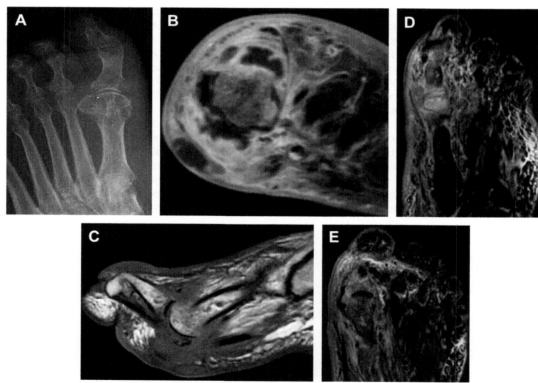

Fig. 11. A 67-year-old woman with a history of diabetic neuropathy. She noted a callus on the plantar aspect of her great toe, which subsequently opened into a nonhealing ulcer. She was initially treated with empiric antibiotics, but she developed chills, increased white blood cell count, CRP level, and ESR without improvement in the foot ulcer. Radiograph findings include extensive soft tissue swelling. The radiopaque marker sits at the site of a shallow plantar-based ulcer near the first metatarsophalangeal (MTP) joint. There is a focal calcification along the MTP as well as demineralization of the medial aspect at the base of first proximal phalanx. (A) Axial T1 FS with contrast and sagittal T1 image show a soft tissue ulcer and abscess extending into the first MTP joint. (B, C) Long-axis STIR images reveal moderate to large first MTP joint effusion, thick enhancement noted on contrast images, and there is associated bone marrow edema of the base of proximal phalanx as well as the head of the first metatarsal. These findings were consistent with septic arthritis complicated by osteomyelitis (D, E). (Case contributed by Dr Scott Schiffman, University of Rochester Medical Center.)

Complications of septic arthritis include cartilage and bony damage, osteomyelitis, and systemic sepsis/shock (**Figs. 11** and **12**). Nongonococcal septic monoarthritis has a reported mortality as high as 10% in adult patients; older age is associated with higher mortality.[47]

Plain radiograph and joint ultrasonography are preferred initial studies to assess for septic arthritis, although the diagnosis is made clinically.[48]

Initial radiographs may be nondiagnostic for septic arthritis but are considered as a baseline assessment for joint damage. Radiographs of the acute septic joint are likely to show joint effusion and may show chondrocalcinosis. Bacteria within the joint space create an acute inflammatory response, hyperplasia of synovial lining, and large joint effusion with widening of the joint space (**Fig. 13**). Cytokines released by inflammatory cells promote the degradation of cartilage and impede chondrocyte synthesis of cartilage. As the disease progresses, articular cartilage is damaged, and marginal erosions become apparent. Superimposed osteomyelitis, as shown by periosteal reaction, bony destruction, and osteonecrosis, result in sequestrum formation. Sequestra are pieces of bone that are separated from vascularized bone via resorption of intervening necrotic bone (**Fig. 14**).

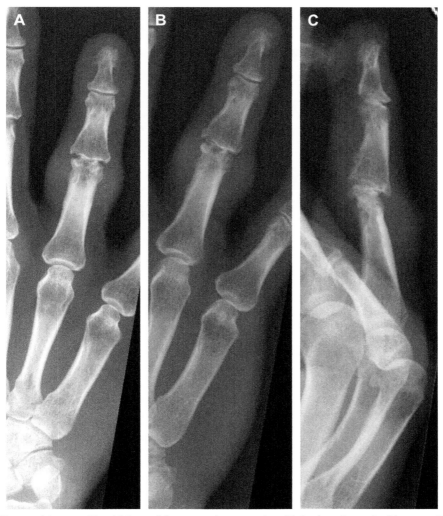

Fig. 12. A 53-year-old man with a history of Down syndrome and multiple chronic medical issues, with right ring finger pain. Right fourth digit radiographs (PA [*A*], oblique [*B*], lateral [*C*] projections) reveal soft tissue swelling at the fourth proximal interphalangeal joint with erosions involving the head of the proximal phalanx and the base of the middle phalanx, best appreciated on the lateral view (*C*). These findings were found to be consistent with septic arthritis and chronic osteomyelitis. (*Case contributed by* Dr Scott Schiffman, University of Rochester Medical Center.)

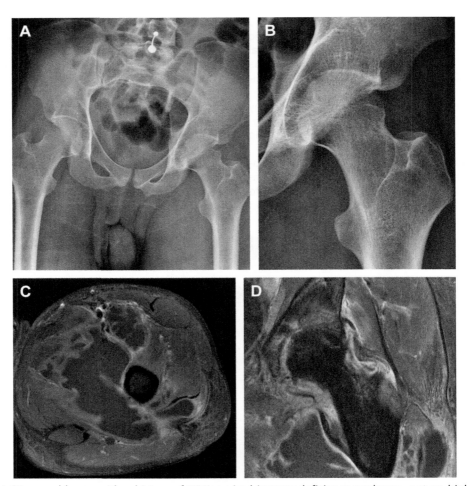

Fig. 13. A 24-year-old man with a history of HIV/acquired immunodeficiency syndrome, not on highly active antiretroviral treatment, who presented after 1 week of left hip and thigh pain, no trauma, and the inability to walk. He had a fever and CD4 count of 206 cells/mm³. Imaging revealed a left iliopsoas abscess extending into the thigh and hip. Pelvic (A) and AP left hip (B) radiographs show severe joint space loss of the left hip. Axial and coronal T1 FS with contrast MR images (C, D) with a large rim-enhancing fluid collection consistent with abscess noted in the adductor musculature of the proximal thigh. Moderate left hip effusion with enhancing synovium consistent with synovitis. Severe loss of articular cartilage without significant erosive changes. (*Case contributed by* Dr Scott Schiffman, University of Rochester Medical Center.)

MR imaging is typically not recommended for initial diagnosis of septic arthritis; however, it may be helpful if underlying osteomyelitis is suspected. The contrast agent gadolinium increases the sensitivity of MR imaging for detection of early osteomyelitis and associated soft tissue disease (see **Fig. 11**).

Bone scan may be considered; it is highly sensitive but not specific in the presence of existing bone disorder, prosthetic joint, recent surgery, or trauma. A 3-phase bone scan has sensitivity and specificity of 95%. Radionuclide indium-111–labeled leukocytes improved the specificity of identifying osteomyelitis in patients with prosthesis or underlying disorder.

COMPLEX REGIONAL PAIN SYNDROME
Simone Montoya (University of Rochester Medical Center; Rochester, New York)

Complex regional pain syndrome (CRPS) is a condition with a long and controversial history. It is characterized by chronic pain and a combination of sensory, motor, vasomotor, and/or sudomotor findings after trauma, surgery, or other noxious event. Previous names used for this spectrum of conditions include Sudeck atrophy, algodystrophy, and reflex sympathetic dystrophy. The current terminology arose as a result of a consensus conference held by a special task force of the International Association of the Study of Pain in 1994,[49]

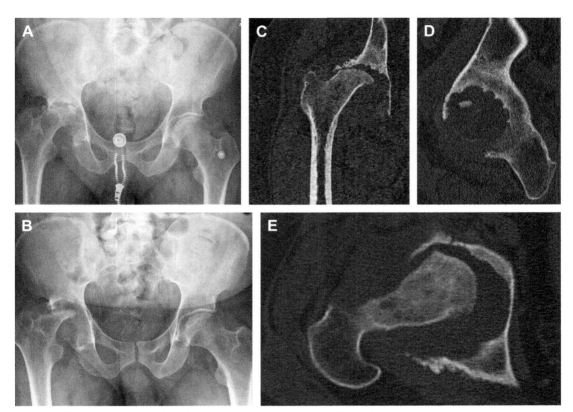

Fig. 14. A 39-year-old man with a history of follicular lymphoma after autologous stem cell transplant associated with septic shock. He was found to have a right iliopsoas muscle abscess with associated right hip septic arthritis, and right acetabular osteomyelitis. He required operative washout. Cultures were positive for methicillin-sensitive *S aureus*. He was treated with 12 weeks of IV nafcillin, with improvement in his CRP and ESR values. There are 2 pelvic radiographs (*A, B*); the second is 9 months after the first. There are advanced erosive destructive changes of the right hip compared with the left hip. There is flattening of the femoral head and interval progression of acetabular protrusion. AP (*C*), sagittal (*D*), and axial (*E*) CT images of the right hip show involvement of both the femoral head and the acetabulum, suggestive of septic arthritis/osteomyelitis (*C*). On CT, the acetabular thinning and scalloping is better appreciated. There is osteochondral fracture of the inferior acetabulum (*D*). Evidence of periostitis of the superior acetabulum. Several intra-articular bodies were noted within the joint, likely resultant sequestra. (*Case contributed by* Dr Scott Schiffman, University of Rochester Medical Center.)

with the goal of creating a name that would encompass the wide range of presentations (complex) and also allude to the hallmark finding (regional distribution of pain). Type 1 represents almost all cases and is what was historically referred to as reflex sympathetic dystrophy, and type 2 refers to what was previously known as causalgia; both have the same set of criteria but type 2 has a known nerve injury, whereas type 1 does not. Specific diagnostic criteria (the Budapest criteria[50]) were proposed in 2007 and were recently revised in 2013.[51] Notably, current criteria still do not include imaging, although distinctive findings have been described with several modalities over the years. Findings on radiographs, bone scans, and MR imaging may be characteristic but do not necessarily correlate temporally with the clinical picture. Thus,

imaging remains of limited utility for diagnosis but can be used for confirmation.

Over the years, CRPS has been known colloquially as Sudeck atrophy. Paul Sudeck, a German surgeon and early adopter of radiography, described in his 1900 article "Acute Inflammatory Bone Atrophy" several examples of increased bone lucency after an inflammatory event, suggestive of an active process of bone loss.[52] Radiography in CRPS may be normal but many cases show osteopenia out of proportion to the expected amount for disuse; this is usually seen late in the disease process. Many groups have described patchy osteopenia seen several weeks (ie, >8 weeks) after the initial insult[53]; this is by far the most common finding. It is usually more pronounced in the periarticular regions (**Fig. 15**)

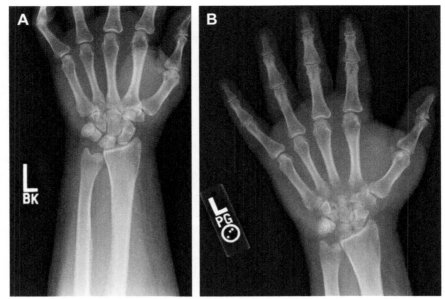

Fig. 15. (*A*) Plain radiographs of the left wrist taken immediately after a hyperextension injury shows no osseous abnormality. (*B*) After 1 month, there is marked periarticular osteopenia of the distal radius and ulna, multiple carpals, and the bases of the metacarpals. There is also diffuse soft tissue swelling of the entire left hand.

but is not accompanied by other prominent joint changes such as joint space loss and intra-articular erosions seen in arthritides.[54] Other findings that can be seen include soft tissue swelling, cortical bone resorption, and erosions.[55] Differentiating CRPS from posttraumatic disuse osteopenia can be difficult[56]; it has been postulated that the two may arise from a similar pathogenesis, which is hastened or augmented in CRPS.[57]

There are 3 stages described for CRPS, with significant overlap and time variability.[58,59] First, within several weeks of the initiating trauma there is pain and swelling out of proportion to the degree of injury, associated with hyperalgesia/allodynia. Second, occurring over several months, the edema becomes more thick and firm, and there is notable joint stiffness. Third, over a year from the initial insult, pain is less severe (but still persistent), and there are signs of atrophy and osteopenia. Scintigraphy classically shows increased uptake in the affected limb on all phases (blood flow, blood pool, and delayed static), diffusely throughout the limb but particularly at the joints (**Fig. 16**). Findings can be bilateral, but are more severe in the affected limb. Demangeat and colleagues[60] described 3 stages of CRPS with different patterns. Up to 20 weeks there is hyperperfusion (blood flow/velocity), increased vascularity (blood pool), and hyperfixation on delayed images. From 20 to 60 weeks there is normalization of blood flow and blood pool, but persistent hyperfixation. After 60 weeks there is usually decreased blood flow and blood pool along with normalization on delayed images; scintigraphy may be overall normal late in

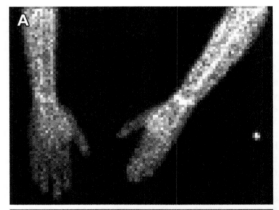

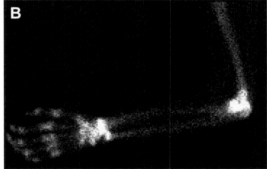

Fig. 16. Triple-phase bone scintigraphy after right elbow dislocation, obtained in the posterior projection (right arm is on the right in the image). There is increased perfusion to the distal right upper extremity on blood flow phase (not shown), diffuse hyperemia of right extremity relative to the left on blood pool phase (*A*), and increased polyarticular radiotracer uptake after a 3-hour delay (*B*).

the disease. However, these scintigraphic stages do not necessarily correlate with the clinical stages, and, although findings are highly specific, they are not sensitive to CRPS. Thus CRPS remains a clinical diagnosis, with triple-phase bone scintigraphy (TPBS) being used as a confirmatory test.

MR imaging has proved useful in CRPS because of its ability to characterize the bone as well as the soft tissues. Findings include (periarticular) bone marrow edema (**Fig. 17**), soft tissue edema, skin changes, joint effusions, skin and intra-articular contrast enhancement, muscle atrophy, and fibrosis of periarticular structures.[53–56] There is a typical pattern of bone marrow signal (decreased on T1-weighted sequences, increased on T2-weighted sequences, and contrast enhancing) that indicates bone marrow edema, likely caused by a combination of hyperemia, increased bone metabolism, and inflammation.[54] MR imaging also shows different stages, each with characteristic findings.[61] Stage 1 has skin thickening (with or without enhancement) and soft tissue edema. Stage 2 has skin thinning, usually without enhancement. Stage 3 has muscle atrophy. Joint effusions are seen early, in stages 1 and 2. MR imaging abnormalities often correspond with the same areas of increased scintigraphic uptake. MR imaging, like TPBS, remains an ancillary test; however, the avoidance of radiation and additional information about nonosseous structures may favor the utility of MR imaging rather than TPBS.

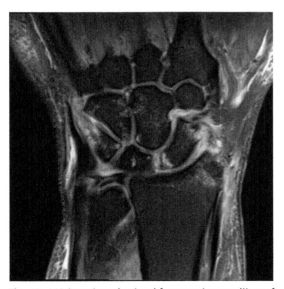

Fig. 17. MR imaging obtained for ongoing swelling of the left hand and left arm pain after nonspecific wrist injury 2 months prior. Proton density image in the coronal projection reveals periarticular edema at multiple carpal bones.

CANCER MIMICKING ARTHRITIS
Usa Cain (University of Rochester Medical Center; Rochester, New York)

There are several instances in which cancer can mimic the appearance of arthritis. Primary imaging modalities for musculoskeletal disorders include plain film radiography, CT, and MR imaging.

Plain film is the initial choice of modality because it is the most useful for characterization of neoplastic margins. The zone of transition is useful to distinguish between benign and malignant lesions. It is limited for evaluation of soft tissue tumors. CT is most helpful for detection of juxta-articular lesions, which are not well seen on radiographs. CT is more sensitive for further evaluation of the bone, including cortical invasion, periosteal reaction, and pathologic fracture. Soft tissue involvement on CT is better seen with the use of IV contrast. MR imaging is useful for preoperative planning; because it is most helpful in assessing soft tissue, it is used to delineate the tumor in relation to neurovascular structures, as well as for medullary and extracortical spread. Bone scintigraphy takes advantage of the increased uptake of technetium-99m–labeled methylene diphosphonate in processes that increase bone turnover, such as infection, neoplasm, trauma, and arthritis. It can be useful in documenting the presence of metastatic disease and arthritis because it is more sensitive than CT; however, findings are nonspecific and bone scan is usually performed in conjunction with other imaging modalities.

There are several benign intra-articular tumors and tumorlike lesions that can mimic the symptoms and appearance of arthritis, including synovial osteochondromatosis, pigmented villonodular synovitis (PVNS; also known as tenosynovial giant cell tumor), lipoma arborescens, and an intra-articular ganglion cyst. Malignant intra-articular diseases include synovial sarcoma and synovial chondrosarcoma. Several of these intra-articular processes are caused by disorders of the synovium, which is the connective tissue that lines the inner surface of joint capsules; it is responsible for maintaining synovial joint fluid.[62–65]

PVNS is a benign idiopathic process characterized by synovial hypertrophy with hemosiderin deposition, primarily seen in young and middle-aged adults. On plain film there may be a joint effusion and erosive changes without significant osteophyte formation. On MR imaging, there are nodular intra-articular masses with low T1, T2, and STIR signal intensity caused by hemosiderin deposition. Furthermore, there are bony erosions and possible extra-articular extension (**Fig. 18**).

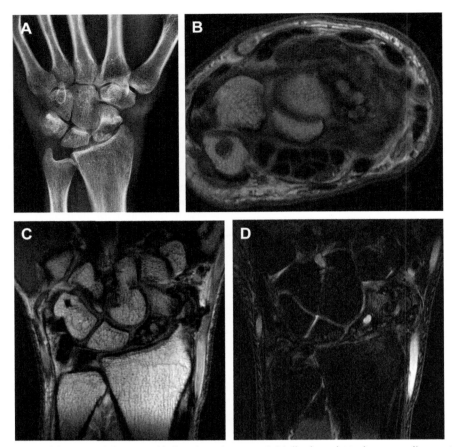

Fig. 18. A 23-year-old man with history of left wrist volar mass, initially thought to be a ganglion cyst with teno-synovitis. Progressive problems with movement and heavier activities. Found to have a scaphoid lucency on wrist radiographs. Subsequent MR imaging consistent with PVNS with erosions of the proximal pole of the scaphoid. PA left wrist radiograph (*A*) shows a lucency of the proximal pole of the scaphoid with sclerotic changes; this could be the appearance of an old healing fracture with cystic degeneration. Axial proton density (*B*) as well as coronal proton density and coronal intermediate T2 MR imaging images (*C, D*) reveal a pressure erosion in the distal radius and distal scaphoid along with chondral loss in the radiocarpal joint. There is extensive cystic change in the proximal pole of the radius. The joint space is filled with multiple lobulated areas of low T1/T2 signal intensity, consistent with PVNS. (*Case contributed by* Dr Scott Schiffman, University of Rochester Medical Center.)

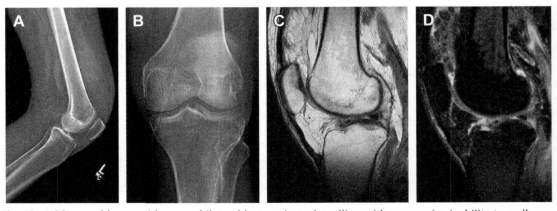

Fig. 19. A 56-year-old man with severe bilateral knee pain and swelling with progressive inability to walk over the course of 1 year. AP and lateral left knee radiographs (*A, B*) primarily notable for suprapatellar soft tissue fullness and joint effusion with some joint space narrowing. Sagittal proton density (*C*) and FS (*D*) images show a multilobulated villous synovial mass, which shows fat suppression, within the joint space. Patient underwent extensive synovectomy and tumor removal of the bilateral knees. Pathology diagnosis of lipoma arbores-cens with extensive gouty tophi, fat necrosis, and chronic inflammatory changes. (*Case contributed by* Dr Scott Schiffman, University of Rochester Medical Center.)

Likewise, synovial osteochondromatosis is a benign disorder of the synovial lining with the presence of intra-articular cartilaginous bodies that ossify in most cases. Secondary osteoarthritis is usually present because of damage from loose bodies.

Lipoma arborescens is an idiopathic intra-articular process characterized by benign lipomatous proliferation of the synovium. It may arise as a response to chronic inflammation caused by an alternate disease, such as rheumatoid arthritis or gout. Lipoma arborescens is most commonly

seen in the knee, usually in men in their fourth or fifth decade[66] (**Fig. 19**).

Skeletal metastases are the most common malignant tumor of the bone, and can mimic erosive changes of arthritis if there is involvement of the joint space (**Figs. 20** and **21**). Synovial sarcoma and chondrosarcoma are rare tumors arising from the synovium and usually present with joint pain and soft tissue mass. Primary soft tissue sarcomas may present as a painless mass that may or may not involve bone.

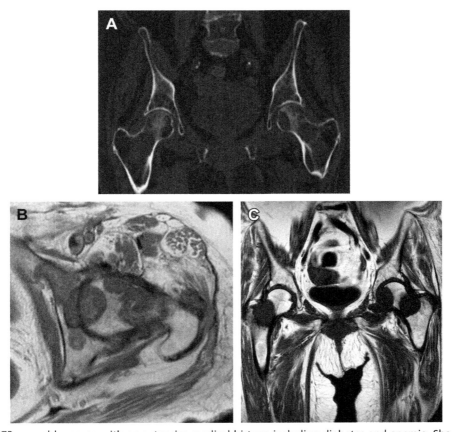

Fig. 20. A 73-year-old woman with an extensive medical history, including diabetes and anemia. She presented with progressive left hip pain and was found to have multiple lytic lesions of her left hip. Biopsy revealed lambda light chain multiple myeloma and amyloidosis. Coronal CT with bilateral femoral neck lytic lesions and left femoral head lytic lesion (*A*), axial proton density (*B*), and coronal T1 (*C*) MR images reveal low T1 marrow replacing lesions of the bilateral femoral necks and a left femoral head lesion with soft tissue component extending into the joint space. Patient went on to get a bone scan, which was negative. Biopsy was inconclusive. She underwent left hip arthroplasty, and pathology found clonal plasma cell infiltrate and extensive acellular amyloid deposition consistent with amyloidoma. Amyloidosis can occur alone or in association with multiple myeloma; it is a plasma cell dyscrasia caused by extracellular deposition of monoclonal protein derived from immunoglobulin light chain fragments. Amyloid deposition in muscles can result in pseudohypertrophy, stereotypically macroglossia with scalloping of the lateral tongue.[45,46] Amyloid arthropathy tends to occur in the shoulders, knees, wrists, metacarpophalangeal joints, and proximal interphalangeal joints, and less commonly in the elbows and hips. Symptoms include joint pain and morning stiffness. Osteolytic tumors of the bone are at increased risk of pathologic fracture. (*Case contributed by* Dr Scott Schiffman, University of Rochester Medical Center.)

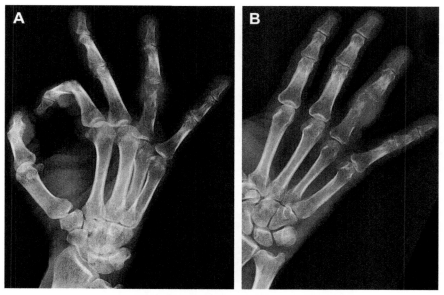

Fig. 21. A 44-year-old man with history of stage IV lung adenocarcinoma presenting with right ring finger pain. On oblique and PA radiographs of the right hand (*A*, *B*), there are extensive erosive changes of fourth proximal interphalangeal joint with overhanging edges, periarticular osteopenia, and significant soft tissue swelling; this could be the appearance of gout. Given the osteolysis, infection could also be considered. However, in this patient with metastatic bronchogenic carcinoma, metastases would also have this appearance. Pathology was consistent with poorly differentiated carcinoma. (*Case contributed by* Dr Scott Schiffman, University of Rochester Medical Center.)

REFERENCES

1. Buckwalter JA, Felson DT. Post-traumatic arthritis: definitions and burden of disease. In: Olson SA, Guilak F, editors. Post-traumatic arthritis: pathogenesis, diagnosis and management. New York: Springer Media; 2015. p. 8–13.
2. Louden K. Investigations show new link between trauma and arthritis. In: AAOS Now. 2009. Available at: http://www.aaos.org/news/aaosnow/may09/research4.asp. Accessed February 26, 2017.
3. Pickering RD. Post-traumatic arthritis. Can Fam Physician 1984;30:1511–3.
4. Punzi L, Galozzi P, Luisetto R, et al. Post-traumatic arthritis: overview on pathogenic mechanisms and role of inflammation. RMD Open 2016;2(2):e000279.
5. Martin JA, Buckwalter JA. Post-traumatic osteoarthritis: the role of stress induced chondrocyte damage. Biorheology 2006;43(3–4):517–21.
6. Ostałowska A, Kasperczyk S, Kasperczyk A, et al. Oxidant and anti-oxidant systems of synovial fluid from patients with knee post-traumatic arthritis. J Orthop Res 2007;25(6):804–12.
7. Anderson DD, Chubinskaya S, Guilak F, et al. Post-traumatic osteoarthritis: improved understanding and opportunities for early intervention. J Orthop Res 2011;29(6):802–9.
8. McKinley TO, Tochigi Y, Rudert MJ, et al. The effect of incongruity and instability on contact stress directional gradients in human cadaveric ankles. Osteoarthritis Cartilage 2008;16(11):1363–9.
9. Goldring SR. Pathophysiology of post-traumatic arthritis. Osteoarthritis and Cartilage 2012;20:S7.
10. Jacobson JA, Girish G, Jiang Y, et al. Radiographic evaluation of arthritis: degenerative joint disease and variations. Radiology 2008;248(3):737–47.
11. Parsons B, Reddy S, Ramsey M. Elbow arthroplasty. In: Garino JP, Beredjiklian PK, editors. Adult reconstruction and arthroplasty: core knowledge in orthopedics. Philadelphia: Elsevier Science; 2007. p. 211–44.
12. Peters AC, Lafferty PM, Jacobson AR, et al. The effect of articular reduction after fractures on posttraumatic degenerative arthritis. JBJS Rev 2013;1(2):e4.
13. Hartley BR, Roberts CS, Giannoudis PV. Current treatment and outcomes of intra-articular fractures. In: Olson SA, Guilak F, editors. Post-traumatic arthritis: pathogenesis, diagnosis and management. New York: Springer Media; 2015. p. 269–83.
14. Omoumi P, Mercier GA, Lecouvet F, et al. CT arthrography, MR arthrography, PET, and scintigraphy in osteoarthritis. Radiol Clin North Am 2009;47:595–615.
15. Kijowski R, Roemer F, Englund M, et al. Imaging following acute knee trauma. Osteoarthritis Cartilage 2014;22(10):1429–43.
16. Ravaud P, Giraudeau B, Auleley GR, et al. Radiographic assessment of knee osteoarthritis:

reproducibility and sensitivity to change. J Rheumatol 1996;23:1756–64.

17. Tochigi Y, Vaseenon T, Heiner AD, et al. Instability dependency of osteoarthritis development in a rabbit model of graded anterior cruciate ligament transection. J Bone Joint Surg Am 2011;93(7):640–7.

18. Laird A, Keating JF. Acetabular fractures: a 16-year prospective epidemiological study. J Bone Joint Surg Br 2005;87:969–73.

19. McBride MT, Muldoon MP, Santore RF, et al. Protrusio acetabuli: diagnosis and treatment. J Am Acad Orthop Surg 2001;9(2):79–88.

20. Goodman SB, Schurman DG. Miscellaneous disorders. In: Steinberg ME, editor. The hip and its disorders. Philadelphia: Saunders; 1991. p. 683–6.

21. Reddy S, Pedowitz D, Okereke E. Ankle arthroplasty. In: Garino JP, Beredjiklian PK, editors. Adult reconstruction and arthroplasty: core knowledge in orthopedics. Philadelphia: Elsevier Science; 2007. p. 157–79.

22. Gartsman GM, Edwards TB. Chapter 6 - Indications and contraindications. In: Shoulder arthroplasty. Philadelphia: Saunders Elsevier; 2008. p. 45–60.

23. Kramer WC, Hendricks KJ, Wang J. Pathogenetic mechanisms of posttraumatic osteoarthritis: opportunities for early intervention. Int J Clin Exp Med 2011;4(4):285–98.

24. Buechel FF. Knee arthroplasty in post-traumatic arthritis. J Arthroplasty 2002;17(4 Suppl 1):63–8.

25. Marsh JL, Buckwalter J, Gelberman R, et al. Articular fractures: does an anatomic reduction really change the result? J Bone Joint Surg Am 2002;84-A(7):1259–71.

26. Lotz MK. Posttraumatic osteoarthritis: pathogenesis and pharmacological treatment options. Arthritis Res Ther 2010;12:211.

27. Ferri FF. Avascular necrosis. In: Ferri FF, editor. Ferri's clinical advisor 2017. Philadelphia: Elsevier; 2017. p. 155–7.

28. Hanumantharaya GH, Kamala GR. A study on AVN cases attending at a tertiary care hospital: etiological factors and treatment. Indian J Orthopaedics Surg 2016;2(1):69–76.

29. Dunn AW, Grow T. Aseptic necrosis of the femoral head. Treatment with bone grafts of doubtful value. Clin Orthop 1977;122:249–54.

30. Chang CC, Greenspan A, Gershwin ME. Osteonecrosis: current perspectives on pathogenesis and treatment. Semin Arthritis Rheum 1993;23(1):47.

31. Lieberman JR, Berry DJ, Montv MA, et al. Osteonecrosis of the hip: management in the twenty-first century. J Bone Joint Surg Am 2002;84:834–53.

32. Shigemura T, Nakamura J, Kishida S, et al. Incidence of osteonecrosis associated with corticosteroid therapy among different underlying diseases: prospective MRI study. Rheumatology 2011;50:2023.

33. Matsuo K, Hirohata T, Sugioka Y, et al. Influence of alcohol intake, cigarette smoking, and occupational status on idiopathic osteonecrosis of the femoral head. Clin Orthop 1988;234:115–23.

34. Cruess RL. Steroid-induced osteonecrosis. J R Coll Surg Edinb 1981;26:69–77.

35. Zizic TM, Marcoux C, Hungerford DS, et al. The early diagnosis of ischemic necrosis of bone. Arthritis Rheum 1986;29:1177.

36. Jawad MU, Haleem AA, Scully SP. In brief: Ficat classification: avascular necrosis of the femoral head. Clin Orthop Relat Res 2012;470(9):2636–9.

37. Lee GC, Khoury V, Steinberg D. How do radiologists evaluate osteonecrosis? Skeletal Radiol 2014;43(5):607–14.

38. Mazieres B. Osteonecrosis. In: Hochberg MC, Silman AJ, Smolen JS, et al, editors. Rheumatology. London: Mosby; 2003. p. 1877.

39. Beltran J, Herman LJ, Burk JM, et al. Femoral head avascular necrosis: MR imaging with clinical-pathologic and radionuclide correlation. Radiology 1988;166:215–20.

40. Stevens K, Tao C, Lee SU, et al. Subchondral fractures in osteonecrosis of the femoral head: comparison of radiography, CT, and MR imaging. AJR Am J Roentgenol 2003;180(2):363–8.

41. Zurlo JV. The double-line sign. Radiology 1999;212(2):541–2.

42. Glickstein MF, Burk DL, Schiebler ML, et al. Avascular necrosis versus other diseases of the hip: sensitivity of MR imaging. Radiology 1998;169:213–5.

43. Mont MA, Carbone JJ, Fairbank AC. Core decompression versus nonoperative management for osteonecrosis of the hip. Clin Orthop Relat Res 1996;(324):169–78.

44. Morgan DS, Fisher D, Merianos A, et al. An 18 year clinical review of septic arthritis from tropical Australia. Epidemiol Infect 1996;117:423.

45. Goldenberg DL, Reed JI. Bacterial arthritis. N Engl J Med 1985;312(12):764–71.

46. Shen CJ, Wu MS, Lin KH, et al. The use of procalcitonin in the diagnosis of bone and joint infection: a systemic review and meta-analysis. Eur J Clin Microbiol Infect Dis 2013;32(6):807–14.

47. Gavet F, Tournadre A, Soubrier M, et al. Septic arthritis in patients aged 80 and older: a comparison with younger adults. J Am Geriatr Soc 2005;53(7):1210–3.

48. Beaman FD, von Herrmann PF, Kransdorf MJ, et al, Expert Panel on Musculoskeletal Imaging. ACR Appropriateness Criteria® suspected osteomyelitis, septic arthritis, or soft tissue infection (excluding spine and diabetic foot). Reston (VA): American College of Radiology (ACR); 2016. p. 15.

49. Stanton-Hicks M, Jänig W, Hassenbusch S, et al. Reflex sympathetic dystrophy: changing concepts and taxonomy. Pain 1995;63:127–33.

50. Harden RN, Bruehl S, Stanton-Hicks M, et al. Proposed new diagnostic criteria for complex regional pain syndrome. Pain Med 2007;8:326–31.

51. Harden RN, Oaklander AL, Burton AW, et al. Complex regional pain syndrome: practical diagnostic and treatment guidelines, 4th edition. Pain Med 2013;14:180–229.

52. Iolascon G, de Sire A, Moretti A, et al. Complex regional pain syndrome (CRPS) type I: historical perspective and critical issues. Clin Cases Miner Bone Metab 2015;12:4–10.

53. Albazaz R, Wong YT, Homer-Vanniasinkam S. Complex regional pain syndrome: a review. Ann Vasc Surg 2008;22:297–306.

54. Borré GE, Borré DG, Hofer B, et al. Sudeck's dystrophy of the hand. Clin Imaging 1995;19:188–92.

55. Cappello ZJ, Kasdan ML, Louis DS. Meta-analysis of imaging techniques for the diagnosis of complex regional pain syndrome type I. J Hand Surg 2012; 37A:288–96.

56. Schürmann M, Zaspel J, Löhr P, et al. Imaging in early posttraumatic complex regional pain syndrome. Clin J Pain 2007;23:449–57.

57. Bickerstaff DR, O'Doherty DP, Kanis JA. Radiographic changes in algodystrophy of the hand. J Hand Surg 1991;16:47–52.

58. Lee GW, Weeks PM. The role of bone scintigraphy in diagnosing reflex sympathetic dystrophy. J Hand Surg 1995;20A:458–63.

59. Fournier RS, Holder LE. Reflex sympathetic dystrophy: diagnostic controversies. Semin Nucl Med 1998;28:116–23.

60. Demangeat J-L, Constantinesco A, Brunot B, et al. Three-phase bone scanning in reflex sympathetic dystrophy of the hand. J Nucl Med 1988;29:26–32.

61. Graif M, Schweitzer ME, Marks B, et al. Synovial effusion in reflex sympathetic dystrophy: an additional sign for diagnosis and staging. Skeletal Radiol 1998;27:262–5.

62. Frick MA, Wenger DE, Adkins M. MR imaging of synovial disorders of the knee: an update. Radiol Clin North Am 2007;45:1017.

63. Resnick D. Tumors and tumor-like lesions of bone: imaging and pathology of specific lesions. In: Resnick D, editor. Diagnosis of bone and joint disorders. Third editon. Philadelphia: W.B. Saunders; 1995. p. 3939–81.

64. M'bappé P, Grateau G. Osteo-articular manifestations of amyloidosis. Best Pract Res Clin Rheumatol 2012;26:459.

65. Dhir V, Shukla S, Haroon N, et al. Medical image. Arthritis and macroglossia. Multiple myeloma complicated by amyloidosis causing arthropathy. N Z Med J 2007;120:U2534.

66. Vilanova JC, Barceló J, Villalón M, et al. MR imaging of lipoma arborescens and the associated lesions. Skeletal Radiol 2003;32:504.

Imaging of Childhood Vasculitis

Claudio Granata, MD[a], Maria Beatrice Damasio, MD[a], Federico Zaottini, MD[b],
Sonia Airaldi, MD[b], Clara Malattia, MD[c], Giovanna Stefania Colafati, MD[d],
Paolo Tomà, MD[d], Gianmichele Magnano, MD[a], Carlo Martinoli, MD[b],*

KEYWORDS

- Children • Ultrasound • Computed tomography • MR imaging • Vasculitis

KEY POINTS

- Childhood vasculitis is a challenging and complex group of conditions that are multisystem in nature and often require an integrated multi-imaging approach.
- Diagnostic imaging has a pivotal role in the diagnosis of vasculitis. Selection of the most appropriate imaging modality to help proper diagnosis of pediatric vasculitis is of the upmost importance.
- In large and medium vasculitis, conventional DSA has been replaced in most cases by CT and MR angiography, whereas in small-vessel vasculitis cross-sectional imaging with ultrasound, CT, and MR imaging has a pivotal role in the evaluation of target organ damage.

INTRODUCTION

Primary childhood vasculitides are a complex group of rare multisystem diseases associated with significant morbidity and mortality with an estimated annual incidence of approximately 23 to 50 per 1 million.[1,2] These conditions account for approximately 2% to 10% of all disorders that are pertinent to pediatric rheumatology clinics.[3] Generally speaking, the term vasculitis refers to changes occurring in the vessel wall induced by inflammation. Initially, symptoms may be insidious and nonspecific, including fever, malaise, increased erythrocyte sedimentation rate and C-reactive protein, and diffuse regional pain. As damage progresses, aneurysmal dilatation, stenosis, and occlusion may occur and there may be onset of specific symptoms depending on the target organs, type and size of vasculature, and extent of vascular involvement. The pathogenesis of primary childhood vasculitis is not fully understood, although abnormal regulation of immunocomplex formation, impaired lymphocyte regulation, and antecedent infections have been variably implicated depending on the disease condition. Some ethnic difference in prevalence (eg, higher incidence in Asian and Turkish children) suggests that genetics and environment may play a pathogenetic role. In children, secondary vasculitis may be encountered following hepatitis B or C infection, drug therapies (eg, antithyroid agents, tumor necrosis factor-α inhibitors), other autoimmune diseases (eg, systemic lupus erythematosus, juvenile dermatomyositis, juvenile idiopathic arthritis), and malignancies.[3]

Nomenclature and Classification

Childhood vasculitis encompasses a wide range of subcategories that are mainly defined based on vessel size including predominantly large, medium, and small blood vessel vasculitis

Disclosure: The authors have nothing to disclose.
[a] Radiologia, IRCCS Gaslini Children Hospital, Via Gerolamo Gaslini 5, I-16147, Genova, Italy; [b] Radiologia III, IRCCS San Martino-IST, DISSAL, Università di Genova, Via Pastore 1, I-16132, Genova, Italy; [c] Pediatria II, Reumatologia, IRCCS Gaslini Children Hospital, Via Gerolamo Gaslini 5, I-16147, Genova, Italy; [d] Radiologia, IRCCS Ospedale Pediatrico Bambino Gesù, Piazza S. Onofrio 4, I-00165, Roma, Italy
* Corresponding author. Department of Health Science, Ospedale Policlinico San Martino, University of Genoa, Viale Pastore 1, Genova I-16132, Italy.
E-mail address: carlo.martinoli@unige.it

(granulomatous and nongranulomatous).[4] Clinical presentation and patient management significantly differ between adult and childhood vasculitis. Thus, in 2006, the vasculitis working group of the Pediatric Rheumatology European Society issued specific classification criteria for some of the most common childhood vasculitides, including IgA vasculitis (formerly Henoch-Schönlein purpura), childhood polyarteritis nodosa, childhood granulomatosis with polyangiitis (formerly Wegener granulomatosis), children Takayasu arteritis, and Kawasaki disease.[3] These criteria were modified and validated using a large international World Wide Web–based registry (PRINTO) and finally recognized and endorsed by the European Society of Pediatric Nephrology and the European League Against Rheumatism (http://ard.bmj.com/content/65/7/936.long).[5,6]

Diagnostic Work-up

The diagnostic work-up in childhood vasculitis requires thorough analysis of the patient's history and physical examination because presenting symptoms may be subacute, nonspecific, and can vary widely depending on the size and location of involved vasculature.[4] As damage progresses with more specific clinical features (eg, onset of purpuric rash; evidence of organ involvement, such as glomerulonephritis), careful auscultation for arterial bruits and palpation of four-extremity peripheral pulses is mandatory, as is extensive examination of the skin, fundoscopy, and nailfold capillaroscopy. Antinuclear antibodies and antineutrophil cytoplasmic antibodies (ANCA) and complement should also be assessed.[4]

Diagnostic imaging plays a critical role in securing the diagnosis of vasculitis affecting large- and medium-sized vessels, and in evaluating organ involvement in small vessel forms. In childhood vasculitides affecting predominantly large- and/or medium-sized blood vessels, ultrasound (US) complemented with Doppler techniques, MR angiography, and computed tomography angiography (CTA) are the imaging modalities of choice to provide an early detection of vessel changes.[7–9] All of these investigations are also used as outcome measures to monitor the efficacy of treatment and the evolution of damage in longitudinal studies.[4] In many instances, US is considered the first-line technique because of its excellent spatial resolution and ability to detect mural thickening and luminal changes without exposure to ionizing radiation. In the thorax, however, US has intrinsic limitations related to problems of access and when a vessel is deep-seated in the abdomen, its spatial resolution may

be suboptimal to reveal initial wall abnormalities. CTA has excellent vascular resolution and three-dimensional rendering capabilities, but repeated studies using this modality should be avoided in children because of radiation exposure.[10,11] Although MR angiography has lower spatial resolution than CTA, its sensitivity is almost equal to conventional angiography in detection of luminal changes in large blood vessels.[12,13] In addition, by means of whole-body technique, MR imaging has proved to be a fast and accurate method for detecting, mapping, and monitoring vascular abnormalities throughout the body in systemic childhood vasculitides avoiding exposure to ionizing radiation.[14,15] As a rule, the use of intravenous administration of iodinated or gadolinium (Gd)-based contrast media has to be restricted to the real needs in these patients because renal function impairment may be an issue. Digital subtraction angiography (DSA) should be regarded as a challenging procedure in children in view of its invasive nature, radiation exposure, use of iodinated contrast material, and operator-dependence.[8] Although still considered as the gold standard for the diagnosis of pediatric vasculitides, it does not provide any direct information regarding the vessel wall. Its role is therefore limited as a guide for interventional procedures in cases of vasculitis-related complications and to map the extent of collateralization.[9] Fluorine-18-fluorodeoxyglucose positron emission tomography (PET) is able to detect increased metabolic activity in the wall of inflamed vessels.[8,16,17] Nevertheless, its ultimate role in childhood vasculitis has still to be defined. Aneurysms are typically encountered in vasculitis of medium-sized blood vessels. Most are localized in the coronary, mesenteric, and renal arteries. For evaluation of the coronary arteries and cardiac function, echocardiography plays a pivotal role.[18] In small-vessel disease, the role of diagnostic imaging to detect tissue damage related to microvasculature and perfusion abnormalities is limited because of insufficient resolution of imaging and restrictions for use of microbubble-based ultrasonic contrast agents in the pediatric age group.

LARGE-VESSEL VASCULITIS
Takayasu Arteritis

Takayasu arteritis is a granulomatous vasculitis of unknown cause that predominantly affects the aorta with its major branches (eg, the subclavian, and more rarely, the pulmonary, carotid, renal, and coronary arteries).[19,20] This condition has a definite female predominance (3:1) and is diagnosed during adolescence (peak age at onset,

13 years).[21] Takayasu arteritis is characterized by granulomatous inflammation of the vessel wall that may lead to concentric wall thickening and fibrosis with subsequent stenosis, occlusion, and aneurysm formation.[21] Arterial stenosis is observed in approximately 53% of children with Takayasu disease, whereas aneurysm formation is encountered in only 10%. Depending on the location of the affected vasculature, the disease is classified into five types: type I (supraortic); type II (IIa, ascending aorta and aortic arch; IIb, descending aorta); type III (ascending aorta, aortic arch, descending aorta, and renal arteries); type IV (abdominal aorta or renal arteries); and type V (generalized involvement).

Initial symptoms are nonspecific and include headache, dizziness, fever, and weight loss.[22] With development of arterial stenosis, hypertension secondary to renal artery involvement (66%–93% of affected children), peripheral diminished pulses and claudication (pulseless disease), abdominal angina, and cardiac insufficiency is observed.[4,20,21] Involvement of the aortic arch and/or its major branches may be associated with central nervous system (CNS) manifestations including ischemic strokes, cerebral aneurysms, and seizures.

In Takayasu arteritis, US and Doppler techniques can reveal segmental uniform thickening of the vessel wall, stenotic lumen, and intravascular blood flow velocity changes (**Figs. 1** and **2**).[21,23] Main limitations of this technique include limited field of view, poor access for a comprehensive analysis of intrathoracic vasculature, and inability to assess disease activity. MR imaging and CTA offer a panoramic view of large vessels and their branches, allowing detection of early disease changes (**Fig. 3**). Different from CTA, MR imaging allows identification of inflammatory changes in the arterial wall as a sign of active vasculitis before wall thickening becomes apparent and is able to distinguish between stenoses caused by inflammation and

fibrosis. In our institution, the MR imaging protocol includes fat-suppressed T2-weighted sequences to detect wall edema, Gd-enhanced gradient-recalled echo three-dimensional T1-weighted angiographic images to assess stenoses, and "black-blood" Gd-enhanced T1-weighted images (electrocardiogram-gated spin-echo sequences with presaturation pulses) to evaluate wall inflammation (**Fig. 4**). The sensitivity and specificity of MR angiography for the diagnosis of Takayasu arteritis is high, although some overestimation of the degree of stenosis may occur with possible misdiagnosis of vessel occlusion (**Fig. 5**).[8,12] Several studies have shown that MR angiography has a comparable accuracy with DSA in the assessment and follow-up of vascular lesions in Takayasu arteritis with an average sensitivity greater than 90%.[12,13] The major disadvantage of MR imaging seems to be related to its limitation in assessing the extent of collateralization and the poor visualization of vascular calcifications. Recently, fluorodeoxyglucose PET has been proposed as an alternative modality to assess vessel wall inflammation, although its sensitivity (70.1%) and specificity (77.2%) in demonstrating the extent and degree of inflammation is moderate in terms of diagnostic test performance.[16–24] Overall, challenges remain in distinguishing between the active phase of the disease in which immunosuppressive treatment is required and the chronic phase, where tissue ischemia derives from progressive arterial narrowing. In this latter state, treatment involves revascularization procedures (eg, angioplasty, stenting) or more invasive surgery, such as aortic bypass grafting.[25,26]

MEDIUM-VESSEL VASCULITIS
Kawasaki Disease

After Henoch-Schönlein purpura (IgA vasculitis), Kawasaki disease is the second most common

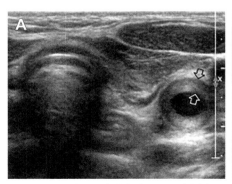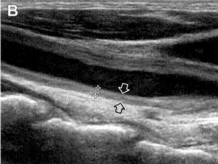

Fig. 1. Takayasu arteritis (type I). (*A*) Short- and (*B*) long-axis 12.5-MHz US images of the left common carotid artery demonstrate uniform concentric thickening of the vessel wall (*arrows*) with loss of its layered appearance.

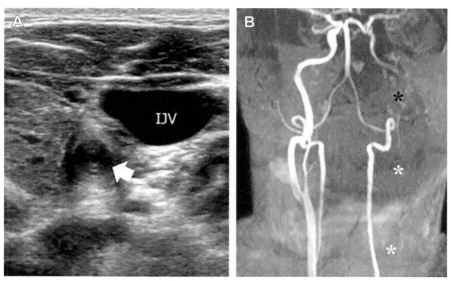

Fig. 2. Takayasu arteritis (type I). (*A*) Transverse 12.5-MHz US image over the left major neurovascular bundle of the neck shows occlusion of the common carotid artery (*arrow*), which appears reduced in size and characterized by concentric wall thickening and critical narrowing of the lumen. IJV, internal jugular vein. (*B*) Maximum intensity projection MR angiogram confirms complete occlusion (*asterisks*) of the left common, internal, and external carotid arteries. The left vertebral artery is patent.

childhood vasculitis, accounting for approximately 23% of all disease types.[4,27] In the western world, its estimated annual incidence is approximately 20 per 1 million of cases but its prevalence is much

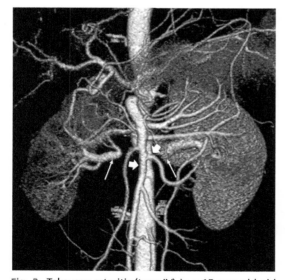

Fig. 3. Takayasu arteritis (type IV) in a 15-year-old girl with severe arterial hypertension. Contrast-enhanced volume-rendered computed tomography image shows aortic stenosis (*thick arrows*) between the origin of the celiac trunk and the renal arteries. The proximal segment of the renal arteries (*thin arrows*) is occluded. Reduced right renal perfusion is observed.

higher in eastern Asia and especially in Japan (100 per 1 million).[28,29] The cause of Kawasaki disease is still unproven, but an infectious agent is suspected to trigger the immune response in a genetically predisposed host.[30] From the clinical point of view, Kawasaki disease is a severe condition with significant morbidity and mortality related to cardiovascular complications. It has a triphasic course consisting of an acute phase that lasts up to 14 days, a subacute phase of 2 to 4 weeks, and a long convalescent phase that lasts months to years.[4]

The acute phase is characterized by persistent high fever (>38.5°) that seems to be secondary to high level of IL-6 and tumor necrosis factor-α and is often refractory to antipyretic drugs.[30,31] Ocular symptoms (eg, bilateral conjunctivitis, anterior uveitis), oral mucosal changes (eg, strawberry tongue and dry and cracked lips), unilateral anterior cervical adenopathies (25% of cases), skin abnormalities with diffuse erythema of the palms and soles, soft tissue swelling of the dorsum of the hands and feet, and rash (often perineal) with macular/target lesions on the trunk and extremities are typically observed.[4,32,33] Nondestructive arthritis affecting the knees, ankles, and hips and gastrointestinal complaints including diarrhea, vomiting, abdominal pain, and hydrops of the gallbladder may be variably associated. During the acute phase, cardiovascular disease may include valvulitis, myocarditis,

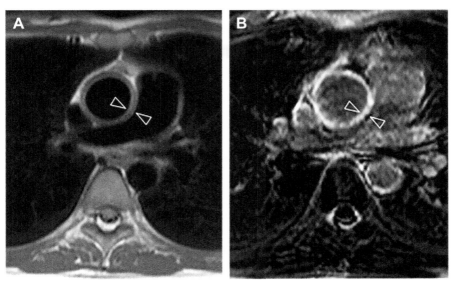

Fig. 4. Takayasu arteritis (type II). (*A*) Axial T1-weighted MR image reveals concentric wall thickening (*arrowheads*) of ascending aorta. (*B*) Late Gd-enhanced black blood axial T1-weighted image shows wall enhancement (*arrowheads*) suggesting active inflammation.

and pericarditis. Coronary artery involvement is a typical disease feature, but other large-sized (eg, humeral, iliac, and femoral) and medium-sized arteries (eg, mesenteric, renal) may be affected with stenotic segments and aneurysms.[18] Regarding coronaries, most aneurysms tend to develop during the subacute/convalescent phases despite normalization of clinical symptoms. The risk for aneurysms is higher in children younger than 1 year of age and is substantially reduced by early

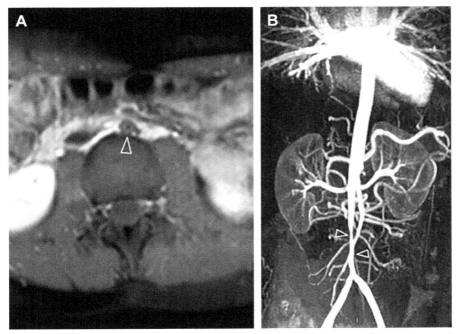

Fig. 5. Takayasu arteritis (type IV). (*A*) Axial fat-suppressed T1-weighted MR image of the abdomen shows significant wall thickening and lumen narrowing of the distal abdominal aorta (*arrowhead*). (*B*) Maximum intensity projection MR angiogram identifies a long stenotic segment (*arrowheads*) of the infrarenal abdominal aorta.

recognition of the disease and administration of intravenous immunoglobulin in the acute phase. Large aneurysms may thrombose and lead to ischemic heart disease, whereas small aneurysms (<5 mm in diameter) may regress (Fig. 6).[18]

Although imaging does not have a critical role in the early diagnosis of Kawasaki disease, its use is important in the assessment of complications.[8] Echocardiography is the imaging technique of choice to provide serial follow-up checks and monitor the heart status throughout the disease duration. This technique has proved able to identify myocarditis and pericarditis, depressed vascular contractility, abnormal pericoronary echogenicity in early phases, and coronary aneurysms in subacute and convalescent phases.[8] Transesophageal echocardiography has a limited application in challenging cases.[4] Because of its high spatial resolution, CTA has diagnostic accuracy comparable with DSA for evaluation of coronary involvement and detection of wall thickening, calcification, and thrombosis. Its use is limited, however, because of the high radiation exposure (especially relevant to assess myocardial perfusion and ventricular function) and the need to perform repeated follow-up studies. Electrocardiogram-gated dual-source computed tomography (CT) systems seem to be promising in this field because of a lower radiation exposure and excellent anatomic details[34] (see Fig. 6B). However, MR imaging with MR angiography sequences is able to provide information on the proximal and middle segments of the coronary arteries and to assess cardiac function and myocardial perfusion.[35] In the acute phase, MR angiography does not provide significant advantages over echocardiography, particularly in case of mild vascular changes. Early and delayed Gd-enhancement images have a value to differentiate myocardial inflammation from ischemic necrosis. Early myocardial enhancement is related to increased membrane permeability or capillary blood flow, whereas a late uptake (15–20 minutes after injection) of contrast indicates the slower wash-out from fibrotic/necrotic tissue.[36] In chronic phase, coronary MR angiography is reliable to detect coronary artery stenoses, clots, and intimal hyperplasia in difficult-to-scan locations, such as the circumflex artery and distal arterial segments.[37]

Childhood Polyarteritis Nodosa

Childhood polyarteritis nodosa is predominantly a medium/small-sized ANCA-negative necrotizing vasculitis accounting for approximately 3% of all childhood vasculitides, with a peak age at onset of 9 years.[38,39] Its cause is still unclear, although several reports suggest an immune-mediate process triggered by an infective agent as causative.[4] Two main types of polyarteritis nodosa are observed in children: systemic and cutaneous, with the former the most frequent. In systemic polyarteritis nodosa the vascular supply to any organ (lungs excluded) may be impaired. Clinical symptoms related to vascular insufficiency may vary widely depending on the distribution of vessel abnormalities. Target organ damage may occur with hypertension, ischemic heart disease, abdominal pain, hematuria, and proteinuria. Cutaneous polyarteritis nodosa has a better outcome and is mostly confined to the skin of the lower extremities with painful subcutaneous nodules, rash, livedo reticularis, purpura, and gangrene. In this latter form, the musculoskeletal system may also be

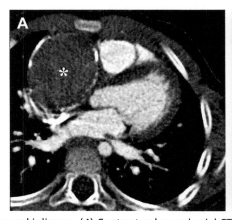
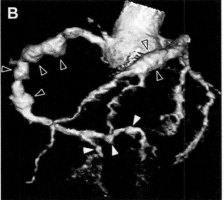

Fig. 6. Kawasaki disease. (A) Contrast-enhanced axial CT image shows a large thrombosed aneurysm (asterisk) of the right coronary artery. (B) Dual-source CT with maximum intensity projection reconstruction of the coronary arteries demonstrates multiple aneurysms affecting proximal (open arrowheads) and mid-distal (solid arrowhead) arterial segments.

involved with arthralgias, myalgias, and nonde-structive arthritis. Although Doppler US and MR angiography are used to detect vessel abnormal-ities in children with polyarteritis nodosa, DSA and CTA are the imaging techniques of choice to depict segmental narrowing, aneurysms, and oc-clusions in medium- and small-sized arteries (**Fig. 7**).[8] DSA still has the highest sensitivity to detect stenoses in smaller vasculature.[39,40]

SMALL-VESSEL VASCULITIS
IgA Vasculitis (Henoch-Schönlein Purpura)

IgA vasculitis (formerly Henoch-Schönlein pur-pura, anaphylactoid purpura, or purpura rheuma-tica) is the most common vasculitis of childhood (49% of all pediatric vasculitides) accounting for approximately 20 per 1 million with a peak age of onset at 4 to 6 years and a definite male (2:1) pre-dominance.[4,5] It is a nongranulomatous ANCA-negative vasculitis resulting from IgA deposition that predominantly occurs in the walls of small blood vessels and renal mesangium.[41] It has been hypothesized that IgA-vasculitis may derive from an infectious episode: group A ß-hemolytic

streptococcus, *Staphylococcus aureus*, and other viruses (eg, influenza, parainfluenza, Epstein-Barr, adenovirus) have been implicated as triggers.[4,42]

Typical symptoms include lower-extremity pur-pura, arthritis, abdominal pain, gastrointestinal bleeding (30% of cases), and glomerulonephritis.[4] Gastrointestinal manifestations may precede the purpura and affect one-half to three-quarters of diseased children.[43] Intussusception (1%–5% of cases, mostly ileoileal in location) and bowel perfo-ration (0.38% of cases) may also occur in these pa-tients.[44,45] Renal disease affects 20% to 60% of children and is characterized by microscopic hema-turia with or without proteinuria, possibly evolving to chronic renal impairment (2%–15% of cases) and end-stage disease (<1% of cases).[46] Among genito-urinary disturbances, scrotal swelling and pain caused by orchiepididymis, spermatic cord inflam-mation, and hydrocele are observed.[47,48]

In IgA vasculitis, US is the most common initial im-aging modality but early disease signs may be nonspecific, such as peritoneal fluid and mesenteric adenopathies. Later in the disease course, US may play a more significant role to evaluate possible complications and target organ damage, typically

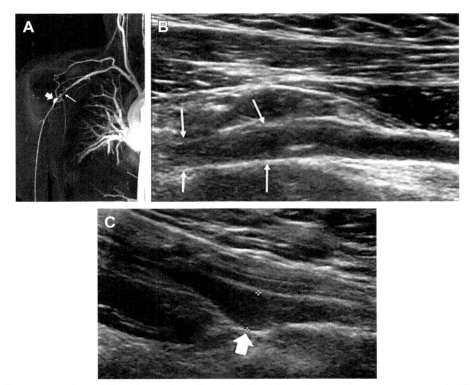

Fig. 7. Polyarteritis nodosa. (*A*) Maximum intensity projection MR angiogram demonstrates stenosis (*thin arrow*) and poststenotic aneurysm (*thick arrow*) of the right axillary artery. Proximal (*B*) and (*C*) distal long-axis 12.5-MHz US images of the right axillary artery show wall thickening leading to a narrowed vessel lumen (*thin arrows*). In the distal image, the small poststenotic aneurysm (*thick arrow*) is seen.

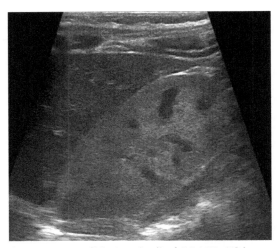

Fig. 8. IgA vasculitis. Longitudinal 5.2-MHz US image shows an enlarged right kidney with diffuse increased echogenicity (grade II) of the renal cortex.

genitourinary or gastrointestinal.[4] Detection of enlarged kidneys with diffusely hyperechoic (grade II-III) parenchyma, segmental bowel wall thickening with hypervascular pattern at Doppler imaging, and intussusception can lead to a conclusive diagnosis (**Figs. 8** and **9**).[49,50] IgA vasculitis is generally self-limited and has a benign course with symptoms lasting 3 to 4 weeks. About one-third of affected children have a relapse in the first 4 months.[48] Long-term prognosis depends on the severity of renal involvement, because chronic nephritis may appear many years after the disease onset.[22]

Granulomatosis with Polyangiitis (Wegener Granulomatosis)

Granulomatosis with polyangiitis, formerly known as Wegener granulomatosis, accounts for less than 3% of all childhood vasculitides.[51,52] This condition is a pauci-immune necrotizing vasculitis leading to inflammation and fibrinoid necrosis of vessel walls with no deposition of complement or immunoglobulins.[4,44] Perivascular and extra-vascular spaces may also be involved.[8] A high titer of myeloperoxidase ANCA or positive perinuclear-ANCA staining is observed in most cases.[53,54] Symptoms are nonspecific and include fever, malaise, and weight loss.[51,55] The nose, paranasal sinuses, upper and lower respiratory tract, and kidneys are primarily affected.[4,55] In the paranasal sinuses, mucosal thickening, nasal septum perforation (with subsequent saddle nose deformity), turbinates, and lateral nasal wall destruction are observed (**Fig. 10**). The orbital cavities may be involved because of their proximity to the paranasal sinuses. Subglottic and bronchial stenosis is also a typical finding.[55]

On MR imaging, early granulomatous tissue appears T1-hypointense and T2-hyperintense, whereas chronic granulomas are hypointense on T1- and T2-weighted sequences and do not show contrast enhancement. Pulmonary manifestations may include nodules (63%–89% of cases), areas of consolidations, ground glass opacities, cavitations, and respiratory failure (**Fig. 11A**).[56–58] Approximately 20% to 30% of patients with granulomatosis with polyangiitis and no respiratory symptoms show lung abnormalities on radiography.[55] CT is considered the modality of choice to depict nasal, paranasal, tracheobronchial, and lung abnormalities.[56–59] The renal involvement may result in necrotizing glomerulonephritis that can cause rapidly progressive glomerulonephritis with hematuria, proteinuria, and kidney failure.[60] The 5-year survival rate is 85% to 100%; relapse is observed in 75% of cases. Similar to

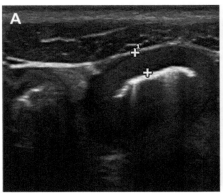
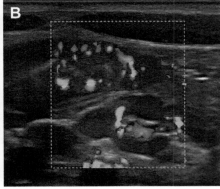

Fig. 9. IgA vasculitis in a 9-year-old boy with abdominal pain and melena lasting for 3 days. Gray-scale (*A*) and color Doppler (*B*) 12.5-MHz US images demonstrate marked wall thickening (distance between *calipers*) of a bowel loop with loss of its multilayered appearance and signs of intramural hyperemia. In *B*, regional mesenteric adenopathies are also observed.

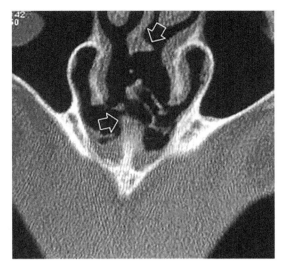

Fig. 10. Granulomatosis with polyangiitis. Coronal CT image of the nasal cavity and maxillary sinuses shows nasal septum perforation (*arrows*). Both inferior turbinates and medial walls of the maxillary sinuses retain a normal appearance.

granulomatosis with polyangiitis, microscopic polyangiitis is an ANCA-associated vasculitis that typically involves lungs and kidneys, possibly resulting in pulmonary-renal syndrome.[4] Its imaging features do not differ as is seen with granulomatosis with polyangiitis.[8]

Eosinophilic Granulomatosis with Polyangiitis (Churg-Strauss Syndrome)

Eosinophilic granulomatosis with polyangiitis, formerly known as Churg-Strauss syndrome, is a granulomatous vasculitis of small- and medium-sized vessels that primarily affects children with asthma or allergies.[4] The onset is insidious and may last years. The most common disturbances

include asthma, pulmonary infiltrates, sinusitis, skin involvement, cardiac disease, gastrointestinal symptoms, and peripheral neuropathy.[61] The renal involvement is usually mild and rarely progresses. High-resolution CT of the lungs can demonstrate ground glass opacities with symmetric peripheral location, areas of consolidation, and septal lines (see **Fig. 11**B).[62,63]

CENTRAL NERVOUS SYSTEM VASCULITIS

CNS vasculitis may be either part of a systemic inflammatory disease or a primary disorder restricted to the CNS. This latter condition, which is referred to as childhood primary angiitis of the CNS, is considered one of the most important causes of acquired neurologic deficits in children.[64,65] Clinical criteria for childhood primary angiitis of the CNS include an acquired neurologic deficit that remains unexplained after a thorough initial basic evaluation, either classic angiographic or histopathologic features of angiitis within the CNS, and no evidence of systemic vasculitis or any other condition to which the angiographic or pathologic features could be secondary. The disease includes three different subtypes that differ in terms of clinical presentation, imaging findings, and treatment: (1) nonprogressive medium-large vessel, (2) progressive medium-large vessel, and (3) small-vessel CNS vasculitides.

Nonprogressive Medium-Large-Vessel Central Nervous System Vasculitis

Nonprogressive medium-large vessel CNS vasculitis typically presents with focal neurologic deficits including movement disorders, cranial neuropathies, and headache.[65] Imaging findings are highly variable and nonspecific. DSA still remains the gold standard to make the diagnosis showing focal or multifocal segmental narrowing, occlusion

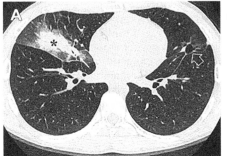
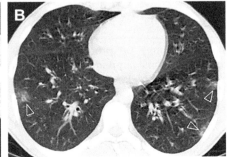

Fig. 11. (*A*) Granulomatosis with polyangiitis (Wegener granulomatosis). Axial CT scan of the lungs shows a small pulmonary cavitation with thin walls (*arrow*) on the left and a consolidation (*asterisk*) in the middle lobe on the right, associated with thickened bronchial walls. (*B*) Eosinophilic granulomatosis with polyangiitis (Churg-Strauss syndrome). CT scan reveals ground glass opacities (*arrowheads*) with symmetric peripheral distribution.

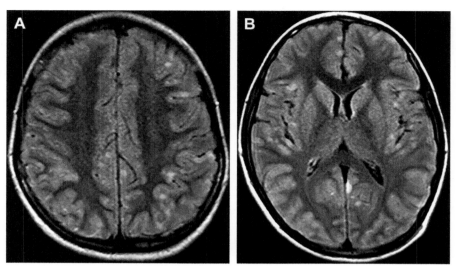

Fig. 12. (*A,B*) CNS vasculitis. Axial FLAIR MR images of the brain reveal diffuse cortical-subcortical high-intensity signal foci related to multiple small infarctions affecting different vascular territories.

or irregularities of small- and medium-sized parenchymal and leptomeningeal blood vessels, collateral formation, and prolonged circulation time. Abnormalities typically involve the upper carotid arteries and the proximal segments of the anterior and middle cerebral arteries. Microaneurysms are rarely seen. Interpretation of angiographic findings should be careful and especially to distinguish vasospasms from real stenotic segments.[66] CTA may reveal ischemic events in the territories supplied by occluded vessels and hemorrhagic lesions.[67] MR imaging is sensitive but not specific, showing supratentorial and infratentorial lesions involving the deep and superficial white matter, basal ganglia, and the lateral lenticulostriate territory. These lesions show T2-hyperintensity (chronic phase) or diffusion-weighted imaging restriction (acute phase) and exhibit contrast enhancement (90% of cases) (**Fig. 12**).[68]

Progressive Medium-Large-Vessel Central Nervous System Vasculitis

Large-vessel disease may be progressive with additional vascular lesions appearing over time. Several bilateral lesions of large-sized cerebral vessels are typically observed at DSA, along with bilateral cerebral infarctions.[69,70] Rarely, MR imaging reveals nonspecific space-occupying lesions, which are characterized by central necrosis, surrounding edema, infiltration and displacement of adjacent structures, and variable contrast enhancement. Treatment is based on cyclophosphamide and corticosteroids. With steroid therapy, children with progressive medium-large

vessel CNS vasculitis do not acquire new neurologic deficits.[69]

Small-Vessel Central Nervous System Vasculitis

Small-vessel CNS vasculitis is characterized by lymphocytic inflammatory infiltrates within the walls of arterioles, capillaries, and venules of the brain and meninges.[69,70] Typical symptoms include seizures, encephalopathy with diffuse neurologic dysfunction, and behavioral changes.[4] Cognitive deficit and mood disorders may be associated. Affected children show increased erythrocyte sedimentation rate and C-reactive protein levels and, in most cases, abnormal cerebrospinal fluid with pleocytosis, increased protein levels, or both.[71] The von Willebrand factor antigene level has reported to be an indicator of disease activity.[72] No abnormality is detected with angiographic techniques, including DSA, CTA, and MR angiography, and the diagnosis requires brain biopsy.[73] On MR imaging, detection of leptomeningeal enhancement is regarded as a disease-specific sign, especially considering demyelinating diseases in the differential diagnosis list. MR imaging can also depict parenchymal punctate enhancement in the spinal cord and optic nerve.

REFERENCES

1. Gardner-Medwin JM, Dolezalova P, Cummins C, et al. Incidence of Henoch-Schoenlein purpura, Kawasaki disease, and rare vasculitides in children of different ethnic origins. Lancet 2002;360:1197–202.

2. Jennette JC, Falk RJ, Andrassy K, et al. Nomenclature of systemic vasculitides: the proposal of an international consensus conference. Arthritis Rheum 1994;37:187–92.

3. Ozen S, Ruperto N, Dillon MJ, et al. EULAR/PReS endorsed consensus criteria for the classification of childhood vasculitides. Ann Rheum Dis 2006;65: 936–41.

4. Weiss P. Pediatric vasculitis. Pediatr Clin North Am 2012;59:407–23.

5. Ozen S, Pistorio A, Iusan SM, et al. EULAR/PRINTO/PRES criteria for Henoch-Schönlein purpura, childhood polyarteritis nodosa, childhood Wegener granulomatosis and childhood Takayasu arteritis: Ankara 2008. Part II: final classification criteria. Ann Rheum Dis 2010;69:798–806.

6. Ruperto N, Ozen S, Pistorio A, et al. EULAR/PRINTO/PRES criteria for Henoch-Schonlein purpura, childhood polyarteritis nodosa, childhood Wegener granulomatosis and childhood Takayasu arteritis: Ankara 2008. Part I: overall methodology and clinical characterisation. Ann Rheum Dis 2010; 69:790–7.

7. Khanna G, Sargar K, Baszis KW. Pediatric vasculitis: recognizing multisystemic manifestation at body imaging. Radiographics 2015;35:849–65.

8. Soliman M, Laxer R, Manson D, et al. Imaging of systemic vasculitis in childhood. Pediatr Radiol 2015;45:1110–25.

9. Pipitone N, Salvarani C. Role of imaging in vasculitis and connective tissue diseases. Best Pract Res Clin Rheumatol 2008;22:1075–91.

10. Hausleiter J, Meyer T, Hermann F, et al. Estimated radiation dose associated with cardiac CT angiography. JAMA 2009;301:500–7.

11. Apfaltrer P, Hanna EL, Schoepf UJ, et al. Radiation dose and image quality at high-pitch CT angiography of the aorta: intraindividual and interindividual comparisons with conventional CT angiography. AJR Am J Roentgenol 2012;199:1402–9.

12. Kumar S, Radhakrishnan S, Phadke RV, et al. Takayasu's arteritis: evaluation with three-dimensional time-of-flight MR angiography. Eur Radiol 1997;7: 44–50.

13. Yamada I, Nakagawa T, Himeno Y, et al. Takayasu arteritis: diagnosis with breath-hold contrast-enhanced three-dimensional MR angiography. J Magn Reson Imaging 2000;11:481–7.

14. Weckbach S. Whole-body MR imaging for patients with rheumatism. Eur J Radiol 2009;70: 431–41.

15. Eutsler EP, Khanna G. Whole-body magnetic resonance imaging in children: technique and clinical applications. Pediatr Radiol 2016;46: 858–72.

16. Cheng Y, Lv N, Wang Z, et al. 18-FDG-PET in assessing disease activity in Takayasu arteritis: a meta-analysis. Clin Exp Rheumatol 2013;31: S22–7.

17. Karapolat I, Kalfa M, Keser G, et al. Comparison of F18-FDG PET/CT findings with current clinical disease status in patients with Takayasu's arteritis. Clin Exp Rheumatol 2013;31:S15–21.

18. Newburger JW, Takahashi M, Gerber MA, et al. Diagnosis, treatment, and long-term management of Kawasaki disease: a statement for health professional from the Committee on Rheumatic Fever, Endocarditis and Kawasaki Disease, Council on Cardiovascular Disease in the Young, American Heart Association. Circulation 2004;110: 2747–71.

19. Cakar N, Yalcinkaya F, Duzova A, et al. Takayasu arteritis in children. J Rheumatol 2008;35:913–9.

20. McCulloch M, Andronikou S, Goddard E, et al. Angiographic features of 26 children with Takayasu's arteritis. Pediatr Radiol 2003;33:230–5.

21. Brunner J, Feldman B, Tyrrell P, et al. Takayasu arteritis in children and adolescents. Rheumatology 2010;49:1806–14.

22. Barut K, Sahin S, Kasapcopur O. Pediatric vasculitis. Curr Opin Rheumatol 2016;28:29–38.

23. Kissin EY, Merkel PA. Diagnostic imaging in Takayasu arteritis. Curr Opin Rheumatol 2004;16: 31–7.

24. Spira D, Kötter I, Ernemann U, et al. Imaging of primary and secondary inflammatory diseases involving large and medium-sized vessels and their potential mimics: a multitechnique approach. AJR Am J Roentgenol 2010;194:848–56.

25. Endo M, Tomizawa Y, Nishida H, et al. Angiographic findings and surgical treatments of coronary artery involvement in Takayasu arteritis. J Thorac Cardiovasc Surg 2003;125:570–7.

26. Miyata T, Sato O, Koyama H, et al. Long-term survival after surgical treatment of patients with Takayasu's arteritis. Circulation 2003;108:1474–80.

27. Bowyer S, Roettcher P. Pediatric rheumatology clinic populations in the United States: results of a 3 year survey. Pediatric Rheumatology Database Research Group. J Rheumatol 1996;23:1968–74.

28. Yanagawa H, Nakamura Y, Yashiro M, et al. Results of the nationwide epidemiologic survey of Kawasaki disease in 1995 and 1996 in Japan. Pediatrics 1998; 102:E65.

29. Nakamura Y, Yashiro M, Uehara R, et al. Epidemiologic features of Kawasaki disease in Japan: results of the 2007-2008 nationwide survey. J Epidemiol 2010;20:302–7.

30. Yeung RS. Kawasaki disease: update on pathogenesis. Curr Opin Rheumatol 2010;22:551–60.

31. Leung DY. The potential role of cytokine-mediated vascular endothelial activation in the pathogenesis of Kawasaki disease. Acta Paediatr Jpn 1991;33: 739–44.

32. Kumagai N, Ohno S. Kawasaki disease. In: Holland G, Wilhelmus K, editors. Ocular immunity and infection. St Louis (MO): Mosby; 1996.

33. Sung RY, Ng YM, Choi KC, et al. Lack of association of cervical lymphadenopathy and coronary artery complications in Kawasaki disease. Pediatr Infect Dis J 2006;25:521–5.

34. Yu Y, Sun K, Wang R, et al. Comparison study of echocardiography and dual-source CT in diagnosis of coronary artery aneurysm due to Kawasaki disease: coronary artery disease. Echocardiography 2011;28:1025–34.

35. Kim JW, Goo HW. Coronary artery abnormalities in Kawasaki disease: comparison between CT and MRI coronary angiography. Acta Radiol 2013;54: 156–63.

36. Abdel-Aty H, Boye P, Zagrosek A, et al. Diagnostic performance of cardiovascular magnetic resonance in patients with suspected acute myocarditis: comparison of different approaches. J Am Coll Cardiol 2005;45:1815–22.

37. Greil GF, Seeger A, Miller S, et al. Coronary magnetic resonance angiography and vessel wall imaging in children with Kawasaki disease. Pediatr Radiol 2007;37:666–73.

38. Ozen S, Anton J, Arisoy N, et al. Juvenile polyarteritis: results of a multicenter survey of 110 children. J Pediatr 2004;145:517–22.

39. Eleftheriou D, Dillon M, Brogan P. Advances in childhood vasculitis. Curr Opin Rheumatol 2009; 21:411–8.

40. Schmidt WA. Use of imaging studies in the diagnosis of vasculitis. Curr Rheumatol Rep 2004;6: 203–11.

41. Brogan B, Bagga A. Leukocytoclastic vasculitis. In: Cassidy JT, Laxer RM, Petty RE, et al, editors. Textbook of pediatric rheumatology. 6th edition. Philadelphia: WB Saunders; 2011. p. 483–97.

42. Weiss PF, Klink AJ, Luan X, et al. Temporal association of streptococcus, staphylococcus, and parainfluenza pediatric hospitalizations and hospitalized cases of Henoch-Schönlein purpura. J Rheumatol 2010;37:2587–94.

43. Saulsbury FT. Henoch-Schonlein purpura. Curr Opin Rheumatol 2010;22:598–602.

44. Glasier CM, Siegel MJ, McAlister WH, et al. Henoch-Schönlein syndrome in children: gastrointestinal manifestations. AJR Am J Roentgenol 1981;136: 1081–5.

45. Yavuz H, Arslan A. Henoch-Schönlein purpura-related intestinal perforation: a steroid complication? Pediatr Int 2001;43:423–5.

46. Narchi H. Risk of long term renal impairment and duration of follow up recommended for Henoch-Schönlein purpura with normal or minimal urinary findings: a systematic review. Arch Dis Child 2005; 90:916–20.

47. Ben-Sira L, Laor T. Severe scrotal pain in boys with Henoch-Schönlein purpura: incidence and sonography. Pediatr Radiol 2000;30:125–8.

48. Tmka P. Henoch-Schönlein purpura in children. J Paediatr Child Health 2013;49:995–1003.

49. Ozdemir H, Işik S, Buyan N, et al. Sonographic demonstration of intestinal involvement in Henoch-Schönlein syndrome. Eur J Radiol 1995;20:32–4.

50. Shirahama M, Umeno Y, Tomimasu R, et al. The value of colour Doppler ultrasonography for small bowel involvement of adult Henoch-Schönlein purpura. Br J Radiol 1998;71:788–91.

51. Cabral DA, Uribe AG, Benseler S, et al. Classification, presentation, and initial treatment of Wegener's granulomatosis in childhood. Arthritis Rheum 2009; 60:3413–24.

52. Siomou E, Tramma D, Bowen C, et al. ANCA-associated glomerulonephritis/systemic vasculitis in childhood: clinical features-outcome. Pediatr Nephrol 2012;27:1911–20.

53. Hoffman GS, Specks U. Antineutrophil cytoplasmic antibodies. Arthritis Rheum 1998;41:1521–37.

54. Bohm M, Gonzalez Fernandez MI, Ozen S, et al. Clinical features of childhood granulomatosis with polyangiitis (Wegener's granulomatosis). Pediatr Rheumatol Online J 2014;12:18.

55. Akikusa JD, Schneider R, Harvey EA, et al. Clinical features and outcome of pediatric Wegener's granulomatosis. Arthritis Rheum 2007;57:837–44.

56. Levine D, Akikusa J, Manson D, et al. Chest CT findings in pediatric Wegener's granulomatosis. Pediatr Radiol 2007;37:57–62.

57. Ananthakrishnan L, Sharma N, Kanne J. Wegener's granulomatosis in the chest: high-resolution CT findings. AJR Am J Roentgenol 2009;192: 676–82.

58. Connolly B, Manson D, Eberhard A, et al. CT appearance of pulmonary vasculitis in children. AJR Am J Roentgenol 1996;167:901–4.

59. Mujagic S, Sarihodzic S, Huseinagic H, et al. Wegener's granulomatosis of the paranasal sinuses with orbital and central nervous system involvement: diagnostic imaging. Acta Neurol Belg 2011;111: 241–4.

60. Allen SD, Harvey CJ. Imaging of Wegener's granulomatosis. Br J Radiol 2007;80:757–65.

61. Zwerina J, Eger G, Englbrecht M, et al. Churg-Strauss syndrome in childhood: a systematic literature review and clinical comparison with adult patients. Semin Arthritis Rheum 2009;39:108–15.

62. Lanham JG, Elkon KB, Pusey CD, et al. Systemic vasculitis with asthma and eosinophilia: a clinical approach to the Churg-Strauss syndrome. Medicine 1984;63:65–81.

63. Castaner E, Alguersuari A, Gallardo X, et al. When to suspect pulmonary vasculitis: radiologic and clinical clues. Radiographics 2010;30:33–53.

64. Hajj-Ali RA, Calabrese LH. Primary angiitis of the central nervous system. Autoimmun Rev 2013;12:463–6.

65. Salvarani C, Brown RD Jr, Hunder GG. Adult primary central nervous system vasculitis: an update. Curr Opin Rheumatol 2012;24:46–52.

66. Probert R, Saunders DE, Ganesan V. Reversible cerebral vasoconstriction syndrome: rare or under-recognized in children? Dev Med Child Neurol 2013;55:385–9.

67. Ay H, Sahin G, Saatci I, et al. Primary angiitis of the central nervous system and silent cortical hemorrhages. AJNR Am J Neuroradiol 2002;23:1561–3.

68. Bouhaouala MH, Charfi M, Saîd W, et al. Nervous system vasculitis. In: Hendaoui L, Stanson AW, Bouhaouala MH, et al, editors. Systemic vasculitis: imaging features. Medical radiology/diagnostic imaging series. Berlin: Springer-Verlag; 2012. p. 415.

69. Twilt M, Benseler SM. Childhood inflammatory brain diseases: pathogenesis, diagnosis and therapy. Rheumatology (Oxford) 2014;53:1359–68.

70. Twilt M, Benseler SM. CNS vasculitis in children. Mult Scler Relat Disord 2013;2:162–71.

71. Benseler SM, Silverman E, Aviv RI, et al. Primary central nervous system vasculitis in children. Arthritis Rheum 2006;54:1291–7.

72. Cellucci T, Tyrrell PN, Pullenayegum E, et al. Von Willebrand factor antigen: a possible biomarker of disease activity in childhood central nervous system vasculitis? Rheumatology (Oxford) 2012;51:1838–45.

73. Benseler SM, deVeber G, Hawkins C, et al. Angiography-negative primary central nervous system vasculitis in children: a newly recognized inflammatory central nervous system disease. Arthritis Rheum 2005;52:2159–67.

Printed and bound by CPI Group (UK) Ltd, Croydon, CR0 4YY

08/05/2025

01864703-0013